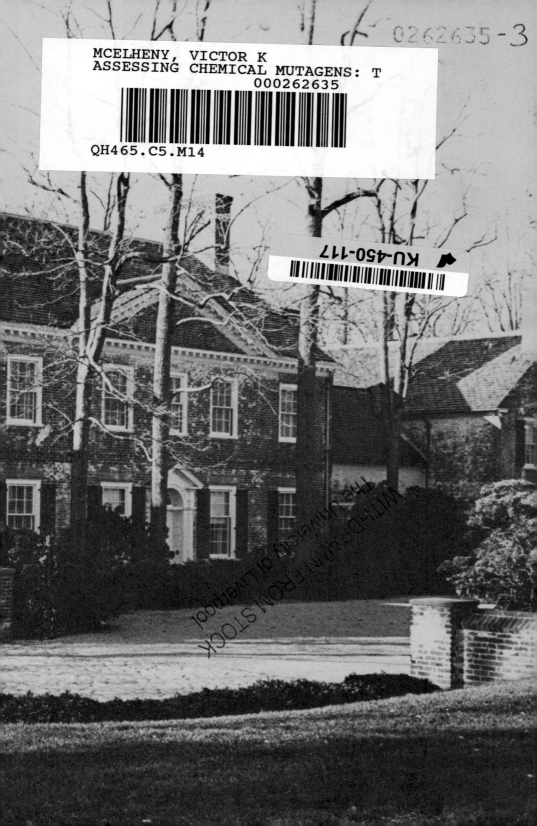

ASSESSING CHEMICAL MUTAGENS:
The Risk to Humans

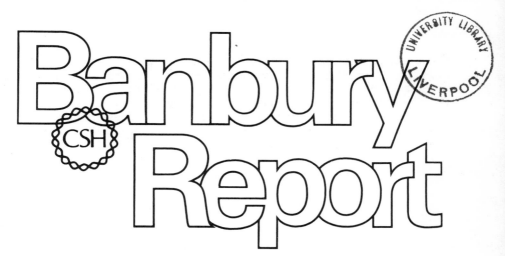

1
ASSESSING CHEMICAL MUTAGENS:
The Risk to Humans

Edited by

VICTOR K. McELHENY
Banbury Center

SEYMOUR ABRAHAMSON
University of Wisconsin

COLD SPRING HARBOR LABORATORY
1979

This project has been funded at least in part with Federal funds from the U.S. Environmental Protection Agency under contract number 68-01-4813. The content of this publication does not necessarily reflect the views or policies of the U.S. Environmental Protection Agency, nor does mention of trade names, commercial products, or organizations imply endorsement by the U.S. Government.

Banbury Report 1
ASSESSING CHEMICAL MUTAGENS:
The Risk to Humans

Printed in the United States of America

Cover design by Emily Harste

Library of Congress Cataloging in Publication Data

Main entry under title:

Assessing chemical mutagens.

    (Banbury report ; 1)
    Edited proceedings of a meeting sponsored by the Office of Toxic Substances of the U.S. Environmental Protection Agency in May 1978 at Banbury Center, Lloyd Harbor, N.Y.
    1.   Chemical mutagenesis--Congresses.
    2.   Mutagenicity testing--Congresses.
I. McElheny, Victor K. II. Abrahamson, Seymour. III. United States. Environmental Protection Agency. Office of Toxic Substances.
IV. Series: Banbury Center. Banbury report ; 1.
QH465.C5A85   615.9   79-998
ISBN 0-87969-200-6

Participants

SEYMOUR ABRAHAMSON, Department of Zoology, University of Wisconsin

JOHN W. BAUM, Safety and Environmental Protection Division, Brookhaven National Laboratory

J. GRANT BREWEN, Biology Division, Oak Ridge National Laboratory

JOHN DOULL, FIFRA Scientific Advisory Council, Environmental Protection Agency (University of Kansas Medical School)

LARS EHRENBERG, Wallenberg Laboratory, Stockholm University

ERIC EISENSTADT, Departments of Microbiology and Physiology, Harvard University School of Public Health

ERNEST FALKE, Office of Toxic Substances, Environmental Protection Agency

W. GARY FLAMM, Division of Toxicology, Bureau of Foods, Food and Drug Administration

RICHARD N. HILL, Office of Toxic Substances, Environmental Protection Agency

DAVID HOEL, Biometry Branch, National Institute of Environmental Health Sciences

ALEXANDER HOLLAENDER, Associated Universities, Inc.

VILMA HUNT, Science Advisory Board, Environmental Protection Agency (Pennsylvania State University)

PETER INFANTE, Carcinogen Identification and Classification, Occupational Safety and Health Administration

WILLIAM R. LEE, Department of Zoology and Physiology, Louisiana State University

VICTOR K. McELHENY, Banbury Center, Cold Spring Harbor Laboratory

JAMES V. NEEL, Department of Human Genetics, University of Michigan Medical School

ROBERT OSTERBERG, Public Health Service, Bureau of
    Foods, Food and Drug Administration
RUTH PERTEL, Food and Drug Administration (then with
    Environmental Protection Agency)
VERNE RAY, Medical Research Laboratory, Pfizer, Inc.
RICHARD SETLOW, Biology Department, Brookhaven Nation-
    al Laboratory
MICHAEL D. SHELBY, National Institute of Environmental
    Health Sciences
ELDON SUTTON, University of Texas
LAWRENCE R. VALCOVIC, Public Health Service, Bureau of
    Foods, Food and Drug Administration
GRAHAM C. WALKER, Biology Department, Massachusetts
    Institute of Technology
JAMES D. WATSON, Cold Spring Harbor Laboratory
DAVID ZIPSER, Cold Spring Harbor Laboratory

Preface

GENESIS OF THE BANBURY REPORTS

In the spring of 1976, Mr. Charles S. Robertson gave to the Cold Spring Harbor Laboratory his fine Georgian-style house, together with the surrounding forty-five acres of fields, gardens, woods, and beach. Located at the end of Banbury Lane in Lloyd Harbor, Robertson House looks over Cold Spring Harbor and occupies one of the finest sites on Long Island's north shore.

In transferring his home and land to us, Mr. Robertson was aware that we planned to utilize it as a site (The Banbury Center) for small meetings on biological topics. Our first step in the creation of this center was the restoration of the Georgian garage into a meeting place, with offices, a library, and a conference room designed for thirty-two participants. The decision was then made that we would focus many of our meetings on the risks to humans of the now multitudinous agents that might damage our genetic material and create the mutations that can allow cancers to arise. We saw such meetings as a means of providing factual data which should help the public to make rational responses to the dangers that these agents may or may not present. Toward this end, we decided that each meeting should be transcribed and the edited proceedings made available to a potentially broad audience as a Banbury Report.

We thus proceeded to look for a Director who would help to bridge the gap between the informed scientist and the responsible citizenry, and so we sought out a leader in scientific journalism. Happily we were able to persuade Victor McElheny, then the Technology Correspondent of the New York Times, to join us as soon as we obtained the start-up support to let him assemble the appropriate staff.

The funds became available in the spring of 1978 through most substantial grants from the Klingenstein Fund and the Sloan Foundation. This allowed Victor McElheny to assume the Directorship of the Banbury Center in early May, just before our first Banbury Conference brought together many of the authorities on chemical mutagens to assess how we might measure the potential harm of such mutagens to humans.

This meeting was to serve as the prototype for many conferences on biological risk assessment to be held at the Banbury Center in future years. For 1979 we already have solid agendas for four such meetings, and plans are being made for a similar number in 1980.

We hope that they and the Banbury Reports that they will generate will live up to the high expectations which were created through Charles S. Robertson's most generous benefaction.

J.D.   WATSON
February   1979

Contents

x/ Contents

Foreword

The Banbury conference in May 1978 on the scientific basis for estimating risks to humans from chemical mutagens was the first of a series of meetings to be held at Banbury on potential health hazards from substances in the natural or man-made environment. I wish to thank the Environmental Protection Agency most warmly for its enlightened support of a conference that addressed itself to many of the central issues in biological risk assessment.

As the conference participants considered how to estimate the hazards from chemical mutagens to future generations, two themes were dominant.

1. <u>Confidence in basic knowledge of genetics</u>. A basis, stronger than existed 25 years ago for ionizing radiation, exists for estimating the risks to humans of chemically induced mutations. Data exist on the spontaneous or background frequency of mutations in people. Test systems ranging from bacteria and fungi to fruit flies and laboratory mice and rats exist for gathering data on the mutagenic potential of chemicals. Hence, genetic data are beginning to provide a measure of support for regulations restricting exposure to certain chemicals.

2. <u>The need for further research</u>. A continuous and vigorous research program is an essential underpinning for health-protection regulations.

The conference discussed, in a way considered fruitful by its participants, several points of direct, practical importance where present knowledge may be expanded. Among these were the actual consequences of mutations in germ cells and somatic cells; the differential sensitivity of germ cells, spermatogonia and spermatozoa and, especially, female germ cells; the differential senstitivity of male and female germ cells; the identification of populations at risk through monitoring, including sensitive subpopulations; and the impact of low doses of chemicals.

Gradual establishment of more accurate values for the background of spontaneously occurring human mutations was considered crucial for the long-term solidity of assessments of risks from environmental chemicals. Thus, wide-ranging, expensive, and time-consuming programs of monitoring human populations, such as an international sample of newborns or of the children of workers exposed to high levels of chemicals already identified as mutagens or carcinogens, need to be designed and started promptly. Increasing the amount and solidity of the human data can only strengthen the health-protecting intent of regulations controlling chemicals that are deemed crucial to production of food or energy.

The growing number of diseases being identified with a genetically caused lack or abnormality of specific proteins was of interest to attendees. The hope was expressed that intensified monitoring of such disorders, as well as chromosomal aberrations, might afford early warning of the genetic impact of synthetic chemicals.

The meeting explored other questions requiring further research. How robust are the mechanisms of repair of damage to DNA in animal or human germ cells? In dealing with the potential risks of very low doses of mutagenic chemicals, should we follow the same conservative path that was adopted with radiation (assuming that there is no threshold below which no risk is run)? How can we measure the true level of individual exposure to a mutagenic chemical? In extrapolating animal data to humans, what do we know about the comparative metabolism of a compound that is metabolized rapidly to other compounds of greater or lesser potential for damaging DNA? To what extent can animal data for the rate of elimination from tissues and detoxication of a compound such as ethylene oxide, which rapidly spreads throughout the body, be applied to humans? What exactly happens to DNA when mutagenic chemicals operate on it? How similar are these effects to those from radiation?

The conference attendees seemed to make a strong link between the continued robustness of regulations designed to shield the public from present and potential health risks and continuous research efforts to support and expand the data base for these regulations. The conference was reminded several times that prolonged research did not necessarily imply more and more onerous regulations. Some of the early estimates of risk from radiation have been revised downward with advancing knowledge.

While emphasizing areas of ignorance, and repeatedly counseling great caution in quantifying the mutagenic risks of chemicals, those attending the conference inclined to the view that genetic research does provide support today for a rational process of reviewing the risks of genetic damage to workers or the general population from chemicals.

We wish to acknowledge, with warmest thanks, our appreciation for the unflagging intellectual contribution of Dr. Ruth Pertel, formerly of the Environmental Protection Agency and now of the Food and Drug Administration, in the organization of the meeting and the editing of its proceedings.

It is a pleasure to recognize the absolutely essential contributions to the production of this book by Nancy Ford, director of publications of the Cold Spring Harbor Laboratory, who gave long hours over several months to editing the manuscript and seeing it through composition and printing; by Marie Moschitta, word-processing system operator in our Demerec laboratory, who produced both the final draft for comment and the camera-ready pages of this book; and by Lynda Moran, editor at Banbury Center, who cleared up innumerable unresolved questions in the manuscript and references during the weeks before the book went to the printer.

VICTOR K. McELHENY

ASSESSING CHEMICAL MUTAGENS: The Risk to Humans

Introduction

RICHARD N. HILL

Office of Toxic Substances
Environmental Protection Agency

We are pleased to have been the first group to meet at Banbury Center to consider the subject of risk assessment, a topic which will undoubtedly be the focus of many future conferences in this setting. At EPA we have gone through a transition period in our approach to risk assessment and the regulation of chemicals. In the past, chemicals were identified as producing a certain type of adverse effect in humans or on the environment. When a hazard was defined, action was often initiated to ban the chemical. It then became apparent that we could not go on restricting all chemicals in the environment. Instead, it was determined that the risk of occurrence of the effect in individuals exposed to a particular chemical should be determined. The first effect the Agency dealt with was carcinogenicity. For about two years we have been performing risk assessments of carcinogenicity in a two-step process: the first step is a determination of the likelihood that a given chemical may pose a carcinogenic hazard; the second is a quantitative estimate of the magnitude of risk if the chemical does in fact pose a carcinogenic hazard to humans. The Agency now recognizes there are many other end points besides carcinogenicity upon which risk assessments should be performed, but it needs to learn about methods for performing these assessments.

The EPA's Office of Toxic Substances administers two Acts, the Federal Insecticide, Fungicide and Rodenticide Act, which controls the use of pesticides, and the new Toxic Substances Control Act. Under both Acts programs are being initiated to look at the mutagenic effects of chemicals; these programs are reviewed below.

All pesticides must be registered by the EPA before they can be used. Registration involves the review of tests on the environmental fate and effects of the substance, in

1

addition to toxicological tests. In generating a set of test-ing guidelines to be employed by potential pesticide registrants, Pesticide Programs has received from an expert study group of the EPA Science Advisory Board a set of mutagenicity tests which evaluate the ability of substances to produce DNA damage and point and chromosomal muta-tions. The study group also developed criteria for defining mutagenic and nonmutagenic substances based on the results of testing. (The testing guidelines were published [EPA, Pesticide Programs, 1978] in August, and public comment was received through November.) After evaluating the comments, the Agency will decide whether to include mutagenicity tests in its final guidelines, and if it does, which tests it will utilize for the registration of pesticides.

The second activity of Pesticide Programs involves the Rebuttable Presumption Against Registration (RPAR) process. Whenever information is received by the Agency which suggests a chemical may produce unreasonable adverse effects, the Program initiates a formal review of the evidence against use of the chemical. Following a presump-tion against a chemical, the general public has a period of time to rebut our presumption of hazard. If there is successful rebuttal, the effect is not considered further. If the presumption remains, the Agency attempts to balance the risks of using the pesticide against the benefits of usage. Regulatory decisions vary from continued use of the chemical because the benefits outweigh the risks, to some sort of control of exposure of humans or the environ-ment to the pesticide, to cancellation of the registration and, thus, of the use of the chemical.

Pesticide Programs has initiated RPAR's on several chemicals on the basis of mutagenicity. The regulatory clock has been set. The Agency now needs to know methods for estimating risks from mutagens.

In the Toxic Substances Control Act, mutagenicity is identified as a toxicological end point of concern. An Interagency Testing Committee has already identified existing industrial chemicals that they recommend for mutagenicity testing under the Act. Another part of the Act deals with new chemicals entering production for the first time; schemes must be devised for evaluating the toxicity and risk of these chemicals.

In summary then, EPA has two Programs in the Office of Toxic Substances that need to decide on testing methods for mutagenicity. Should we employ these tests, we must be prepared to evaluate risks from chemicals that may pose mutagenic hazards to humans. At this point we are unable to evaluate adequately mutagenic risk--that was the reason for this conference.

Certain points need to be made with regard to the EPA position. When we speak of mutagenicity, we mean the potential risk to future reproductive generations; thus, we are talking about mutations occurring in germ cells. At the present time our concern is with the potential risk to humans, not to the totality of biological forms. In addition, there is a growing body of information dealing with the correlation between mutagenicity and carcinogenicity. This relationship is of great interest to the EPA, but it was not our intention to develop that subject at this conference, because carcinogenesis is a separate end point and should be dealt with separately.

Lastly, we assembled to consider the scientific issues associated with mutagenic risk, and in no way should this conference be interpreted as setting policy for the regulation of chemicals. We invited participants from other regulatory agencies (Occupational Safety and Health Administration, Consumer Product Safety Commission, and Food and Drug Administration) in addition to the EPA scientific advisory groups to share in the information generated at the conference. Any policy that may develop in the aftermath of this meeting will be formulated within the respective agencies.

The purpose of this meeting was to discuss means of evaluating mutagenic risks to humans from exposure to chemicals. Because most of the information on mutagenicity will be generated in experimental test systems, we need means for concluding whether or not a human germinal risk is expected from chemicals defined as mutagenic. Thus, a chemical may be called a mutagen because it is positive in the Ames test and in Drosophila, but how does one bridge the gap from test results to humans in general and human gonads specifically?

The second area of concern flows from the first. Some indication of the test systems that can be utilized for extropolating risk needs to be developed. Lastly, what models should be used for extrapolating risks from high experimental dosages to the lower expected human exposure levels? It is the consideration of models that led to the inclusion in the conference of radiation-induced carcinogenicity, chemically induced carcinogenicity, and radiation-induced genetic effects because people have already tackled dose-response data in these fields and have developed models for estimating risks.

The purpose of the conference, then, was to develop a scientific summary of the state-of-the-art in mutagenic risk assessment. It was hoped that this would include not only what can be done today but also what needs to be done to improve our knowledge in this field for tomorrow.

SUGGESTED BACKGROUND INFORMATION

Before we turn to the formal presentations, I should mention the group of scientific papers selected by some of the conference participants to serve as background for the prepared talks and discussions. From examination of the subject areas included, the impact that radiation studies have had on all aspects of hazard evaluation, including dosimetry, types of effects produced, and risk extrapolation methodology, becomes apparent. The National Academy of Sciences (1972)[1] study on the Biological Effects of Ionizing Radiation (BEIR report) recommends the linear, no-threshold extrapolation for radiation-induced mutagenic and carcinogenic effects. A paper by Crump et al. (1976)* shows that various models for carcinogenic risk estimation for chemicals become linear at low exposure levels.

Several differences between radiation and chemically induced mutagenic effects are laid out in a review by Lee (1975). Certainly, one big difference is accounted for by the difficulty in determining effective gonadal dose from exposures to chemical mutagens. Methods for estimating these exposure levels are given in papers by Lee and his colleagues (Lee, 1976; Aaron, 1976; Aaron and Lee, 1978). Ehrenberg and coworkers have chosen another means for evaluating chemical mutagenic risk by utilizing physical-chemical information and expressing hazard in terms of equivalent radiation doses (Ehrenberg et al., 1974; Osterman-Golkar et al., 1976). A third approach to estimating mutagenic risk for various effects, including chemicals inhibiting the cell-division spindle, is provided in a paper by Seiler (1977).

Abrahamson et al. (1973)* have pointed out an interesting relationship between genome size among biological forms and the induction of mutations by radiation. They observed a proportionality between mutation rate and haploid DNA content. The same connection between mutation and exposure has been reported for the chemical mutagen ethyl methanesulfonate (Heddle and Athanasiou, 1975).* Both the radiation and chemical relationships have been challenged, and critiques have been provided (Schalet and Sankaranarayanan, 1976; Schalet, 1978).

Some of the problems in setting up point mutagenesis test systems in mammals have been developed in a paper by Malling and Valkovic (1977).

---

[1]For complete bibliographic information on works cited, consult the cumulative Reference list given at the end of the book. Starred (*) citations are reprinted in their entirety in the Appendix.

In addition to the papers mentioned above, the reader may also find it helpful to examine the battery of muta-genesis tests proposed by the EPA Pesticide Programs (1978).

Mutation and Disease in Humans

JAMES V. NEEL

Department of Human Genetics
University of Michigan Medical School

My assignment is to generate an estimate of the contribution the mutational process makes to the ill health to be experienced by a human cohort, however defined, as it travels through life. This figure has a basic biological interest as the price a human population pays for generating the variation on which human evolution is ultimately based. In recent years it has become of practical interest as a figure that can be altered by human exposure to radiation and chemical pollutants, leading us to a variety of cost-benefit analyses. Finally, with the recent realization of the extent to which repair mechanisms can dull an initial insult to DNA or recoup a molecular slip, the figure comes to have another meaning, as a target for manipulation once we understand repair mechanisms better.

Unfortunately, efforts over the past 25 years to generate this estimate of mutational contribution to disease have not fared well. The superficial reason is a lack of adequate statistics on the prevalence of genetic entities in populations. Even if we had good figures for all the well-defined genetic entities, there would remain a major source of difficulty--the same difficulty that arises whenever an effort is made to estimate the prevalence of "disease in general" in a population.

What is the standard of reference? Do we, in the Mullerian tradition, try to define a genetic superhuman, whose attributes we all fail to match to some degree or

---

This is a modified version of a paper presented elsewhere (Neel 1978).

The author gratefully acknowledges support from Department of Energy Contract EY-77-C-02-2828.

other because of the erosions of mutation (Muller, 1950), or do we take a kind of genetic average and define disease as a certain number of standard deviations below the functioning of that average? In the latter case, the genetic load imposed by mutation would in theory certainly appear to be much less than in the former case.

Although this is an important conceptual point, with which we must ultimately deal, in the present state of the art it does not greatly influence how we proceed. This is because in medicine we are still working at a very gross level--in general, diagnosing disease only when the disability is plainly apparent. Thus, for the present, no matter which of the two viewpoints one espouses, a person is in practice forced to diagnose disease in identical terms. The implications of the distinction between the two views will become apparent when, if ever, medical genetics progresses to the point of assigning handicap or advantage to heterozygosity and homozygosity for a whole array of biochemical traits for which human beings are known to differ.

Putting aside the foregoing philosophical point, geneticists, in attempting to define the contribution of mutation to disease, can pursue either a direct or an indirect approach. In the indirect method, we estimate as well as possible the frequency of those diseases in the population which have a defined genetic basis, inferring from what we know of the negative selection to which individuals with the diseases in question are subject that the diseases must be maintained by mutation. In this approach, we usually tacitly assume that the population is in an approximate equilibrium between the input of disease-producing genes through mutation and the loss of these genes through early mortality or impaired fertility; for recessives we also assume that there is no heterozygote advantage. In the direct method, the approach is more conservative and much more exacting. Now one attempts an enumeration of specific diseases whose frequencies are demonstrably maintained by mutation, accepting as evidence for mutation the absence of the allele in question in both parents of an affected individual, but with subsequent transmission of the trait by the affected person, and accepting a disease as maintained by mutation pressure only when there is substantial evidence for that pressure. The total impact is estimated by summing across diseases. Let us consider where we stand in the application of these two approaches.

SOME RESULTS OF THE INDIRECT APPROACH

The most frequently cited estimates of the types and frequency of hereditary disease and congenital malformations

TABLE 1
Estimates of Frequency of Genetic Disorders in a Birth Cohort; Cases per 100 Liveborn (UNSCEAR, 1977)

Disease category	Northern Ireland (Stevenson, 1959)	UNSCEAR (1962, 1966)	British Columbia (Trimble and Doughty, 1974)		UNSCEAR (1977)
			minimal	adjusted	
Dominant	3.32[a]	0.95	0.06	0.08	1.0[e]
Recessive	0.21	0.21	0.09	0.11	0.1
X-linked	0.04	0.04	0.03	0.04	—[f]
Chromosomal	—[b]	0.42[c]	0.16	0.20[d]	0.4
Congenital malformations	1.41 ⎰	2.50 ⎰	3.58 ⎰	4.28 ⎰	9.0
Other multifactorial	1.48 ⎱	1.50 ⎱	1.58 ⎱	4.73 ⎱	
Unknown	—[b]	—[b]	(0.60)[g]	(2.70)[g]	—
Total[d]	6.46	5.62	5.50	9.44	10.5

[a] Including both trivial and serious anomalies.
[b] No information.
[c] Including Down's syndrome (0.15), other autosomal trisomies (0.05), Klinefelter's syndrome (0.17), Turner's syndrome (0.03), and Cri-du-chat syndrome (0.02), but excludes XXX females (0.12) and individuals with translocations (0.50).
[d] All but about 3% are due to Down's syndrome.
[e] Including X-linked disorders.
[f] Included in the dominant category.
[g] Frequency of unknown diseases is not included in the total.

9

in a defined population are those of Stevenson (1959) for Northern Ireland and Trimble and Doughty (1974) for British Columbia. The results of these two studies, as well as the results of certain manipulations of these data in 1977 by the United Nations Scientific Committee on the Effects of Atomic Radiation (UNSCEAR), are summarized in Table 1. Note the considerable differences between the two estimates. Both are rather soft, as the authors of the papers themselves recognize, and all of the efforts of UNSCEAR cannot turn soft data into hard. UNSCEAR estimated that 1,500 out of a cohort of 100,000 newborn infants would sooner or later be affected by serious dominant, recessive, or sex-linked traits or chromosomal abnormalities maintained by mutation pressure, and that 5% of the "congenital malformations" and "other multifactorial" traits, these together amounting to 9,000 per 100,000, were also so maintained. Thus, the frequency of disease ultimately maintained in human populations by mutation pressure was taken to be 1,950/100,000 individuals--about 2%.

Earlier, in 1972, the U.S. National Academy of Sciences Advisory Committee on the Biological Effects of Ionizing Radiations--the so-called BEIR committee (NAS, 1972)--took a somewhat more cautious approach, as shown in Table 2. Their estimates of the frequency of dominant and sex-linked traits are similar to those of UNSCEAR; their report preceded UNSCEAR which apparently adopted the BEIR estimates. The BEIR committee was so unhappy with our knowledge of how recessive and multifactorial traits and congenital malformations are maintained in popula-

TABLE 2
Estimated Effects of Radiation for Specific Genetic Damage

Traits	Current incidence per million live births	Number that are new mutants	Effect of 5 rem per generation	
			first generation	equilibrium
Autosomal dominant	10,000	2,000	50−500	250−2,500
X-chromosome-linked	400	65	0−15	10−100
Recessive	1,500	?	very few	very slow increase

The range of estimates is based on doubling doses of 20 and 200 rem. The values given are the expected numbers per million live births (NAS, 1972).

lations that it decided not to produce precise numerical estimates of the mutational component in these latter categories.

Figures on the frequency of a variety of genetic diseases are not easily translated into the burden of these diseases for their bearers and for society. The social impact of a child with trisomy 13 who dies shortly after birth is very much less than the impact of an adult who develops Huntington's chorea. Trimble and Smith (1977), employing as their point of departure the well-known British Columbia program, have begun to translate "disease" into "days of hospitalization." Their studies reveal that children with identified dominant or recessive disorders are admitted to hospital five to ten times more frequently than the average child, and the days of hospitalization are at least ten times the average. This brief review of efforts to develop an estimate of the mutational contribution to ill health fails to convey the full flavor of the sometimes strong disagreements that have characterized the interactions of committee members. Most of this centers around the role of mutation in maintaining recessives and multifactorial traits in humans.

SOME RESULTS OF THE DIRECT APPROACH

A much more rigorous approach, which sets an absolute minimum for the contribution of mutation to disease, stems from summing up the frequency of those entities that are demonstrably maintained by mutation. This demonstration entails a determination of how frequently individuals with specific syndromes usually inherited as dominant traits, or with chromosomal abnormalities, are born to normal parents (i.e., entails direct determinations of mutational events). Also, because of the improbability that sex-linked traits which are essentially genetic lethals are maintained by heterozygote advantage, indirect estimates of mutation rates for such sex-linked recessive traits are usually felt to be rather reliable, and such traits can be included among those maintained by mutation. Edwards (1974), specifying some but not all the abnormalities involved, suggested that in England the dominants with serious consequences for which there is clear evidence of maintenance by mutation pressure have a collective frequency of 60/100,000 newborns, and the sex-linked recessives, a collective frequency of 50/100,000. Vogel (1975) in his comprehensive review of human mutation rates identified 18 estimates (5 for sex-linked traits) he considered reliable; the average of these estimates is approximately 2×10^{-5}/locus/generation. The censuses and other studies that resulted in these estimates suggest that approximately 100-120 per 100,000 (0.1%) liveborn children are destined to develop one or the other of just these 18 diseases, so that Edwards's estimate appears to be on the low side. With respect to diseases due to major chromosomal abnormalities, we will for the moment adopt the same figure used by UNSCEAR--that they afflict approximately 400/100,000 (0.4%) newborns each generation; all of these appear to be afflicted by chromosomal disease due to mutation. Thus, at present, we can be rigorous in our identification each generation of some 500-520 per 100,000 newborn infants who either have or will later exhibit disease maintained by mutation pressure.

FUTURE DEVELOPMENTS

Three developments may be expected to increase the estimate rather dramatically in the next decade, in consequence of which even the UNSCEAR estimate will appear to have been conservative. First, medical genetics will develop a strong case for identifying a number of other syndromes whose etiology is now unknown as maintained by dominant mutation. For the recognition of a syndrome as dominantly inherited, it must satisfy Mendelian expectations. Unfortunately, there are two conditions under which a genetic test is impossible: where one aspect of the syndrome is infertility or early death and where one aspect is mental deficiency so severe as to preclude a marriage partner. Several quite distinctive syndromes that almost always occur as isolated events in sibships meet one or the other or both of these criteria. Among these should be mentioned the Rubinstein-Taybi syndrome, the Williams syndrome, and the Prader-Labhart-Willi syndrome. Other rare syndromes occur as isolated events and do not always preclude reproduction, but there are as yet inadequate data on the transmission of the trait; these include the Hallerman-Streiff and the aglossia-adactylia syndromes. Still other of the rare syndromes are characterized by some handicap where affected sibs are reported, suggesting rare recessives, but the data do not meet Mendelian ratios, and one wonders about a mixture of dominant mutation and recessive inheritance; the deLange syndrome would be an example of this. Finally, a visit to any state institution for the retarded reveals a collection of symmetrically dysplastic children without affected siblings, and here, too, one wonders about dominant mutation. If a characteristic biochemical defect could be identified for any of these syndromes, most geneticists would accept that the syndrome is due to dominant mutation. I would suggest that the combination of this type of evidence with standard genetic evidence where this can be obtained will lead us during the next decade to attribute to dominant mutation at least another 50-100 defective individuals out of each 100,000 live births, for a total of 150-220/100,000 births with dominant or sex-linked disease clearly maintained by mutation pressure.

Second, and a development needing little comment, our ability to define chromosomal lesions as a cause of disease will probably continue to improve, increasing substantially the number of defects attributable to such causes. As shown in Table 1, the figure for the frequency of chromosomal abnormalities at birth accepted by UNSCEAR was 400 per 100,000. This figure has since crept up to at least 500 per 100,000 liveborn infants (rev. in Jacobs, 1975; Carr and Gedeon, 1977). The demonstration that in humans approximately 50% of all early abortuses have chromosomal abnormalities (rev. in Carr and Gedeon, 1977), with the implication that nearly 5% of all conceptuses are cytologically abnormal, has surely been one of the very unexpected developments during recent years. It would be hazardous to guess how far these figures may be extended with improvements in cytological techniques.

. The third development in our ability to generate a direct estimate of the impact of mutation is of a rather different sort, to which I shall devote the major portion of this presentation. Recent years have witnessed the recognition of a wide range of diseases attributable to the absence of activity of an enzyme or a transport or receptor protein. For instance, many of the so-called inborn errors of metabolism, both classical and updated (rev. in Harris, 1963; Kirkman, 1972), are associated with the absence or near absence of enzymatic activity, as are some of the bleeding disorders, thyroid disorders (rev. in Stanbury, 1974), and a class of nonspherocytic hemolytic anemias which are due to the absence or near absence of such enzymes as pyruvate kinase, hexose kinase, glucose phosphate isomerase, etc. (rev. in Miwa, 1973). The defects in DNA repair mechanisms now documented in the various forms of xeroderma pigmentosum and in ataxia telangiectasia and Fanconi's anemia are the result of enzyme deficiencies. Familial hypophosphatemic rickets, Hartnup disease, and a dozen other rare entities are probably due to the absence or malfunction of a transport protein (rev. in Scriver, 1973), and testicular feminization and the severe form of familial hypercholesterolemia are due to the absence or malfunction of a receptor protein (Attardi and Ohno, 1974; Meyer, Migeon, and Migeon, 1975; Goldstein and Brown, 1977). These are all the result of what in the past have been termed "null" mutations--characterized by complete or nearly complete loss of function, usually with, in classic terminology, a recessive form of inheritance, although heterozygotes, where studied properly, show impaired activity as well. Just which of the wide range of phenomena encompassed under the term immunodeficiency diseases result from null mutants remains to be seen, but our knowledge of the many different polypeptides comprising the immunoglobulins suggests that the latter should become a fertile area for the delineation of such mutants. The ultimate biochemical basis for these nulls may range from a single amino acid substitution in a polypeptide to total loss of the polypeptide; in theory, the latter may reflect mutation of either structural or controller genetic elements. A distinction between the two possibilities in humans seems possible with somatic-cell hybridization studies, as described by Siciliano, Bordelon, and Kohler (1978).

Because it is rather difficult to visualize heterozygote advantage for these null mutants, it seems likely that most, if not all, are maintained by mutation pressure. Some hints of the possible total impact of this type of mutation emerge from the following somewhat devious reasoning. Using an indirect approach, Neel and Rothman (1978) have estimated that in Amerindians, mutations resulting in electrophoretic variants of a series of 25 proteins found in blood serum and erythrocytes occur at a rate of 1.6×10^{-5}/locus/generation. Mukai and Cockerham (1977), based on a study of five enzymes in Drosophila, have, with a direct approach, estimated that such mutations have a frequency of 0.2×10^{-5}/locus/generation. These same authors also report that "null" mutations, characterized by loss of enzyme activity, occur with a frequency of 1.0×10^{-5}/locus/generation. (As noted above, these nulls can result from mutation at either a structural or a controller locus, so that these rates cannot be compared with those based on defined polypeptides.) O'Brien (1973) pointed out that none of the 14 then-known null mutations in Drosophila were lethal when homozygous and argued for the relatively benign nature of null mutations. This is certainly not the case for humans. I suggest that the apparent difference may be an artifact of ascertainment. Flies with the degree of impairment experienced by many of the humans homozygous for the nulls will usually not make it to the "counting block," and so it is the least severe among the nulls with which the Drosophila geneticist would become familiar. To obtain an unbiased view of the phenotypic impact of the nulls, we must ascertain them as was done by Mukai and Cockerham (1977); unfortunately, these authors do not report on the effects of their null mutations when homozygous.

What I regard as a very conservative calculation of the possible impact of these null mutations on human health proceeds as follows. If the rate of mutation to electrophoretic variants in humans were only 1.0×10^{-5}/locus/generation in humans (i.e., less than our actual estimate for Amerindians), and if in humans the ratio of nulls to electrophoretic variants is only 2:1 rather than the 5:1 of Drosophila, then, with allelism, persons with nulls of a specific protein should be encountered with a frequency of 2×10^{-5}. There must be at least 5000 proteins in humans the absence or failure of function of which can lead to diseases such as those mentioned above. This assumption is, of course, not tantamount to assuming that the loss of activity of each human protein leads to disease. If homozygosity for a null mutation were in general incompatible with reproduction (i.e., genetic lethality) and if there were no heterozygote advantage or disadvantage--the simplest possible assumptions--then (assuming allelism and neglecting linkage) the probability that a zygote would be homozygous for at least one of the various nulls affecting these 5,000 proteins is approximately $1.0 - 0.99998^{5000}$, or 0.095; in other words, at conception 9.5% of all zygotes will be homozygous for one or more of these nulls. I hasten to emphasize that this calculation must be viewed with many, many reservations, but it does illustrate the potential for disease in this class of mutations. In particular, if absence of a particular protein may result from mutation at more than one locus, this calculation is an overestimate. Further, if there is selection against the heterozygote, this is a high estimate--but that selection will have contributed to the disease burden we are trying to estimate. The message is clear: this class of so-called recessive mutations may far outweigh in impact the dominants of the type discussed earlier.

We are thus led to postulate that future studies will reveal that roughly (5,000 + 9,500 + 200) zygotes /100,000 conceptions, or 14.7%, will have serious disease potentialities maintained by mutation pressure. As mentioned, most fetuses with cytological abnormality die early in pregnancy, and the same may be true for fetuses homozygous for null mutations. Note that this very rough calculation has not yet brought into the picture the possible contribution of mutation to other types of monogenic recessive inheritance or to the "constitutional" or "degenerative" diseases or the mental diseases; I shall not even begin to attempt to deal with them in this brief presentation. Incidentally, it remains an unexplained mystery why intrauterine mortality is so high for such aneuploids as the trisomy 21's and XO's, when postnatally they do relatively well. A 10% shift in either direction in the intrauterine mortality of fetuses with karyotypic abnormality would have roughly the same effect as doubling or halving the mutation rate. We do not yet know whether similar considerations apply to the null mutants, but, if so, understanding the mechanisms of prenatal selection has the same practical implications as understanding genetic repair mechanisms.

SOME GENERAL GENETIC CONSIDERATIONS

This observation concerning the possible frequency of null mutations, together with the other data on genetic disease in humans, will undoubtedly serve to reawaken Mullerian-type concerns over "our load of mutation." Kimura's hypothesis (1968) that a high proportion of genetic variation is selectively neutral, which seemed to ease concerns over the impact of mutation, can scarcely be applied to null mutations, and the suggestion that truncate selection can make the elimination of deleterious alleles highly efficient (King, 1967; Milkman, 1967; Sved, Reed, and Bodmer, 1967) also cannot be applied to lethals, which, in the genetic sense, many of the nulls known in humans are. It is tempting to postulate that these nulls play an important role in the relatively high fetal death rate in humans, but the demonstration, alluded to above, that as much as 50% of human fetal loss is due to a chromosomal abnormality preempts a large part of that selective arena. Because the accumulation of nulls in the gene pool should facilitate the expression of classic recessive genes, we cannot by invoking intrauterine selection against most of them dismiss the nulls as scarcely contributing to the social burden of mutation.

How can we proceed to direct estimates of the frequency of these null mutations in the human species? Strains of Drosophila and mice have been developed in which the standard phenotype is characterized by heterozygosity at some six to eight isozyme loci. A null mutation is thus detected by the absence of an expected enzyme band. Such a contrived situation is, of course, not possible in human genetics, but it has been demonstrated that individuals who are obligate heterozygotes with respect to such null traits as acatalassemia, Lesch-Nyhan syndrome, pyruvate kinase deficiency, and many other conditions exhibit approximately half-normal levels of the enzyme involved. On this basis, Harvey Mohrenweiser of our group has embarked on an effort to employ the miniature centrifugal-type fast analyzer (Burtis et al., 1972; 1973) in a screening program looking for half-normal enzyme activities in appropriate family studies to determine mutational status when such an activity variant is found

(Fielek and Mohrenweiser, 1978). This effort is part of a larger effort to carry the study of mutation to the protein level in humans, an effort that also searches for variant proteins on the basis of changes in electrophoretic mobility, in thermostability, and in kinetic parameters (Neel et al., 1978). We are collecting placental cord blood samples from all infants born in the University of Michigan Maternity Hospital, as well as blood from their fathers and mothers. Thus, when a variant is discovered in a child, the material is immediately at hand for a family study. In addition to collecting data on spontaneous mutation rates, the operation is seen as piloting out approaches to monitoring for changing mutation rates. In this connection, we are attempting to develop the most cost-effective system possible, beginning with the collection of the sample and extending to a data storage and retrieval system that will permit calling up any part of the data on a moment's notice.

Further technical developments may have great impact on our ability to detect both null phenotypes and mutations that result in reduced amounts of protein. Klose (1975; 1977) described two-dimensional polyacrylamide gel electrophoresis involving isoelectric focusing in the first dimension followed in a second dimension by electrophoresis, and O'Farrell (1975) described a similar technique in which separation in the second dimension is according to molecular weight on the basis of sodium dodecyl sulfate electrophoresis. This technique can already satisfactorily resolve some 1,100 components of $\underline{E}$. $\underline{coli}$. Anderson and Anderson (1977) have introduced innovations that render the technique more suitable for a screening procedure, and they have made substantial progress in identifying the various components in a human serum sample. The preparations have such high reproducibility that the prospects appear good for automating the scoring of at least a subset of the components. This machine scoring should present a lesser challenge than the machine scoring of a karyotype because the position of each normal component can be specified in isometric coordinates.

It is clear that the component of the burden of genetic disease attributed to the nulls dominates the estimate of the mutational burden of populations generated earlier, the degree of dominance depending on the amount of intra-uterine selection. How realistic is this assessment? We really cannot yet reach a judgment. The various rare entities cited earlier as falling under this classification probably do not average out at 2,000 per 100,000 of population, but precise estimates are not available for most of these diseases, and, as noted, there may be intrauterine selection. I suggest that as the screening techniques for half-normal enzyme levels mentioned earlier are applied, we will have a first rough assessment of the validity of this simplified treatment, because with a homozygote frequency of 2×10^{-5}, heterozygote frequencies for nulls of any particular protein should be almost 1% (again, the possible involvement of multiple loci has been neglected). The assessment of the contribution of mutation to disease really cannot be completed until there are direct estimates of the mutation rates for nulls, because, for example, conformity with the 1% heterozygote frequency postulated above could also result from higher mutation rates with some selection against the heterozygote as well as the homozygote.

The demonstration in recent years of the variety and importance of genetic repair mechanisms in coping with DNA lesions clearly prompts speculation concerning our future ability to influence what I shall term realized mutation rates. If we cannot stop primary insults to the DNA and/or if we must live in a world where these insults are increasing, perhaps ways can be found to influence repair mechanisms for the better. At this point in our thinking it becomes very important to understand the molecular basis for the kinds of mutations we have been discussing. The nature of the chromosomal mutations--although not the basic mechanisms--is relatively clear. For none of the dominant mutations supplying that component of the estimate do we yet understand the molecular basis of the trait. For the null-type mutations, substantial progress is being made. As already indicated, the mutations broadly termed nulls can in theory range from single amino acid substitutions to deletions encompassing several cistrons. For humans, the hemoglobin variants represent the most extensively studied example to date of the impact of mutation on a protein molecule. As is well known, these variants are for the most part due to single amino acid substitutions, such as can be attributed to single nucleotide substitutions; the frequency of this type of mutation can presumably be influenced by repair mechanisms. Technically, the thalassemia-type variants (characterized by the absence or a reduced amount of messenger RNA) correspond to null mutants (rev. in Kazazian, Cho, and Phillips, 1977), as do some of the methemoglobins and unstable hemoglobins due to single amino acid substitutions in strategic positions in the molecule. The hemoglobin and thalassemia variants that have been analyzed have, with few exceptions, all survived some measure of selection and so are not an accurate reflection of the primary results of mutation. This same comment applies to the other enzymes and proteins for which the molecular basis of the nulls and seminulls is being elucidated; they do not accurately reflect the spectrum of mutation at the molecular level. For humans, we really can say nothing authoritative at the present time about the relative frequency with which the nulls and the variants consistent with function arise through mutation.

The only study that begins to develop a picture of the primary product of mutation in mammals at the protein level is one by Milstein and colleagues on spontaneous mutants of immunoglobulin in mouse myeloma cell lines (rev. in Adetugbo, Milstein, and Secher, 1977). Of the four mutants subjected to detailed biochemical studies, only one was characterized by a single amino acid substitution, apparently due to an A to G transition. The other three all resulted in substantial shortenings of the myeloma protein, one apparently because of a point mutation of the "nonsense" type, one because of an intracistronic deletion, and one because of a frame-shift mutation resulting in an abnormal and shortened sequence of amino acids. The last three mutations, if they affected an enzyme, would almost surely be nulls. Thus, in this small but important series, the ratio of electrophoretic to null variants is very close to that of the Drosophila data. Questions can appropriately be raised about using the immunoglobulins as a model.

The discussion thus far has been entirely directed toward so-called spontaneous mutation. It is appropriate to point out that with respect to any possible increase in mutation rates because of human exposure to radiation or chemical mutagens, it now seems clear that the majority of mutations produced in the mouse by radiation are homozygous lethals, with increasing evidence that many, if not most, are small deletions--that is, they would be classed as nulls (Russell, 1971; Erickson, Eicher, and Glueckson-Waelsch, 1974; Gluecksohn-Waelsch et al., 1974; Russell et al., 1976; Russell and Cacheiro, 1977; Bernstine, Russell, and Cain, 1978). Comparable extensive studies on mammals have not been carried out with respect to the mutations produced by chemical mutagens, but from the results with lower organisms, one might anticipate a higher proportion of transition- and transversion-type mutations (rev. in Drake, 1970).

Clearly it will be some time before the molecular basis of mutation in humans and the repair mechanisms that operate on it are so well understood that we can consider whether mutation rates might be influenced by any manipulations of the genetic system or environment (other than the avoidance of mutagens). I would suggest that one of the most important steps toward delving into the potentialities will be better definition of the protein product of mutation in mammals, not only from the type of studies just described, but also for the nulls and other human variants detected by biochemical means. As our understanding of repair mechanisms improves, we can presumably infer from this information what aspects of the repair system are most critical for humans.

SUMMATION

In summary, then, we do not yet know the extent to which mutation contributes to the burden of disease in a human population, although substantial progress is being made. This is not an area of inquiry to which the results of experimental genetics can make a large contribution--we need human data. It appears that the health impact of the mutational events we are just beginning to be able to measure (i.e., the nulls and seminulls and the chromosomal) will far outweigh the impact of those we are more accustomed to trying to measure (i.e., dominantly inherited syndromes). Dominantly inherited syndromes clearly maintained by mutation can be shown to affect 100-200/ 100,000 infants, and the figure may double in the next decade. Chromosomal abnormalities affect some 500/100,000 infants, but at conception the frequency is more like 5,000/100,000; these figures may also increase substantially. A case is developed for something of the order of 9,500/ 100,000 conceptuses being homozygous for one or more null mutations, characterized by the absence or impaired activity of an enzyme or receptor or transport protein. What proportion of these survive to term is unknown, but it is a substantial fraction. Finally, there is undoubtedly a mutational component to a variety of the mono- and multi-factorial traits; this cannot now be estimated even roughly.

DISCUSSION

NEEL: We are here to talk about the quantitative assessment of risks. I am sure that as today and tomorrow unfold, our various positions and prejudices will rapidly become apparent. I would say (with all due respect to the screening studies that will certainly flag the most important mutagens, keeping them off the market) that in the final analysis, geneticists, having created a problem in the minds of people, are not going to be able to get away with merely extrapolating from experimental organisms to humans; we must have human data, and the means are now at hand for beginning to monitor human populations efficiently and effectively for mutation rates.

EHRENBERG: I have a few questions. In the title of Table 1 you used the phrase genetic disorders; in Table 2 the phrase used is genetic damage; in the first column of Table 1 disease, UNSCEAR is calculating the frequencies of diseases resulting from the mutation load. You have talked about the multi-factorial traits; when these are mentioned by the committees, they are called multifactorially conditioned diseases. I think it is rather important--if we are going to estimate the consequences, at our present stage of knowledge, of spontaneous or induced mutation--to consider the degree of change, whether it is a real disease or whether it could be a quantitative change of some kind; these are so difficult to measure epidemiologically. You said you did not want to discuss here constitutional and degenerative diseases, but there you used the word disease. I wonder to what degree these degenerative diseases are changes of a quantitative character. One reason I ask this comes from our work with plants, where we can work with almost completely homozygous strains. We measure drastic (morphological) mutations and then, per drastic mutation observed, find the number of mutations conditioned by polygenic control. This means that a mutation in that factor leads to a slight quantitative change that becomes more and more severe the bigger it is, so that at some level you could start to call it a qualitative change. In plants it has been possible to demonstrate, first of all, that the change goes in the direction against the one that worked at evolution (Brock, 1965; Denic, Dumanovic, and Ehrenberg, 1969). We need not discuss what that would mean to humans. But when we discuss chemical mutagenesis versus radiation mutagenesis, it is of interest that if you now measure per drastic mutation the number of quantitative mutations, you obtain with neutrons a little less than 1, with gamma radiation 2-3 with ethylenimine (which is an effective chromosome-breaking and mutagenic agent) around 10, and with ethyl methanesulfonate, which is more effectively point-mutagenic versus chromosome-breaking as compared to ethylenimine, around 30 (Ehrenberg, 1971). The X-ray-caused mutations that have been investigated so far are mainly deletions--specific-locus mutations.

Could it be that those point mutations in a strict sense are base-pair substitutions, or rather cause quantitative changes, which you would expect if the genes are duplicated? Could it be that this great number of around 10% per conception is a new null mutation involvement? They may also really exist but as quantitative traits due to duplication of genes.

What do you think of mutator genes, especially their importance to cancer in later generations? I refer you to a paper by Tomatis, Hilfrich, and Turusov

(1975) which showed an increased cancer incidence in all loci in the second and third--maybe fourth--generation after treatment with a chemical mutagen.

NEEL: In response to your first question, Table 1 was taken directly from the UNSCEAR report, using their terminology; Table 2 was directly from the BEIR report and uses their terminology. I used them but with many reservations, and I feel we must be more rigorous than either of those committees was.

The impact of mutation on quantitative traits is, of course, a highly controversial subject, the more so because when we say quantitative traits we hide a great deal of ignorance. Quantitative inheritance is a mess. We operate by regression; we postulate many small genes with cumulative effects. Ultimately, those mysterious many small genes have to have some physical counterpart. I think in the end it will be the protein variations that we are able to measure. For the present, it is extremely difficult to be at all rigorous in talking about the impact of changing mutation rates on quantitative traits. I think my intuition is in the direction of yours. Given what we can postulate for the ultimate genetic basis, mutation is going to impair rather than improve most quantitative traits to the extent that in some human diseases we simply cut off the tail of a distribution and call that "disease"--like hypercholesterolemia, or impaired glucose metabolism, or high blood pressure; mutation in quantitative systems is also going to alter disease frequencies. I do not think that the end results of specific-locus-mutation studies, as in the Russell system, will be too different, when we finally understand them, from the results of studies on quantitative traits.

You asked me about mutator genes. If I were planting questions, I could not have planted better. It just so happens that in the summers of 1940 and 1941, while I was in an interval between completing my Ph.D. and doing medicine, I spent two lovely summers at the Cold Spring Harbor Laboratory, when Demerec was director, working on a Drosophila strain that had suddenly gone mad. I started out teaching at Dartmouth, miles from anybody's Drosophila stocks that could have contaminated my strain, and suddenly mutants were literally coming out of the woodwork. I brought the problem first to Columbia on an NRC fellowship, and then out here. I believe firmly that this was one of the first well-documented cases of a mutator event in <u>Drosophila</u>. We never got a clear resolution of the genetic basis of the phenomenon, I am sorry to say, but the fact was pretty apparent. I have no doubt that we must begin to try to recognize those phenomena in human populations, but it is going to be a lot more difficult, and I think if we ever do work successfully with them, it will be somatic-cell-genetics rather than the kinds of germ-cell genetics that I am talking about here. I do not doubt high mutator lines exist in humans; I do not see why they should be an exception.

EHRENBERG: I was thinking of retinoblastoma.

NEEL: Well, that is one that I have worked on quite a bit; I feel at home with that. We published some of the basic estimates. I do not see (you know Knudson's papers--e.g., 1971) why you want to invoke a mutator gene for retinoblastoma. Knudson's hypothesis for hereditary retinoblastoma involves two mutations: one in a germ cell and one that occurs later in a somatic cell. I think he has corrected the germ-cell rate down to about 0.8×10^{-5}, which is a reasonable mutation rate. His somatic-cell rate is not too far off that when you put it per cell generation rather than per life cycle. So I do not see why we need to invoke a mutator gene there, unless you are using that for the second somatic-cell mutation that permits the germ-cell mutation to express itself. I do not think of that in the mutator gene context.

PERSON: I have heard, but cannot point to a paper, that children with retinoblastoma who are not treated with radiation do have a high frequency of other types of tumors; at one time these were attributed to radiation therapy, but this obviously cannot be.

NEEL: This is correct. Knudson and I were on the same panel last week. You do get an increase of malignancy in the radiation field, but aside from that there is now evidence of osteogenic sarcoma having an increased frequency in children with retinoblastoma. I do not know whether this is from a mutator gene or whether the mutation resulting in retinoblastoma in the eye is expressed differently in different tissues.

PERSON: Are you saying there is an increase in tumors in other sites outside the radiation field for children treated for retinoblastoma?

NEEL: This is now accepted for retinoblastoma, and the reference would be Knudson.

EHRENBERG: May I just make one very short remark to clarify a small difference between us? If you define as an end point a 5% decrease of intelligence, or something like that, it is a quantitative trait, which could, of course, become qualitative if you could find out what was behind this on the biochemical level. In any case, this is something we cannot measure today; there are no methods to find such a thing. It would be catastrophic if we had a high mutation frequency with such consequences. You can see it in plant models where we measure as the end point the yield of seeds, or the reproductivity, or something like that.

NEEL: Yes, I think I understand the thrust of what you are saying. I try to be hard-nosed in human genetics, and I restricted my presentation to developments where I believe we can be on fairly firm ground. The moment we begin to talk about the quantitative traits we run into all kinds of difficulties with quantitation. I accept what you are saying but I do not think we are able to handle that problem with any authority.

EHRENBERG: We have to recognize that it is there, and I shall not say anything more about it.

NEEL: I agree with you that it is there, so there is no difference of opinion.

PERSON: Is that same problem present in electrophoretic patterns? Are the proteins either there or not there, or is there a whole range of being there?

NEEL: Let me divide your question into two parts. Electrophoresis, as you know, picks up charge differences between various forms of a protein, and if you are working with a reasonable-sized protein, of molecular weight of 60,000, say, and mutation results in an amino acid substitution that adds or subtracts one or two charges, you can usually detect it, yet no single electrophoretic method is going to pick up all the substitutions; this is an empirical observation. In experimental animal systems, you can also be pretty sure whether, as a result of mutation, the animal is completely lacking a protein. You set up an experimental design where the expectation in the absence of mutation is two electrophoretic bands because the animal is heterozygous. In humans we have more trouble; we cannot set up such systems. But electrophoresis in the hands of a good person is more reliable than your question would suggest.

EHRENBERG: There is one more aspect to this problem--

the deletions as reasons mainly behind the X-ray- or gamma-ray-induced specific-locus mutations. In the analysis of <u>Neurospora</u> mutations by Malling and de Serres (1973), there is an astonishingly high percentage of base-pair transitions, the same as we see in bacteria and other organisms. Where are they, if they are induced? They must lead to something, but they are not seen as recessive mutations.

NEEL: I hope that in due time the study of induced mutations in the mouse will be carried to the biochemical level. It <u>is</u> being carried to the biochemical level now. One paper out of Oak Ridge on hemoglobin mutants shows four induced mutations, I think, and every one of these looks to be a deletion.

BREWEN: It is five now, and they are all chromosomal.

NEEL: In the mammal--in the mouse--more and more it looks as though X-rays are producing deletions, and there is this genuine difference from the <u>Neurospora</u> data.

BREWEN: There has also been a study done at NIEHS (the National Institute for Environmental Health Sciences), I understand, where they have looked for enzyme variants and uncovered four or five and they have all been nulls, but this has not been published.

NEEL: I wish they would get that study written up; there have been some administrative problems, and we only hear about it by word of mouth.

VALCOVIC: We presented a portion of that; it was published last year (Malling and Valcovic, 1977).

HOEL: Gene Saures has done some work on this.

ABRAHAMSON: One thing always bothered me about Fred de Serres's work, which showed that 30% of them were gross chromosomal and the other 70% he claimed to be intragenic changes; but most of the studies that analyzed the intragenic changes came from a low dose of 1,000 R, and the doubling dose for that system was well over 1,000 R. My complaint has always been that a good proportion of those, if not more than 50% of them, could have been spontaneous in origin, from that very low dose component, so that he would have had the intragenics of a spontaneous nature; the gross chromosomals could have been from the induced ones at higher doses.

NEEL: Incidentally, I have just written L. B. Russell (at Oak Ridge) to find out whether they ever tested their spontaneous mouse mutants for their lethality when homozygous.

ABRAHAMSON: They did.   They are about 68% homozygous lethal.

NEEL: Are the data clearly published?

ABRAHAMSON: That is what Russell told me a number of times.

NEEL: I have never been able to find that in the literature.

HOLLAENDER: It is not in the literature.

NEEL: Hell, there is a very important observation to get into the literature.   This may imply that two-thirds of the spontaneous mutations measured in the Russell program correspond to the nulls I have been discussing, and, extrapolating to man, as homozygous lethals would usually be characterized by intrauterine loss rather than gross phenotypic effects in populations of liveborn infants.

Strengths and Weaknesses of Tests for Mutagenesis

W. GARY FLAMM

Division of Toxicology, Bureau of Foods
Food and Drug Administration

A benchmark for chemical mutagenesis was the Gabridge and Legator paper (1969) on the host-mediated assay. They placed various Salmonella strains (histidineless mutants) in the peritoneum of mice or rats. They injected drugs such as dimethylnitrosamine that require mammalian metabolic activation. They showed that the mammalian host metabolized the nitrosamine to its active mutagenic form. That active mutagenic form then mutagenized the bacteria placed in the peritoneum of the animal.

There was considerable discussion of that system and its utility for measuring the capacity of chemicals that require activation to produce mutations in mammals. Over several years, approximately 25 to 30 chemicals were tested: alkylating agents, nitrosamines, aromatic amines, and polycyclic aromatic hydrocarbons. Apart from the alkylating agents, which do not require metabolic activation, and a handful of substances such as dimethylnitrosamine, most of the agents did not function as expected. That is, while metabolic activation might well have been going on in the mammal, the active mutagenic forms of that molecule were not reaching the peritoneum in sufficient concentrations to produce a significant number of mutations.

The statistical patterns being generated with dimethylnitrosamine or with alkylating agents made it clear that the statistical unit of the experiment was the treated animal, not the total number of organisms that had been injected into the peritoneum of the test animals. Instead of being able to inject, say, 5 to 15 animals for a reasonably reliable test, 25 to 30 animals would be required. Janet Springer and colleagues (Green and Springer, 1973) of the FDA concluded this as they struggled to interpret information from the host-mediated assay.

Heinrich Malling, then at Oak Ridge, demonstrated the

27

same kind of activation in a test tube (Malling, 1967), starting with dimethylnitrosamine. He used a liver microsomal system and added coenzymes and other appropriate supplements. After one year of struggling, he had his first successful in vitro activation. After experiments with bacteria, he tried yeast and Neurospora.

Bruce Ames (Ames, Lee, and Durston, 1973) also was learning that by immobilizing the microsomes of his liver S-9 fraction in agar, he could enhance the stability and functionality of the microsomal enzymes. He found that the same biochemical metabolizing mixtures useful for examining such simple things as dimethylnitrosamine actually activate many chemicals from different major chemical classes. Malling believed that this in vitro procedure would have very limited utility because it would be necessary to fashion a metabolizing mixture for each new substance. He felt it unlikely that anyone would hit upon a reasonably universal procedure. Clearly, the work by Ames, McCann, and Yamasaki (1975) has shown that this is not an enormous problem.

Thus, we had methods for deducing mutagenic activity of chemicals requiring metabolic transformation. We also had systems that would utilize essentially naked DNA, taking a chemical, activating it with a liver S-9 fraction, and observing whether it reacted to form DNA adducts. The first indication that aflatoxin B_1 interacted with nucleic acids was the work by Sporn and colleagues (1966). Their UV spectrophotometric information indicated that aflatoxin was combining irreversibly to form new covalent bonds with DNA. Today, with high-pressure liquid chromatography, the possibility of conducting highly sensitive studies with DNA is greater. Several people are studying DNA repair replication, not so much to look at mutagens as to understand repair itself.

DNA repair in human cells can be established so that it certainly rivals gene mutational systems in mammalian tissue culture cells for sensitivity. Indeed, it is probably five to ten times more sensitive in terms of measuring genetic effects than most of the HGPRT (hypoxanthine guanine phosphoribosyl transferase) and TK (thymidine kinase) systems.

Once the hurdle of metabolic activation was overcome, a whole variety of in vitro systems could be used to study whether a substance or its metabolic product was mutagenic. Along with naked DNA or DNA repair in human tissue culture cells and in a variety of bacterial systems about which we will hear more later, we have mitotic recombination and gene conversion in yeast. This may eventually prove especially interesting. It may also correlate with the work Heidelberger is doing with either 10T½ or 3T3 cells. He is looking at promotional activities, using the phorbal esters as his basic standard of comparison. His results involve substances that may prove to be promoters, not just of skin cancer, but also of systemic cancer.

Plants have been used very extensively in the radiation field, but not to any great extent for chemical mutagens. Prior to 1968, an enormous number of herbicidal and pesticidal substances were studied in barley and onion. The 1969 Mrak Commission report lists about 500 pesticides and herbicides alleged to have mutagenic activity because they produced chromosomal aberrations in the somatic cells of barley and onion. Much of the evidence comes from onion root tips. The onion roots apparently have the capacity to pump the chemical into the growing meristematic portions of the plant, causing considerable chromosomal disruption in these rapidly dividing cells. Do these observations forecast heritable mutations in mammalian organisms? The answer is not clear.

Around 1967 Chu was developing at Oak Ridge a forward mutational assay in Chinese hamster cells. He studied both the spontaneous mutation rates and the X-ray-induced rates at different dose rates and at different total doses. With some encouragement from Malling, Chu began to utilize the HGPRT X-linked locus of Chinese hamster cells (Chu and Malling, 1968). Such chemicals as EMS (ethyl methanesulfonate) and MMS (methyl methanesulfonate) induced about a two- or threefold increase above the spontaneous mutation frequency of these cells, or around 2×10^{-5}. That rate was about 1,000 times higher than their mutation rate per locus per cell generation. Chu was unable to clean the culture of many HGPRT$^-$ mutants apparently carried along in every effort to clone and to grow up a clean culture. But he could demonstrate an increase in the spontaneous mutation frequency of about two- to fourfold when he used very high concentrations-- about 10 mM of EMS and about 1 mM MMS. This was really slugging the cells very hard.

In the early 1960s Szybalski, Ragni, and Cohn (1964) claimed that this would not happen in somatic cells. Their figure for gene mutations in a human cell line was around 10^{-3}. They obtained no increases at all by using high concentrations of mutagenic substances. Somatic cells, they said, had an extremely high mutation rate because of mitotic recombination. There was so much mitotic recombination going on that they despaired of ever being able to elevate the rate above 10^{-3} by using chemical mutagens. Most structural genes in mammalian cells, such as HGPRT and APRT loci, appear to have mutation rates around 10^{-8} to 10^{-7}, although Bob DeMars of Wisconsin insists that HGPRT in human cells has a rate of 10^{-6} (as discussed in Clive, Flamm, and Patterson, 1973).

These rates are all a very far cry from the 10^{-3} that

led many of us to believe that mammalian tissue culture cells would be a hopeless material for the study of chemically induced mutation, as was indicated by Szybalski. That turns out <u>not</u> to be the case. When Clive and I worked up the TK locus of the L5178Y mouse lymphoma system that was originally isolated and described by Glen Fischer, we found initially that we had frequencies as low as 10^{-7} (Clive et al., 1972); actually, the rates were less than that-- around 10^{-8}. Our initial experience led us to induced rates per rad that were quite comparable to what Chu and DeMars reported (as discussed in Clive, Flamm, and Patterson, 1973). Examining EMS and MMS, we found induced rates comparable to theirs, even though some differences in spontaneous mutation rates existed, as mentioned earlier.

We lost our original line, unfortunately. It was different from any that has been isolated since; we could never get a nonrevertible mutation. Every mutant that we isolated from a whole series of X-irradiations at high doses from 90 R per minute all the way up to 500 R per minute-- which should have given us many deletions and nonrevert- ible mutations--had no revertible mutations. Everything (all mutants) was revertible, which is no longer true today with the other lines.

We can only speculate what might have been the original situation (as opposed to the lines that Clive has today, where the spontaneous rates are more like 10^{-6}). To be sure, we had a heterozygote situation. The TK is definitely autosomal, and we were using a heterozygote that underwent mutation to the TK minus minus condition. But we speculate that the complementing chromosome was probably carrying not much more than a functional TK gene. Everything else in that complementing chromosome was probably in very bad shape. Deletion mutations in the chromosome were probably creating a situation in which genes vital for viability were lacking within that particular cell line. But we will never know the truth. All we know is that once we had a line from which we could not produce a nonrevertible mutant; now many of the mutations pro- duced are nonrevertible.

At present it can be said that, in general, four loci usable for chemical mutagenesis exist in about five different cell lines. These are HGPRT, TK, probably methotrexate resistance, and ouabain resistance. Methotrexate and ouabain resistance may be measuring only base substitu- tions. The theoretical basis for assuming that metho- trexate-resistant mutants are simply a product of base-pair substitution relates to the view that mutation to metho- trexate resistance affects the K_i for methotrexate with the enzyme tetrahydrofolate reductase. Methotrexate normally binds the enzyme 100,000 times more strongly than its normal counterpart, folic acid. Base substitution affects the part of the enzyme molecule that changes the K_i so that methotrexate does not bind as avidly to the enzyme molecule, but leaves the tetrahydrofolate reductase as a functioning enzyme molecule. With base-pair deletions or additions in the structural gene, one would assume a non-functioning enzyme molecule would be produced, rendering the tetrahydrofolate reductase an amorphic mutation, and you would not accrue methotrexate resistance.

We studied TK and methotrexate resistance in L5178Y with a series of chemicals, some of which clearly produce primarily base addition and deletion as opposed to clean base-pair substitutions. Hycanthone and other substances produce principally frame shifts (additions and deletions). With these agents there are few, if any, mutations for methotrexate resistance, but there is good induction of TK mutants. Ultraviolet light and EMS, which frequently induce base-substitution mutations, produce a large number of methotrexate-resistant mutants. Ouabain resistance has not been looked at nearly as carefully as methotrexate resistance.

Frantz, Malling, and others have tried to couple metabolic activation to lymphoma cells--with some success. A difficulty with assessing the data and the total body of information on these particular cells obtained using the TK locus is that less than 10% of the information has been published. Much may never be published, because much of the work is being done in support of regulatory petitions concerning the safety of drugs and food additives. Over the next couple of years the National Cancer Institute plans to study carcinogens and related noncarcinogens at Litton Bionetics and Stanford Research Institute, using the TK locus. The plan is to study 60 to 80 known carcinogens and approximately 30 substances claimed to be noncarcinogens but closely allied structurally to known carcinogens. The resulting information will be critical to our understanding of the capability of the methodology.

Our richest experience with an intact mammalian system is the dominant lethal test (Sheu et al., 1978). This simply measures fetal wastage. Male rats or mice are treated either acutely or chronically and are then mated weekly. In some instances the males are treated throughout spermatogenesis--generally before they are mated to virgin females. At about midterm in pregnancy the females are sacrificed and dead implants are searched for and counted. Early attempts to look at preimplantation loss through a comparison of the number of corpora lutea and the number of total implants caused so many difficulties that the idea has been dropped.

The sensitivity and robustness of the dominant lethal

test and the limits on its reliability were studied carefully, but the work quickly became a statistical nightmare. We had to use concurrent controls; we could not rely on historical controls for fetal wastage rates. The control rates varied from one lab to another, from one supplier to another, from one season to another. Many parameters seemed to affect the rates of spontaneous fetal wastage in both rats and mice. By the end of an experiment, there would generally be eight to ten matings and a couple of hundred implants per mating. Typically, three dosage levels were used. We would have as many as 30 different groups with 200 implants per group being compared to our matched concurrent control groups. We tried at first to test food-additive-like compounds referred to as GRAS (generally recognized as safe). But we found that we really did not know how to cope with the data. If we knew at the beginning of an analysis which group was control and which was treated, then all the treated were positive; if we did not know, then we had a very mixed result. Basically, we had as many values below the control line as we had above, and the magnitudes were about the same.

We tried various statistical approaches. We thought that one approach to enhance the sensitivity of the assay-- appropriate for food-additive-type substances to which we are constantly exposed--would be to expose the male animal on a continuing basis. We would then eliminate the need for ten matings and do only one or two, having covered the whole spermatogenic cycle. Theoretical reasoning told us that there might be a problem because treatment throughout the spermatogenic cycle might result in such extensive damage that we could lose postimplantation effects to preimplantation loss. We feared that the frequency of postimplantation death might be reduced as a consequence.

We used the mutagens EMS and TEM (triethylenemel-amine), both very effective alkylating agents. We exposed males to three or four concentrations of these two sub-stances. But this did not reduce the postimplantation deaths. In fact, it augmented them; an additive effect was noted over weeks of treatment. It was gratifying to find that doses administered throughout spermatogenesis pro-vided essentially an additive effect, and that one or two matings enabled the clear measurement of mutagenicity of these alkylating agents. The work load was reduced from eight to ten weekly matings to just two. We thought we could then add additional dosage levels or expand the size of our groups. Thus, we would still have about the same size of experiment, but would deploy our postimplantation counts in a way we thought might be sounder from a toxicologic point of view.

After variance analysis of our dominant lethal work,

however, our statisticians told us that we had only a 50% chance of picking up a two- to threefold increase in dominant lethals as reflected by fetal wastage. Because fetal wastage is generally around 10%, an increase from 20% to 30% in fetal wastage is detectable only 50% of the time. If this is in fact the case, the lack of sensitivity of the dominant lethal test suggests a very limited utility for this method.

Remember also that the dominant lethal test does not actually measure a heritable genetic event. Thus, from the point of view of heritable mutations, we might be fooling ourselves as well. For instance, the sperm could be carrying the chemical into the egg where a delayed epigenetic effect could result in postimplantation loss. But this seems rather remote.

DISCUSSION

ABRAHAMSON: If you were treating only meiotic germ cells by this procedure, and then you got an increase in dominant lethals, that has to be a heritable change.

FLAMM: Most of the sensitivity is postmeiotic.

ABRAHAMSON: I realize that, but were you getting any premeiotic effects?

FLAMM: A couple of agents, such as 6 mercaptopurine and mitomycin C, gave a premeiotic effect in certain hands; in others they did not.

At any rate, we now understand that substances that induce a 20-30% increase in fetal wastage when the male is treated throughout spermatogenesis are seen as positive only about half the time and negative about half the time. We could test them from now to doomsday, and I suspect the result would be the same. The test really does not offer much sensitivity. Nevertheless, for reasons not understood, we occasionally encounter substances that seem to produce clear and reproducible dominant lethal effects. I wish I could explain this observation adequately.

Two substances have proved interesting in our work with food-related substances. Ammoniated glycyrrhizin used in licorice candy and gum acacia both seem to produce dominant lethals without having any remarkable or dramatic effect in in vitro systems-- the Ames or yeast mutagenicity studies.

EISENSTADT: Isn't acacia used as a carrier for many intraperitoneal injections?

FLAMM: It is a good emulsifying agent, so things that are not soluble but need to be suspended homogeneously can be emulsified with either acacia or gum arabic. Acacia is very commonly used in the cosmetic industry and in pharmacy.

EISENSTADT: How about in carcinogenicity tests as an inert carrier?

FLAMM: It is quite possible; I just do not know; it would not surprise me.

HOLLAENDER: But it could be just serving as an emulsifier in very carcinogenic substances.

FLAMM: BHA (butylated hydroxyanisole) and BHT (butylated hydroxytoluene) are antioxidants commonly used in convenience foods, bakery goods, salad dressing, and so forth.   BHA is fairly ubiquitous in food, and Oak Ridge has a long history of having tested it under a great variety of conditions, primarily because it is in standard animal chow, and one must try to compute any effects this has on one's experiments.   We are now testing these substances for heritable translocations in mice.   I believe that Abrahamson's lab is looking at them in Drosophila as well.

RAY: I would think that for this known lethal effect, which seems related to chromosomal level effect, perhaps some of the in vitro and in vivo cytogenetic tests should have detected these substances as well. Is that information available?

FLAMM: I still do not know how to perform a cytogenetic test in vitro so that I can assure you the findings are relevant to chromosomal anomalies of germinal cells in vivo.   I do not know what will happen in vivo, when in vitro you have produced 90% killing.   Is 20% killing or 50% killing a valid way of running that experiment? I do not know.   That is why we have elected to explore heritable translocations to see whether we can induce them.   The problem with the dominant lethal may not be so much with the biology as with the statistics.   Now Walter Generoso (1979) is beginning to find that different strains, particularly different maternal strains, behave in very different ways.

EHRENBERG: But he gets pretty consistent results with a definite strain?

FLAMM: With a definite strain.   But, of course, he is using a very strong alkylating agent and he is producing dominant lethality as high as 70% fetal wastage.   When you get something like that, you do not have so much of a problem.

   For our purposes in foods, and I daresay for the purposes of many of the regulatory agencies, you must be able to deal with substances that are very weakly mutagenic. Our test systems have to have enough sensitivity to detect the weakly active substances.

In foods, there are two kinds of problems: miniscule exposures to highly toxic substances, such as aflatoxin--as toxic as any substance you can imagine--and enormous exposures to very nontoxic substances. We do not have very much in the middle; we got rid of most of the problems in the middle years ago. So we are looking at those two extreme situations: what to do with an aflatoxin that we cannot entirely remove from corn or peanuts, and what to do with a variety of other unavoidable contaminants where the issue is not banning an additive to food, but banning the food itself.

For instance, saccharin has been tested for carcinogenicity 17 different times in chronic experiments, three times in two-generation experiments.

HOLLAENDER: This is the newest information that just came out from Canada's National Cancer Institute.

PERSON: To reinforce what you are saying, the implications here are quite severe. If, depending on the strain used, you get a 5% dominant lethality one time and 50% another based on strain difference, how do you then move from those data to any realistic consideration of the hazards to humans? If it appears not only in the dominant lethal assay, but also in the heritable translocation assay, this has rather severe implications for the utility of the data for risk assessment.

FLAMM: This does not trouble me greatly because I do not think we really know what it means. We have not done any careful chemical dosimetry. If we did, the chemical dosimetry could take care of that; we just do not know. It is probably too early to worry. What I do worry about is the fact that for many substances the dominant lethal test is not very robust and not very sensitive. Its limits of reliability are such that it troubles me to use it. Yet, it is clearly possible that substances that do not produce mutations in vitro in fact produce dominant lethals. We need additional tests and, just as important, an improved understanding of the meaning of the tests we use. I feel very strongly that one of the foremost goals in the field is better understanding in quantitative terms of the relationship of in vitro systems to in vivo ones. Ultimately, if effective testing is to be done, considerable reliance will have to be placed on in vitro tests. But what do those tests mean quantitatively in terms of in vivo systems?

EHRENBERG: May I ask a question? You say that the statistical analysis is a nightmare. Ray wrote something similar a few years ago. In some cases you get positive, in the next experiment negative, and then again positive, and you do not know what to do with it. May I ask whether you have tried to detect outlayers in the tests by an objective test for independence of events, which you would have if they are mutants? We have done that in tests for dominant lethality from irradiated foods, where there have been such cases, especially in the Indian experiments. You improve the system with respect not only to regularity and robustness, but also to sensitivity. You can detect much smaller effects if you build in this elimination of clusters of interdependent events (see Ehrenberg, 1977). Then there should be, of course, a second analysis to see whether the frequency of clusters has changed. But such an effect probably would have nongenetic causes.

FLAMM: In fact, we attempted to deal with the cluster problem. Bill Russell sort of held our feet to the fire. He and Sid Green obtained different results with regard to hycanthone's ability to induce dominant lethals. Green was using the rat, and Russell was using the mouse; both men were getting exactly the same result for acute doses of hycanthone in a single intraperitoneal administration of the drug. There was no indication that it was positive, but when Green dosed for five days, he saw a dominant lethal effect. He repeated this twice, so that he had three positive effects all occurring in the same week; but they were attributable only to the five doses over a period of five days. Green and Russell discussed it at a meeting, and Russell contended that this was a cluster effect. When the cluster effect was considered, hycanthone was still positive, at least in two of the three, but I think one of the three did drop out. I do not think we have approached it from your point of view. Generoso brought up the possibility that we have not been using the right strain, or the right mother. Quite frankly, when I look at the different strains and their response to different chemicals--I think he used four chemicals; three of them were alkylating agents, all doing a good job with one strain, and one was a nonalkylating chemical doing very poorly--I conclude from his data that when you go from one chemical class to another, you have to shift strains for the mother in order to obtain a high degree of responsiveness.

NEEL: What would be the right strain for extrapolation to human populations?

FLAMM: One would really have to know why you get this variation. Is it a function of the pharmacokinetics or the ability of the agent to get to the germinal cells in an activated form? Generoso has been assuming--and I must say, the way the experiment is constructed, one is almost forced to believe--that the variation is due to different degrees of maternal repair on these zygotes. I would dearly love to see the repair studies done, not necessarily on the zygotes; I would settle for repair studies done on the somatic cells of these mothers, if possible.

RAY: Could I make just a couple of comments, please? One deals with this problem of variation. In a practical sense, most of us in industrial laboratories are subject to commercial production of strains; many of us are using so-called random or outbred stock. If you plot your dominant lethality and control groups over several years, you will see wide fluctuations in this; the greater it becomes, the less sensitive your system becomes for detecting small effects. I suppose we should publish this; I have one study that runs over five years, with periods of interruption where we had to stop doing dominant lethals because the spontaneous rate became so high.

HOLLAENDER: This would apply also to Russell's work. He could never have gotten data with just taking run-of-the-mill mice; the only way he could get any reliable data was with a specific hybrid strain.

RAY: But I am not so sure that in our case it has a genetic basis. At those points of interruption, when you go back to the producer and do some basic microbiology, you find that the strain is carrying some adventitious organism. This infection in fact makes the uterus an extremely sensitive test tube. So issues like that come along to which you have to be sensitive. On the issue of analysis of variance and statistical considerations, most of the data generated on dominant lethals have been expressed on the basis of losses per pregnant female. As commonly done, you take a group of 15 or so males, you collect, as a function of the spermatogenic cycle, the females, and then you express that as the number of dead implantations per pregnant female; in other words, you pool them. A more satisfactory method from a statistical standpoint would identify the progeny from each male. This makes the logistics horrendous, but in that way I think you can get some indication of from where this contribution of variability is coming. In many cases you can identify a male or two that is contributing some of that variation. I think part of the problem in the past has been due to the method of data collection and analysis. Over and above that, we still have a fair degree of variation and control and still are subject to analysis of variance procedures to be able to use those data meaningfully.

FLAMM: One does not normally know what male relates to what postimplantation loss.

RAY: If you have 15 or 20 males, the number of females that came from a male group dosed in a given way is the answer. There has been no collection of the data based on the female progeny from an individual male. A lot of the data are like that in the literature on dominant lethality. Perhaps some of these variations you are talking about can come from that.

You may be able to identify, in certain experiments, contributions from an individual animal which make you wonder about its response--or the response of the chemical in that case--but some individual animal response. You do not need very many of these females with two or three dead implants to set those data into quite a state of variation and make the interpretation of the experiment difficult. But I think an examination of the literature will bear out what I am saying.

EHRENBERG: The danger is that if you have a computer program for variance analyses or significance estimates, without having built in a search for outlayers, you might get false positives. That is what I have shown by an experiment (Ehrenberg, 1977).

HOEL: I am surprised that analysis-variance techniques are used on this kind of data. I am not familiar with it, but I know that at least in the area of teratology it is involved quite a bit. We do not use normal theory-type techniques and look at them trying to identify the proper experimental unit and so on. The same things have been carried over here. Maybe a relook at statistics here would be useful.

FLAMM: We could be just fooling ourselves with respect to what statistics are applicable to these things. But, as I understand it, some time ago when there was already a large data base, the idea was that fetal wastage could be described by a log-normal distribution for both negative-control and positive-control groups.

You would certainly not see this with frank malformation. When you focus on malformation, the statistics are very different. It does not lend itself at all to variance analysis. Is that correct?

Once again, we should evaluate the whole issue. Do others agree with our statisticians that the situation is as hopeless as they say? The last such evaluation was in 1974 at Research Triangle Park, at the symposium that de Serres organized. We contended then that we had serious statistical problems with the dominant lethal test. We worked hard to salvage it, but we have not been very successful to this point.

ABRAHAMSON: One quick question here. You implied in what you said about dominant lethal testing in mice or rats that the treated sperm carry chromosome breaks that are killing the zygote. Fifty years ago that is exactly what you would have looked at; you would have looked at the zygote and said you had found the chromosome breaks cytologically, ergo you induced these dominant lethals. For the compounds you described that gave you consecutive and reproducible positives, did anybody look to see whether there were chromosomal breaks, rearrangements, dicentrics, or acentrics in those four test components?

FLAMM: You mean in the zygote? No, they have been looked at for spermatogonial effects, but to my knowledge no one has looked at the zygote.

BREWEN: What is the effect on the spermatogonium?

FLAMM: I would have to go back and look. That is done mainly to determine whether the drug or any component of that chemical is reaching the germinal tissue. For instance, with many of the nitrosamines (and even nitrosamides and MNNG, which does not need metabolic activation) it seems that these substances are reaching germinal tissue. There is extensive necrosis of the tissue. Yet we still do not see dominant lethality. In fact, it has been tested by a number of labs, and the only laboratory that has reported anything indicated an effect in the first week for late spermatozoa, preimplantation effects, which are a very unreliable measure of dominant lethality.

BREWEN: It may not be.

FLAMM: Well, it may not be, but that was the only thing that anyone was actually able to observe. But if a sperm is carrying a lot of MNNG, it could poison the zygote and lead to early death after a division or two.

One can readily envisage that kind of toxicity. It is a little tricky to accept that as a genetic effect because it would be so easy for the sperm to introduce the chemical to the egg and cause toxicity that does not enable the zygote to implant later and develop.

BREWEN: But in studies on dominant lethality with MMS and EMS, it has been observed that in the first few days after treatment of the male, there is a very high frequency, sometimes as high as 100%, of sterile matings. Females are plugged and they never show up pregnant; they are dissected at midterm, and there are no implants. When we did the cytogenetics, we found an absolute 100% effect cytogenetically on the male genome, but there were no longer recognizable chromosomes; this would lead to very early zygotic death, maybe at the four-cell or eight-cell stage. That is a real dominant lethal effect, but the dominant lethal test, by counting dead implants, turns out negative. You say, well, these females were plugged, but the oocytes perhaps never were fertilized.

EHRENBERG: Does this happen at any dose level, if you lower the dose?

FLAMM: If you lower the dose, you get levels where you get a negative effect or no effect in the dominant lethal test. When you do the cytogenetics, you can barely detect a significant increase in chromosome damage.

PERSON: Does it not allow greater implantation that way?

FLAMM: You get a very low level of dominant lethality, although you may be producing up to 5% or 10%, which is not significant above the 10% spontaneous rate.

PERSON: This is with EMS?

RAY: Do you come to a point where you see relatively nothing cytogenetically and then you see a leap?

BREWEN: No, we see the cytogenetic effect. If we go through and analyze affected embryos as a function of cytogenetic damage, we can show a significant effect. If you extrapolate that to a dominant lethal effect--that is, X embryos carrying chromosome aberrations--you would predict a negative effect because it is only 5-10%. The cytogenetic spontaneous rate is considerably less than 0.1%. So we can say, with some degree of certainty, that when we see five cells with a chromosome aberration out of a hundred, this is significant, but if those five embryos die, they do not contribute to the dominant lethal effect because of the 10% level of background lethals.

FLAMM: It happens that MNNG seems to be quite poor at inducing any kind of chromosomal effects, even in culture. Many of the nitrosamines are also rather poor at doing this. So given the fact that one of our major problems in foods is compounds of this kind, naturally I despair somewhat of the use of the dominant lethal test, which is particularly good at missing these compounds.

About five years ago, Abrahamson and I met with Leo Friedman and came up with a very different approach to testing food-related chemicals that put considerably less reliance on the mouse or the rat dominant lethal and far greater reliance for the first time on looking at sex-linked recessive lethals in Drosophila as well as chromosomal mutations in Drosophila. We are still moving in that direction. In fact, I have indicated to our people in the food additives and GRAS programs that we must take those 194 substances we have tested in in vitro systems, almost all of which came out negative, and begin testing samples of them. They should be selected in different ways, using different criteria, for extensive testing in Drosophila. Even the dominant lethal should be used because of substances such as ammoniated glycyrrhizin. A number of these are being tested or will be tested for the first time in heritable translocations. The heritable translocation test, incidentally, has considerable appeal, if for no other reason than it is clearly a measure of a heritable genetic event. Also, it is one of the few tests in the intact mammal that has a very wide range of response. Let us assume a spontaneous rate for the translocation heterozygote at something like 0.1%, which is a conservative estimate. We can induce up to 50% translocation heterozygotes with things like TEM; we are talking about a range of 500-fold. We do not often work with whole animals having a range anything like that magnitude. There are problems, obviously. If you want to measure the spontaneous rate with reasonable confidence intervals, at 0.1% we are talking about not a thousand, but ten thousand.

ABRAHAMSON: It is a minimum of 7,000 to have significance. Wouldn't the confidence limits on one per thousand be up to 6, down to 0.2? So you would have to get about 6,000 or 7,000 tests going to have at least seven of these events. Or am I saying this wrong?

FLAMM: I would have thought you would need even more animals than that. I would have thought it would be about 100,000. For 1% you need approximately 4,000 to have a reasonable 95% confidence interval for the 1% rate.

NEEL: A change from 1% to what? What do you want to detect?

ABRAHAMSON: You want to establish the value that is the spontaneous value, with accuracy. Isn't that your point?

FLAMM: That is right.

ABRAHAMSON: You have one translocation per thousand-- is that your assumption?

FLAMM: That is right, based on quite a lot of data collected in a variety of ways. Something like 50,000 F1's have been looked at to date, but the data are divided into so many different groups, and the protocols used were so different for detecting the translocation heterozygotes, that none of us feel that the data can actually be used.

EISENSTADT: Is there any correlation between the ability of a chemical to induce mutations in bacteria and its ability to induce chromosomal aberrations? And what is that correlation per assay?

FLAMM: In the heritable translocation test, you have such a paucity of data that it is impossible to determine the degree of concordance.

PERSON: But what do those data look like?

FLAMM: Alkylating agents, which will obviously produce point mutations and gene mutations in prokaryotes, or yeast, or mammalian cells, in culture are literally no problem at all. Whether you are looking at MMS, EMS, TEM, or any of them, you can indeed produce a very high frequency of translocation heterozygotes in mice. But when you get into things such as nitrosamines, polycyclic aromatic hydrocarbons, and aromatic amines, it is a good deal less clear.

EISENSTADT: They do not induce any heritable translocation?

FLAMM: I am not saying that. I am saying that the data base is not adequate to address that definitively.

EISENSTADT: Is it less than you would expect based on the mutagenicity?

FLAMM: I am afraid that any statement I might make would be an overinterpretation of the data that we now have. There just are not enough data for me to comment.

EISENSTADT: How about in the other direction? Are

there many chemicals not mutagenic in the Ames test that can induce heritable translocations?

FLAMM: This is a terribly important question and that is what I was alluding to before with ammoniated gly-cyrrhizin, gum acacia, and BHT. They are being tested now. They seem to be positive for dominant lethal.

EISENSTADT: This is anecdotal in a sense. Are there more, or just those two?

FLAMM: We have four that were far more positive in the dominant lethal than they were in Salmonella, yeast, or any of the in vitro tests we have used. In fact, ammoniated glycyrrhizin did not show any activity at all in the in vitro tests. It and BHT have twice given us a positive effect in dominant lethals. Now we are starting to do the heritable translocation test in Drosophila. One assumes that you are going to be able to measure many more different kinds of genetic events, using sex-linked recessive lethals in Drosophila, than you are going to be able to do with Salmonella strains TA100, 98, and so forth, simply because you are looking at so much of the genome, and one presumes that mutation by virtually any mechanism can be expressed as a sex-linked recessive lethal.

ABRAHAMSON: One quick answer to your question. Captan was tested through EPA. It was questionable as a mutagen. It came up presumably as a positive for inducing translocations in mice.

RAY: It was questionable. The work has not been re-peated.

ABRAHAMSON: There were one or two translocations in-duced, as I recall, in their test system. It is also positive in almost every other test system across the board, including Salmonella.

FLAMM: But, again, that is an alkylating agent.

PERTEL: There are 28 compounds, most of them alkylat-ing.

NEEL: In your presentation of ouabain resistance and methotrexate, you made the point that it now seems that this is detecting only a very small part and a very special part of the mutational spectrum. Some of us who watch somatic rates and try to compare them with germinal rates have always been a little concerned that the somatic rates look pretty high. This would take your 10^{-7} and move it up appreciably, wouldn't it? If you think that test system is getting such a small part of the total mutation in the spectrum, then the total mutational spectrum is an order of magnitude greater.

FLAMM: You misunderstood me. The methotrexate resistance is a couple of orders of magnitude less in rate than the TK; it is about 10^{-9}. When I was talking about 10^{-7}, I was talking about the TK locus, not methotrexate. Ouabain and methotrexate resistance are very low, which would suggest that it is quite a small part of it.

NEEL: So this would bring that rate, if you made a more or less intuitive correction, in line with other rates?

FLAMM: Yes, about 1 to 1/10 of a percent. Incidentally, because of the way the selection medium is being set up, you are not by any means measuring every mutation that occurs. You are measuring only a fraction--in some cases a small fraction--of the total ones that do occur. For instance, with TK and with HGPRT, if you loosen up a bit on this selection medium, you begin to get a lot of very small colonies. If you then grow them up and look at them, you find not only that the enzyme activity seems to be reduced, but also that these things seem to have different K_m's. We are starting to do more and more of that kind of thing--looking at some of these leaky mutants that we are getting both with the BrdU and with the trifluorothymidine, to make sure that most of the events we are witnessing are in fact occurring at the structural gene and not at some controlling site.

ABRAHAMSON: According to Brin (B.A.) Bridges, and I think his interpretation is correct, ouabain-resistant mutants can only be intragenic mutants because X-rays cannot produce any of them. He says X-rays produce deletions; ergo, deletions in that locus or possibly the methotrexate locus cannot survive.

FLAMM: I just surmised that that would be true of ouabain. Certainly our comparison of methotrexate resistance to TK or BrdU resistance would bear that out. Base substitutions seem to be the only thing, and all of them are quite revertible as well.

EISENSTADT: Ouabain resistance always requires a functional enzyme?

FLAMM: Yes.

PERSON: It is just an altered enzyme?

FLAMM: Yes.

ABRAHAMSON: Ouabain is also a membrane-functioning gene isn't it? It is an ATPase. So, if you are destroying the enzyme in the membrane, you may well be destroying the entire cell.

EISENSTADT: That is right.

ABRAHAMSON: Therefore, you do not get any X-ray deletions.

FLAMM: With methotrexate resistance, the whole thing is predicated on methotrexate having a 100,000-fold higher affinity for tetrahydrofolate reductase than folic acid. If you hit that site, apparently that changes. We have seen ratios that are probably down to more like 10:1, so that now they are tolerating enormous amounts of methotrexate they did not tolerate before. It is much more complicated than that, because there are surface proteins that bind methotrexate. It gets to be awfully, awfully complicated, and unless you are aware of all of the aspects, you do not know how to get your cells in a condition for running the assay. It is kind of a tricky assay to run. In answer to your question, the mutation rates are consistent with the notion that there is a restricted target.

FLAMM: Hollaender has suggested that it might be worthwhile for me to indicate those tests that many of us feel hold the greatest promise at the present time. Based on both theoretical considerations and the practical aspects of having a very large data base with some information that suggests that these tests are, in fact, relevant, I am sure none of you will be surprised to hear me say that we feel the Ames test does have considerable utility. We are really beginning to think that some of the gene mutational assays in mammalian cells of the sort that I mentioned earlier also have good utility. I am particularly enamored of DNA replication repair in human cells, because of its sensitivity and likely relevance to the human situation. Unfortunately, for intact animal systems, in terms of what would appear to have practical utility, we are really limited to Drosophila for measuring gene mutations and to translocations in mice for measuring chromosomal mutations.

Bacterial Mutagenicity Testing: Some Practical Considerations

ERIC EISENSTADT

Departments of Microbiology and Physiology
Harvard University School of Public Health

Two projects currently underway in my lab illustrate features of the bacterial mutagenicity system that I am now using--the Ames test. Graham Walker will discuss the importance of DNA repair functions and activities in bacteria in general and how they relate to constructing strains that are particularly sensitive for a wide variety of mutagens. I shall concentrate on some of the practical aspects of mutagenicity testing.

A long-term project is presently underway at the Harvard School of Public Health to study the health effects of occupational exposure to rubber manufacturing processes. We decided to analyze the rubber-industry environment for chemical mutagens to which workers might be exposed. We started with carbon black, a product that constitutes about 50% of the final weight of a tire. Carbon black is essentially soot that is collected after burning certain oils. We extracted carbon black with an organic solvent, methylene chloride, and detected quite a lot of mutagenic activity in that total organic extract (Table 1).

We subjected the extract to a crude fractionation, separating the organic material into neutral, acidic, and basic fractions. The neutral fraction was further separated by silica chromatography into aromatic, polar, and saturated hydrocarbon fractions. We again had a look, with the mutagenicity assay, at how the mutagenic activity was distributed.

INFANTE: Which mutagenicity test was this?

EISENSTADT: The Salmonella typhimurium test with liver microsomal activation developed by Bruce Ames.

INFANTE: How did you separate out the mutagenicity of the methylene chloride?

48/ E. Eisenstadt

TABLE 1
Mutagenicity of Carbon Black Adsorbates

Fraction	Weight (mg)	Revertants/μg
Carbon black (total)	314,000	—
Total organics (CH$_2$Cl$_2$ (extract)	346	14
Neutral		
aromatic	135	38
polar	27	4
saturated hydrocarbon	9	not active
Acidic	49	0.5 nonlinear dose response
Basic	6	not active

EISENSTADT: Methylene chloride blanks have no mutagenic activity.

The distribution of mutagenic activity in the fractions is seen in Table 1. Most of it seems to be in the neutral fraction, and in this fraction predominantly in the aromatic portion. There is some activity in the acidic fraction, which has not been explored, and we have reason to think that this might be very interesting material to look at further.

When we subjected the aromatic fraction to more sophisticated fractionation by high-pressure liquid chromatography, we realized that one component in the mixture accounted for most of the mutagenic activity. In fact, by itself, it can account for all the mutagenic activity in the methylene chloride extract (Figure 1). It was identified as cyclopenta(c,d)pyrene (CPP).

We compared the structure of CPP to that of another polycyclic aromatic hydrocarbon, benzo(a)pyrene (BP). Interestingly, CPP, unlike BP, contained no bay region. Jerina and his colleagues (1977) have been looking for possible structure/function relationships in the microsomal metabolism of polycyclic aromatics. They have developed the concept that the bay-region epoxides of polycyclic aromatic hydrocarbons are the most potent metabolites in terms of their mutagenicity and carcinogenicity. In this view, the bay region is some kind of critical structure or geometric feature of the hydrocarbon that determines where the most potent metabolite of the chemical will be generated. CPP does not have a bay region, but it was mutagenic in

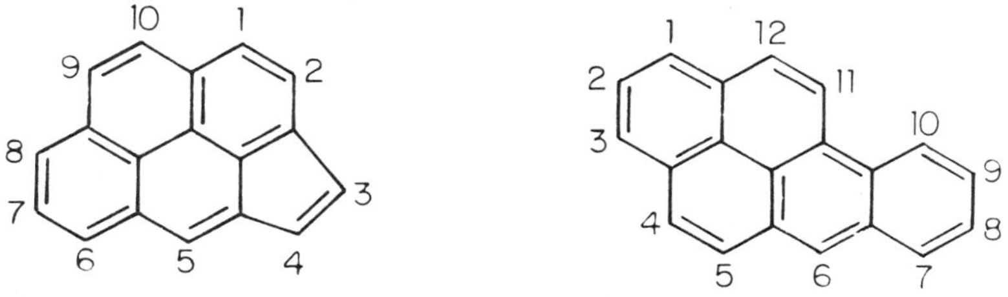

A

B

FIGURE 1
(A) Cyclopenta(c,d)pyrene.   (B) Benzo(a)pyrene.

our hands, and we thought it warranted further study
(Eisenstadt and Gold, 1978).

Theory, as well as some experimental observations as
to the reactivity of the 3,4 double bond in CPP, led us to
predict that CPP could be metabolized to the 3,4-oxide; this
epoxide could open to yield a carbonium ion, which is, by
molecular orbital considerations, indistinguishable from that
formed upon opening of the well-characterized 9,10-epoxide
of the 7,8-hydrodiol metabolite of BP (Figure 2).

By comparing the amount of liver homogenate required
by CPP for optimal mutagenic activity with the amount
required by BP, we found that for CPP optimal mutagenesis
is reached at about 3 µl of S-9, whereas for BP the amount
is 20 µl. As Ames has tried to make clear, the test for any
particular kind of compound really _does_ have to be opti-
mized with respect to microsomal metabolism. What level of
enzymes yields the maximum mutagenic effect? I know of an
instance in which a commercial testing facility failed to
detect the mutagenicity of a chemical because suboptimal
levels of liver homogenate were used.

CPP is equally active against strains TA1537 and
TA100, whereas BP is much less mutagenic toward strain
TA1537 than it is toward TA100. Strain TA1537 carries a
frame-shift mutation in the _his_ operon, whereas TA100
carries the base-pair mutation _hisG46_ and the plasmid
pKM101. Strain TA1537 does not have the pKM101 plasmid.

Table 2 displays the comparative mutagenic activity of
CPP against the five standard Ames strains. Strains TA98
and TA100 are both plasmid-bearing derivatives. The TA98
strain is another of the frame-shift-carrying mutants;
TA100 is a base-pair mutant; TA1537 and TA1538 are
frame-shift mutants; and TA1535 is a _hisG46_ base-pair
mutant. You can see that CPP is potently mutagenic for
four of the strains and not at all for the base-pair-carrying

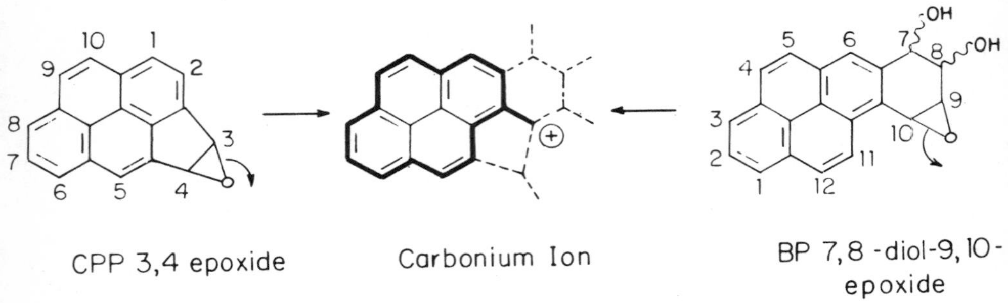

CPP 3,4 epoxide   Carbonium Ion   BP 7,8 -diol-9,10-
                                                         epoxide

FIGURE 2
Benzylic carbonium ion resulting from the opening of CPP
3,4-oxide or BP 7,8-diol-9, 10-oxide.

mutant TA1535. That is very different from the mutational
spectrum you get for BP. It is clear that having the
plasmid present can convert whatever kind of molecular
damage is suffered by DNA to a mutational event, which
can be scored as a base-pair reversion. Graham Walker
discusses in his paper how that plasmid might be functioning.

RAY: This is a pure preparation for the CPP?

EISENSTADT: Yes, it is highly purified.

It would be worthwhile to understand how bulky group
adducts, such as are formed following exposure of DNA to
aflatoxin, BP, or CPP, induce mutations. All of these
compounds are known to form adducts with specific positions on nucleosides. It is important to determine what is
going on at the molecular level: how are bulky group
adducts recognized by DNA repair enzymes and how are
they converted to specific kinds of mutational events? I
know of no systematic studies that have been done to determine the spectrum of mutations induced by bulky group
adducts. They have been done for several low-molecular-
weight alkylating agents, but not, I believe, for the
high-molecular-weight compounds, which include some of the
well-known carcinogens. We now have bacterial systems
(not designed to be test systems in the sense that the Ames
test is a test system) that permit us to explore such
questions. For example, Jeffrey Miller has analyzed the
mutational spectrum of lacI-gene-induced mutations following
UV irradiation and exposure to a number of alkylating
agents (Coulondre and Miller, 1977). Perhaps this analysis
should be extended to some well-known carcinogens to
examine the molecular basis for the mutations they induce.

TABLE 2
Comparison of CPP-induced Mutagenesis in *S. typhimurium* Strains

	Histidine revertants per plate				
Addition	TA98	TA100	TA1537	TA1538	TA1535
S-9	26	95	13	21	14
S-9 + 1 μg CPP	470	523	945	675	10

Liver homogenate (S-9) at 4.5 μl per plate (3 μl per plate for TA1535 plates) was used to determine the mutagenicity of CPP in the experiment. The spontaneous reversion incidence indicated is the average of three plates (two plates for TA1535). The CPP-induced reversion incidence is from the linear portion of dose-response curves.

To study S-9 dependence further, the mutagenicity of another polycyclic aromatic hydrocarbon, perylene, was examined. Perylene mutagenicity increases as a function of S-9 per plate all the way up to 200 μl, or 10 times more than is required for optimal BP mutagenesis and 100 times more than is required for CPP mutagenesis. Thus, we have three polycyclic aromatic hydrocarbons with three very different S-9 optima for mutagenicity. Perylene happens to be a weak mutagen, and at the wrong S-9 concentration it is conceivable that its mutagenicity would have been missed. Again, this emphasizes the importance of optimizing the S-9 concentration when one does mutagenicity testing. Another laboratory has measured the mutagenicity of perylene in a forward mutation assay, developed by William Thilly. Thilly claims that under the conditions used in his system, perylene is just as mutagenic as BP.

Another interesting application of mutagenicity testing uses the bacterial test to detect and identify mutagenic activity in human body fluid samples in an attempt to assess exposure of the human population to mutagens.

Yamasaki and Ames (1977) developed a very simple method for testing human urine for mutagenic activity. They never found mutagenic activity in the urine of nonsmokers, but they readily detected mutagenic activity in the urine of smokers (Figure 3; see also Figure 4). One smoker who did not inhale had no activity in his urine. One low-tar smoker had nothing, and one low-tar smoker had a lot. There is clearly a need for a more quantitative examination of this phenomenon. Yamasaki and Ames also showed that the activity in an evening sample, after a day of smoking, was greater than that in a morning sample, after a night's sleep during which the person did not smoke.

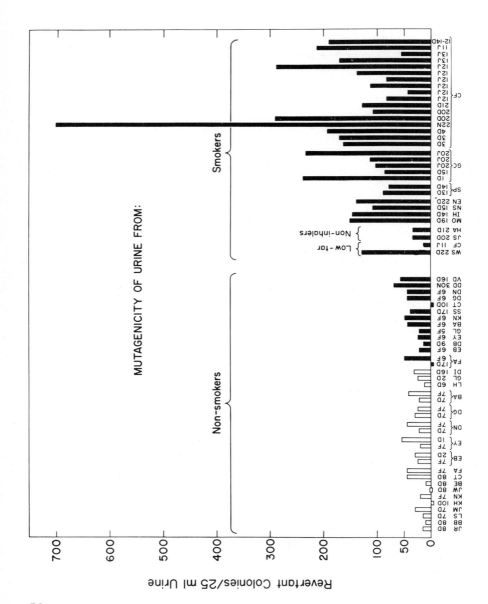

MUTAGENICITY OF URINE FROM:

52

FIGURE 3

Urine samples (usually 200 ml) from 10 smokers and 21 nonsmokers were treated as described in Yamasaki and Ames (1977) and assayed for mutagenicity. In a few samples where less urine was used, the dimethyl sulfoxide was reduced proportionately. The least square line for the control, 50-, and 100-µl points was determined and the mutagenicity (after subtracting the control value) for a 100-µl aliquot (25 ml of urine) is plotted. The results from smokers whose urine samples were assayed on more than one occasion are grouped together. Each bar is identified by the individual's initials, and the data of the sample collection (indicated by the day and the first letter of the month: Nov., Dec., Jan., Feb.). A black bar represents the mutagenic acitivity of a urine sample taken on retiring in the evening (or in A for multiple samples from smokers taken on the same day) and a white bar represents one taken on arising in the morning. (A) Urine voided at various times; (B) evening/next morning samples. (Reprinted from Yamasaki and Ames, 1977).

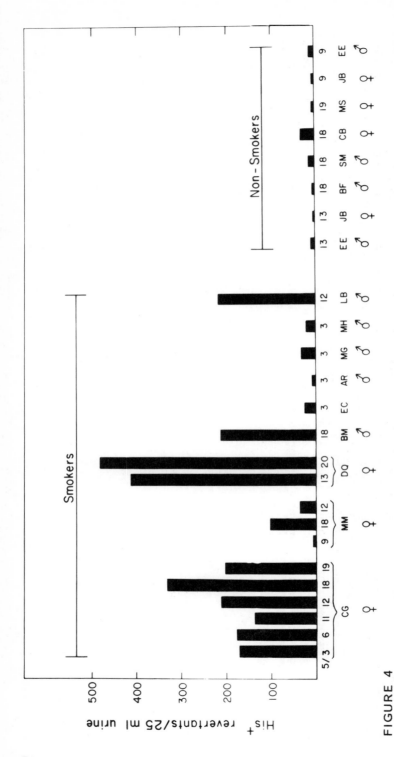

FIGURE 4

Mutagenicity of XAD-2 urine concentrates from cigarette smokers and nonsmokers. Urine concentrates were prepared and assayed as described in Yamasaki and Ames (1977). Letters identify urine donors. Numbers below bars identify the date (in 1977) on which the sample was collected and assayed.

A number of published and unpublished studies have detected mutagenic activity in body fluid samples. I shall briefly discuss four of these studies.

Legator, Truong, and Connor (1978) in a study of Dow Chemical Company workers, used a urine extraction method very different from that used by Ames. The samples he examined consisted of only 40 ml of urine, extracted with organic solvents. It is not surprising that he found no mutagenic activity. But one day some workers in one of the plants cleaned up a spill of epichlorohydrin. Tests of urine samples from these workers, taken a few hours later, showed the presence of mutagenic activity; the activity was not due to epichlorohydrin itself but rather to an epichlorohydrin metabolite.

Mutagenic activity has also been detected in urine samples from anesthesiologists exposed to unspecified levels of halothane (McCoy et al., 1978), which itself is not mutagenic. However, that activity was not enhanced at all by liver microsomal preparations.

ABRAHAMSON: Wouldn't you qualify that? Halothane is not mutagenic in the Salmonella system.

EISENSTADT: It is not detectably mutagenic in the Salmonella system. Do you want to tell us in which system it is mutagenic?

ABRAHAMSON: Drosophila tests by Sobel's group in Leiden have demonstrated a positive effect.

To continue, women taking metronidazole (Flagyl) for some cases of vaginitis are also known to excrete rather high levels of mutagenic activity in their urine (Connor et al., 1977).

WATSON: What is considered high? Twice as much as normal? Five times?

EISENSTADT: Normal is "nothing." You cannot detect mutagenic activity in most people; there is essentially no background. You can demonstrate that the activity is due to Flagyl or Flagyl metabolites in the urine. You can purify them and show that they are mutagenic. "Normal" people do not have Flagyl or Flagyl metabolites in their urine.

Finally, we (and I think others) have looked at cancer patients receiving chemotherapy. Cancer chemotherapeutic agents are known to be mutagenic, and we can detect mutagenic activity in the urine of these patients.

WATSON: Can I go back? In your smoking versus nonsmoking, there seemed to be some level of variation under nonsmoking (see Figures 3 and 4).

EISENSTADT: That has to do with histidine that is trapped on the column. The method involves pouring about 100 ml of urine over a nonionic resin known as XAD-2. When Ames carried out those assays, the columns were not washed with water to remove any trapped histidine--any urine fluid that was trapped in between the resin beads. When you wash those columns with water, you remove all the residual levels of trapped histidine, and you get really nothing above the background.

WATSON: So the curves would be more impressive now?

LEE: When you say "nothing," you mean that the body fluid does not give a rate higher than the spontaneous frequency without body fluid?

EISENSTADT: It gives less than a twofold increase.

LEE: Okay, so it is less than a twofold increase over the spontaneous frequency without body fluid; therefore, the body fluid is considered negative. When you get a body fluid that gives more than a twofold increase over the spontaneous, it is considered a positive "something" added to the body fluid.

HUNT: From an epidemiologic viewpoint, in specifying these normals or the control population it is pretty evident, certainly with industrially exposed people, that there will have to be an at-risk group. I guess my concern is that you are specifying what this normal group is and how you describe them.

EISENSTADT: I think a discussion of these data and Ames's data is relevant. Cigarette smokers constitute an interesting population--a group of people who willingly expose themselves to enormous levels of mutagenic activity. The link between cigarette smoking and cancer is about the clearest link we may ever have between environmental exposure to a carcinogen and cancer incidence. I think it would be worthwhile understanding in as much detail as possible what is going on here, what levels of mutagens do obtain in body fluids, what levels of DNA base alkylation obtain, and can that be correlated at all with the cancer incidence that the people will eventually suffer?

WATSON: Has anyone tried to do . . . I know the messiness . . . arylhydrocarbon hydroxylase studies? I mean what is the significance of that group of people who are smokers but don't have elevated levels of mutagenic activity in their urine.

EISENSTADT: This kind of study has not been done in any systematic way.

WATSON: You do not know why those people don't have elevated levels?

EISENSTADT: I cannot say why they do not; it could be because of how much they smoke. Again, this is very nonquantitative. We do not know how many milligrams of tar they consume. A Japanese study has shown that the mutagenicity per milligram of tar seems to be constant, and so low-tar cigarettes would have the same amount of mutagenic activity per milligram of tar as high-tar cigarettes.

WATSON: Have you tested a urine sample from a person in a room with a lot of heavy smokers?

EISENSTADT: No. But an undergraduate is trying to convince me that we should look at children who live in small quarters with parents who smoke.

ABRAHAMSON: Are you sure? Or are you implying that an organic component in the smoker's urine is responsible for the increased level? There is a literature that suggests that such things as polonium 210 and lead 210, also part of cigarette smoke, might be part of the cancer-inducing mechanism.

EISENSTADT: I am saying that it is an organic component for two reasons. First, XAD-2 extracts it; XAD-2 is a nonionic resin that permits binding of hydrophobic components to its surface. Second, chloroform will extract just as much mutagenic activity from the urine of smokers as XAD-2, although it seems to be pulling out an overlapping organic fraction, not an identical one. It is not identical because you can do dose-response determinations with a chloroform extract and an XAD-2 extract of urine and in general find that with the XAD-2 extract the mutagenic activity is linear with respect to extract over a very narrow concentration range, whereas with the chloroform extract we can go to much higher concentrations and still have a linear response. I am just beginning to understand why this happens. It seems that the XAD-2 is pulling out many substances that are toxic to the bacteria; the chloroform is not doing this. We are pursuing this further in the hope that we can increase the sensitivity of these techniques by about a factor of 10 (I would be happy with a factor of 100 or 1,000) and then we can begin a systematic study of nonsmokers. One nonsmoking population we will look at works in the rubber industry. We have collected urine from that population and hope to examine these samples as we increase the sensitivity. Perhaps every factor of 10 that we go up might warrant another look.

WATSON: Do you need the S-9 for urine?

EISENSTADT: Yes, it is totally S-9-dependent.

HUNT: I have a comment on your sensitivity issue. I was surprised when Abrahamson mentioned the polonium and lead; I thought everybody had forgotten that work that I did back in the early 1960s (Radford and Hunt, 1964).

   The problem we encountered was indeed the problem you are citing here: not knowing the variability within the smoking population. Again, it comes to an epidemiologic problem: the discipline that one must impose on a choice of human subjects is in many respects a bit alien to the laboratory approach that we use. Having transferred from one to the other, I am well aware of the dilemma you are facing, and it is the same problem we experienced 10 or 15 years ago. Somehow, we have to make sure that you are better at identifying your subjects now than we were back then. In the case of polonium 210 and lead 210, when I looked at semen and sperm the central problem was in the identification of subjects. Even though I had a good range of values and the difference between smokers and nonsmokers was evident, I did not have a good idea of the smoking characteristics of those subjects. If I had had that information, I would have felt far more comfortable with the data. I never published the work at that time, but because we are interested in sperm and semen now, I pulled it out, after 10 years, and looked at it again.

ABRAHAMSON: Radford and Martell did publish something more recently on sperm and semen, I believe.

HUNT: I have not seen it.

ABRAHAMSON: At least they have alluded to it.

HUNT: That was probably mine which I did in the mid-1960s (Hunt, 1973).

EISENSTADT: Of course, one would be happy to know the distribution of smokers and nonsmokers for any epidemiologic study to measure incidence.

HUNT: This is what I am trying to get at. To look at smokers and nonsmokers to figure out why the response of some smokers to smoking is different from that of other smokers is a fairly gross approach.

EISENSTADT: I would not make too much of a point of

that now until we have had a chance to look at the data in more detail. These data expressed in terms of creatinine or nicotine levels in the urine or milligrams of tar consumed might be more valuable.

HUNT: That is what I am getting at.

WATSON: How much does each data point cost?

EISENSTADT: Not very much; it is very inexpensive. The hardest thing is to locate people who will participate. Believe it or not, you have to go through human-use committees for this.

WATSON: Do the subjects have to sign, or do you have to get permission from the committee and then not worry about it?

EISENSTADT: You need permission from the committee. You can explain what you are doing, why you are going to do it, and of what benefit it will be to subjects. I always say that the benefit will be to point out how much nasty stuff is in a smoker and that, as a consequence, maybe he or she will stop smoking.

WALKER: You know one of the problems that Ames had was that he could not find a smoker who would stop smoking for longer than about a day.

EISENSTADT: It seems worthwhile to consider doing chemical epidemiology studies on human populations. What is so greatly different chemically about populations that we can pick out--Japanese versus Americans, residents of Wisconsin versus residents of New Jersey? Something like that might be very worthwhile.

WATSON: Is anyone else besides Bob Bruce in Toronto analyzing mutagenicity in human feces?

EISENSTADT: I don't know.

VALCOVIC: There is an awful lot of noise in this system, though. Bruce tried to start out with what he considered normal individuals, who would not be expected to have mutagenic properties in their feces, but they do. He has spent a great deal of time thus far just trying to figure out what may be causing this. He has used various diets and all kinds of things. The system is still a way from having the cleanness of the urine test.

WATSON: You mean it is quite irreproducible?

VALCOVIC: It does vary on days. It varies, but not regularly, with diet. It seems to be somewhat reproducible, but not. In other words, there are mutagenic products in feces of people who are nonsmokers and not occupationally exposed to any known carcinogen.

HUNT: But the critical point is whether it is reproducible within the individual.

RAY: I gathered that one of your standard procedures was diethylether extractions. What happens if it comes down the polarity scale in solvents?

EISENSTADT: I do not know. Bob Bruce has been doing this. What are you driving at?

RAY: In other words, if you used diethylether, if he used chloroform, if he used methylene chloride. You cannot get down too low, obviously, because of the nature of the material.

EISENSTADT: That is right.

HILL: Peter, do you want to make any comments about studies in humans that seem to indicate mutagenic activity on the part of chemicals?

INFANTE: One thing came to mind when the data on epichlorohydrin was being discussed--specifically, for the same population for which Legator had the data on epichlorohydrin I think Dante Picciano has data showing chromosomal aberrations--I think a tenfold difference in chromosomal aberrations, and more if it is exposed to methyl chlorohydrin at pretty low levels.

EISENSTADT: That reminds me of another point that is worth making. W. Nichols, at the Institute for Medical Research in Camden, New Jersey, is now beginning to measure both the mutagenic activity in urine and levels of sister chromatid exchange (SCE) in cultured lymphocytes from smoking individuals. Jack Little and Larry Fine at the Harvard School of Public Health are beginning to do the same thing. Both groups find that smokers tend to have about a twofold higher level of SCE than nonsmokers. Dr. Ehrenberg, do you know of similar studies, or have you been carrying out similar studies?

EHRENBERG: Yes, I have. Lambert and Lindsten (Lambert et al., 1978), in Stockholm, are doing studies. It is a rather remarkable variation, by a factor of five or more.

EISENSTADT: That is SCE among the smoking population.

EHRENBERG: And with a dose-response curve, if you grade the number of cigarettes per day, it is a nice, increasing curve. May I ask one question here? One of the problems is that in some cases you might have short-lived reactive compounds--as in the case of vinyl chloride. The presumed active factor in vinyl-chloride-induced cancer is chlorethylene oxide with an estimated half-life in vivo of about 2 seconds (Osterman-Golkar et al., 1977). It would be very interesting to look at urine samples from PVC workers to see whether there could be something long-lived in addition to this. There are a lot of oligomers about which we know very little. They might be there in addition to chlorethylene oxide.

EISENSTADT: The technique might prove to be important. A priori, with any of these techniques for fractionating and concentrating material from body fluids, you are missing chemicals that are very unstable. They never make it to the petri dish in an active form. Maybe the PVC workers would serve as an appropriate control for that. With this kind of approach (i.e., chemical analysis of body fluids), the hope is that we could identify, out of all the chemicals to which we are exposed in the environment, the ones that we should really worry about. The one-by-one approach that the interagency testing committee has to go through might never lead anywhere. And it is going to cost a lot to get nowhere.

Theory and Design of Short-term Bacterial Tests for Mutagenesis

GRAHAM C. WALKER

Biology Department
Massachusetts Institute of Technology

As a postdoctoral fellow with Bruce Ames in 1974-1976, I got interested in DNA repair and have continued to work on this since I moved to MIT. These short-term bacterial tests seem very important right now. Although there is a tendency to regard them as something that just appeared, it has taken several years to develop them to their present level of sensitivity.

The Ames Salmonella/microsome system actually involves a great many things. We need to review what is known about DNA repair in bacteria--the organisms where DNA repair is probably best understood--to fit the short-term tests into context. In this way, we can have a better feeling for the microbiology that underlies these tests.

Clearly, if a chemical damages DNA, it is possible to get lesions that do not affect the cell greatly. However, it seems that many lesions affecting DNA stop replication. For example, none of the three known E. coli polymerases will polymerize past a thymine dimer. This is a very bad situation in the cell.

Cells seem to have evolved a large number of different repair systems; they have a heavy commitment to maintain the integrity of their DNA. The organism must also maintain the fidelity so crucial for genetic information transfer.

Figure 1 is a diagram of the steps that, at least formally, are thought to occur in excision repair. I am omitting photoreactivation, which is specific for ultraviolet damage and requires light. The representative lesion we will consider is a thymine dimer.

The first step in excision repair is an endonucleolytic cut on the 5' side of the thymine dimer. This is followed by excision of an oligonucleotide that contains the damage. In at least a formal sense, a gap is generated, and a poly-

EXCISION   REPAIR

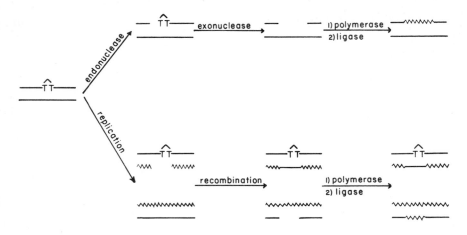

POSTREPLICATIONAL   REPAIR

FIGURE 1
Outline of the current models for excision and postreplication repair of a thymine dimer in DNA.

merase then fills in the missing information by reading off
the opposite strand.   After ligase seals the nick, you are
back to repaired DNA.   These steps are not specific for
thymine dimers.   It seems that most lesions causing a major
distortion in the helix are repaired in this way.
     The process seems to be very accurate.   You get
very, very few mistakes.   It also seems to be constitutive.
Although this is the best-understood repair system, it is
still not completely defined at the biochemical level.
     There seems to be an analogous system for alkylation
damage.   You can imagine a representative base with an
alkyl group hanging from it.   Alkylated bases, in general,
tend to depurinate more readily, producing an apurinic or
apyrimidinic site.   Formally, at least, the process then
seems to be similar to the repair of thymine dimers and
other bulky adducts.   There is an endonucleolytic nick
introduced into the DNA, endonucleolytic excision to
produce a gap, and then repair by a polymerase.   This
process also seems accurate and constitutive.
     Other steps happen in between.   In a number of cases
involving alkylated bases, cells have evolved special glycosylases for removing bases that do not belong in DNA--for
example, uracil resulting from the deamination of cytosine
or hypoxanthine resulting from the deamination of adenine.
Lindahl and colleagues (1978) have isolated one glycosylase

that specifically removes the base 3-methyladenine, generating an apurinic site. The cells carry out these processes in two steps: first, the base is removed; and second, an endonucleolytic cut is introduced at an apurinic or apyrimidinic site.

The first evidence of a third mechanism of excision repair was presented by Linn (1978) at the Keystone Repair Meeting. There seems to be an enzyme that he can isolate from human fibroblasts which will apparently put the correct base into an apurinic site. It will at least put in an A or G. The evidence for this is perhaps a little softer than for some of the other repair systems, but it is an indication of yet another kind of repair system that may be accurate.

A second class of repair illustrated in Figure 1 is postreplication repair. If you get replication of DNA without removal of the damage, then, at least in a formal sense, the polymerizing enzyme does not know what to do when it gets to the dimer. It falls off and initiates somewhere downstream. That gives you a "gap." But the missing information is actually coded for in the other daughter helix. By a recombinational event, you can transfer the information from the complete helix to the deficient one. The gap can be filled in by a polymerase. Such recombination is not really a repair system in the sense that the others are; the damage is not physically excised. Rather, it is a dilution mechanism which gets the cell past the damage and onto another step in the process.

WATSON: Why is it called recombinational?   What recombines?

WALKER: The missing information gets transferred by a recombinational event. What is missing can then be filled in by the polymerase, and presumably in an accurate fashion.

We start to replicate a piece of DNA, and polymerase comes along and generates a gap. One strand of the polymerase can replicate fine. With the other strand, the polymerase does not know what to put in because it is no longer making genetic sense. The equivalent information is in the undamaged strand.

We could draw crossovers. This is much more of a model, I think, than the other. The experimental observation for the model is to UV-irradiate cells, pulse-label the newly synthesized DNA, and check the molecular weight. The newly synthesized DNA seems to be smaller, presumably because of gaps, but, with time, we find that these short pieces of DNA are incorporated in the normal molecular weight DNA.

There seems to be some joining of the gaps, yet we still find a lot of the dimers incorporated in the strands. They end up being evenly distributed between the daughter helices. It does not seem to be a case where you get one good helix and one containing all the damage. It is more of a dilution mechanism at best. For the most part, it is a constitutive process and it seems to be largely accurate. It is certainly complex in E. coli. There are indications of at least five genetic loci that seem to affect the process. It is hard to know whether to call them pathways, but there may be at least five "pathways."

HILL: Is that known outside of prokaryotes?

SETLOW: The recombination events depicted here are easy to follow because one can detect that the dimers that were originally in parental DNA end up in daughter DNA. In mammalian cells, the evidence that dimers in parental DNA end up in daughter DNA is very, very slim and may be an artifact of various measurement procedures. So, at the moment, it would be best to say that what goes on in mammalian cells is uncertain.

WATSON: You mean this might be wrong?

SETLOW: Yes.

PERSON: What about yeast?

SETLOW: I don't know of any data in yeast.

WALKER: There is probably still a little question in bacteria, certainly in conceptual terms.

HILL: I don't know of any data in yeast on this particular.

Another class of repair systems is one on which John Cairns and his colleagues have been working (Schendel et al., 1978). It appears to be an inducible error-free repair system--an inducible accurate repair system. So far, this is known only in E. coli and seems to be induced by a number of alkylating agents such as N-methyl-N'-nitro-N-nitrosoguanidine or methyl methanesulfonate (MMS). If you expose cells to low levels of these compounds, they are mutated for a few minutes, and then, by some process that requires protein synthesis, they stop being susceptible to mutation by these agents. You can swamp it out by putting in a lot more of the mutagen. Mechanistically, I do not think it is too clear what is going on. The last I heard from people in the lab is that they have mutants that apparently knock out the system, and there is at least some suggestive evidence that removal of O-6 methyl guanine may be involved in this process. But this is a fairly recent development, and I do not want to go into it right now.

The other kind of repair differs from the ones that I have been discussing. It is <u>inducible</u> and thus seems to be similar to the Cairns system, but it differs in that it is <u>error-prone</u>. At this point, I may be talking about something that is pretty much a hypothesis. There is still not really any very hard evidence at a biochemical level to justify the use of the term <u>error-prone</u> <u>repair</u>. I plan to use it, but one should have some reservations about it. There seems to be a strong correlation between the existence of the inducibility of the repair and the inducibility of mutagenesis, but they still might turn out to be separable.

One kind of experiment that suggests the existence of such a system is shown in Figure 2. This experiment is termed <u>Weigle-reactivation</u>. Basically, the experiment is to take a phage such as lambda and UV-irradiate it heavily so that the survival comes down a lot, and then look at the survival of the irradiated phage as a function of the dose of radiation given to the bacteria prior to infection with the phage. By irradiating the host before infecting with the damaged bacteriophage, you find an increase in survival of the phage, which can range up to 100-fold without too much trouble. That sort of evidence suggests that there is an inducible repair system. The evidence suggesting that it is an inducible error-prone repair system comes from looking at mutation frequency in terms of something like clear plaque mutants per survivor (instead of looking at the survival of the irradiated phage). This is a real frequency (it is not just more mutants because of more survivors); you get essentially the same curve with the same maximum-- both effects induced at the same time. It is independent of

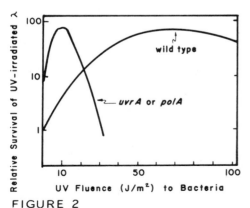

FIGURE 2
Weigle-reactivation of UV-irradiated bacteriophage λ in UV-irradiated <u>E</u>. <u>coli</u> (Radman, 1975).

excision repair. There is some controversy about how you draw these curves, but it is clear that you see some inducible repair in a mutant that lacks excision repair because of a mutation at the uvrA locus. There are three genetic loci in E. coli that knock out this presumptive error-prone repair system. One is called recA, which is required for recombination and has many pleiotropic effects in the cell. LexA is another locus that affects a number of different functions and it seems to be more specific for the error-prone repair system in that it does not affect recombination. Together, there are a lot of functions that are inducible by UV and are dependent on the $recA^+$, $lexA^+$ genotype. These include induction of a prophage such as lambda, filamentous growth, temporary cessation of respiration, control of DNA degradation--a lot of events that can be interpreted after the fact as perhaps promoting cell survival after exposure to a DNA-damaging agent. This may be a structure imposed by the scientist; I do not know--it is possible.

The third genetic locus has recently been reported by Kato and Shinoura (1977). It is called umuC and was identified by looking directly for a nonmutable phenotype. They also found recA's and lexA's, but umuC seems to affect specifically the error-prone repair system. It knocks out Weigle-reactivation--both the induced reactivation and the induced mutagenesis. However, it does not seem to affect any of the other inducible functions--phage induction, filamentous growth, etc. It makes the cells non-mutable by UV light, as do recA and lexA, and makes the cells somewhat sensitive to UV.

One point I want to raise is that UV light, 4-nitro-quinoline-1-oxide, and a large number of compounds are very effective mutagens in bacteria. If you knock out this error-prone repair system, you find that they are no longer mutagenic. UV light is basically nonmutagenic in recA, lexA, and umuC mutants. The same is true for a number of other compounds--I would say for the bulk of the common mutagens. It would seem from this that there must be some kind of processing of damage in order to get mutagenesis, that simply having something hit the DNA does not give damage that is intrinsically mutagenic. But processing must be by some kind of error-prone repair system. Since these same compounds are apparently good mutagens in higher organisms, there is probably some kind of analogous process. I am not going to argue that it is exactly the same, but it is probably analogous.

Radman (1975) and Witkin (1976) have developed much of the theory in this area and I should acknowledge them. Radman has reported a couple of experiments that suggest at least one of the mechanisms by which this error-prone repair may be taking place. One of them is a misincorporation assay. The experiment is basically to take a polymer such as poly(dT) and irradiate it to some extent so as to introduce some UV damage. He then used an oligomer, such as oligo(dA) in this case, as a primer and added unlabeled dATP and labeled dCTP and dGTP so that if he got misincorporation of C's and G's that were not coded for, he could detect it rather easily. He then made extracts from cells in which the error-prone system had been induced and ones in which it had not been induced. There is a certain amount of variability in this assay, but when he turned on the "error-prone" repair system, he found a marked increase in the amount of misincorporation. Radman's latest interpretation is that a polymerase polymerizes past a dimer due to the suppression of its proofreading function. He has reported another experiment that suggests the same sort of thing. Normally when a single-stranded phage replicates, it goes to a double-stranded form. If some thymine dimers are introduced into the phage and the error-prone system is not induced, the newly synthesized DNA never makes it all the way into a circle; it is only made in pieces. If the error-prone repair system is induced, at least some complete DNA is synthesized, again suggesting polymerization past the dimer. Certainly Witkin is pushing the view that this is the more or less complete story of error-prone repair. I think it is more complicated than that. There are a lot of questions as to how frame-shift mutagenesis can take place, etc.

EISENSTADT: It might also be worth stating at this point that Miller's analysis of mutations in the lacI gene following UV irradiation demonstrates that 95% of the mutations occur opposite pyrimidine dimers, 5% are elsewhere; it is probably going to be interesting trying to figure out why they are where they are--not opposite the dimers but somewhere else.

WALKER: That was a quick review of DNA repair. I will now relate it specifically to the Ames test (Ames et al., 1975; McCann et al., 1975; McCann and Ames, 1976).

Most of you are probably familiar with the concept of the Ames test. You take a histidine auxotroph of Salmonella typhimurium LT-2 (i.e., a mutant that cannot make histidine), grow it in rich medium, and put it on a plate with just a trace of histidine and mutagen in it. If you have it set up right, you get a lot of revertants if the chemical is mutagenic and you can do a linear dose-response curve rather nicely for most compounds. There are a number of things you have to do to a system like this to make it as good as the one Ames has now. We estimate that were you to just pick a random histidine mutation and look for reversion to his^+, you would perhaps pick up 20% of the known carcinogens. I have to refer to carcinogens in this case because that is basically how he has calibrated the system.

A number of things went into the design of the current strains. A choice was made very early on whether to go with a back mutational assay from his^- to his^+ or to try to do a forward mutational assay going from some wild-type gene to a mutation--for example, resistance to some compound. At the time, the back mutation was chosen because it seemed to be much cleaner; he could find mutations that gave classes of revertants that all came up together. In forward mutational assays, he tended to find mutants with varying degrees of leakiness so that colonies with a range of sizes appeared, and he never knew quite when to stop. It would seem from some of Jeffrey Miller's experiments, which Eisenstadt has already mentioned, that so much of mutagenesis takes place at hot spots that were you to do a forward mutational assay, much of the time you would be looking at events happening at hot spots anyway (Coulondre and Miller, 1977).

The first thing done by Ames in designing this test was to screen a lot of point and frame-shift mutants (you have to do both mutants because you are doing a back mutation) to find ones that appeared to be at hot spots for mutation. The location of hot spots probably has something to do with the local structure of the DNA. What goes into this is not completely clear, but there are certainly some suggestions in Jeffrey Miller's system that, for spontaneous mutation, the presence of a methyl group on a cytidine may influence it. Two mutations--hisG46 and hisD3052 (hisG46 is the point mutation that is in both TA1535 and TA100 and hisD3052 is a frame-shift mutation that is in TA1538 and TA98)--detect almost all of the mutagens and carcinogens that have shown up. Both are at hot spots.

The second thing done in designing the system was to delete the accurate excision repair system that removes bulky adducts such as thymine dimers from the DNA, the very first repair system I showed you. For many compounds, such as 4-nitroquinoline-1-oxide and the nitroso derivatives of 2-aminofluorene, this resulted in an increase in sensitivity of about 100-fold (Ames, Lee, and Durston, 1973). But the bacteria have been sort of juggled now, so they are particularly sensitive to classes of compounds that were formerly repaired by this very accurate repair system. I once looked at a mutant in Ames's lab that lacked one of the endonucleases that makes a nick at apurinic sites. The strain lacked about 90% of that enzyme activity. I found an increase in mutagenesis for methyl methanesulfonate and for some alkylating agents. That has not been pursued any further, but it is possible that the strains could be manipulated so as to be made more sensitive to various alkylating agents.

Another improvement put in did not have very much to do with DNA repair but was a genetic manipulation. This was to put in the deep rough mutation that removes the lipopolysaccharide from the outside of the bacteria (Ames, Lee, and Durston, 1973). I think this is a fairly important consideration in designing bacterial tester strains of any sort; you have to allow fairly large molecules to get through the membrane. If a tester system does not have such a mutation introduced, you can almost predict right away that certain classes of compounds of a larger molecular weight are just not going to be active.

Chronologically, the next improvement was the intro-duction of the S-9, which Eisenstadt has talked about quite a bit (Ames et al., 1973). But even by 1974, the system had not really caught anybody's attention because it still only detected about 60% of the known carcinogens. One further improvement made the difference between detecting about 60% and detecting about 90%. This was the introduc-tion of an R factor, pKM101, a plasmid that carried a drug resistance derived from a naturally occurring plasmid which protects cells against killing by UV and also increases UV mutagenesis. It was introduced empirically because it was known to increase mutagenesis. On testing, it was found that if pKM101 was present, bacteria became particularly sensitive to mutagenesis by a variety of compounds (McCann et al., 1975).

Figure 3 shows an example of the effect of this plasmid. The tester strain TA1535 has a <u>his</u> point mutation but lacks the plasmid. You can get a reasonable dose-response curve, but you have to go into the next room in terms of dose. With the same strain (TA100) containing the plasmid, you get a really large increase.

Here is another example of the sort of phenomenon that Eisenstadt mentioned. In the frame-shift tester strain (TA1538) without the plasmid, you can weakly detect aflatoxin B_1. In the point-mutation tester strain (TA1535), you cannot see any mutagenesis in the absence of the plas-mid; in the presence of the plasmid, aflatoxin B_1 became an extremely potent mutagen. The frame-shift strain was also elevated to about the same degree of sensitivity by the introduction of the plasmid. Figure 4 demonstrates that this plasmid does increase the resistance of the cell to killing by various agents such as UV. These are equiva-lent strains. One does not have the plasmid; one does; survival is a function of the UV dose.

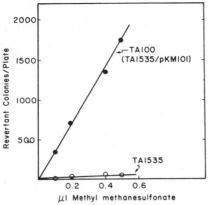

FIGURE 3
Effect of the plasmid pKM101 on the reversion of the standard tester strain TA1535 with MMS. Reversion was determined on petri plates, incorporating mutagen and bacteria directly into the top agar. Revertants were scored after incubation of the petri plates for 48 hours at 37°C. Spontaneous revertants have been subtracted.

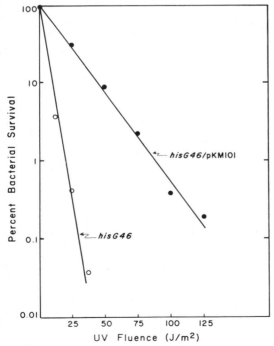

FIGURE 4
UV-protective effect of the plasmid pKM101 in strain hisG46.

ZIPSER: So the implication is that it is saving mutants, rather than heightening...?

WALKER: The implication is that it is doing both repair and mutagenesis because it is increasing the amount of repair going on in the cells and it is increasing the amount of mutagenesis.

ZIPSER: What is the evidence that it increases the amount of mutagenesis?

WALKER: Frequency of the mutation per survivor goes up.

ZIPSER: That is no good; I am sorry. If you argue that the mutagenic event is lethal--that is, lethal to the whole DNA...

WALKER: Can you hold on to that? I will come back to it a little later on and answer more directly with some phage experiments.

So far, I have been concentrating quite a bit on this problem because in the Ames system as it is now used the bulk of the mutations are picked up by TA100 and TA98, both of which contain the plasmid pKM101. How it works was really not known at all when it was introduced. It was pretty much an empirical observation that it worked. I have been looking at it a lot and can summarize it, I think, by saying that the plasmid pKM101 seems to increase the amount of error-prone repair activity in the cell. Thus, the Ames system has two basic things going on. One is the removal of an accurate repair system by allowing the damage to be processed by some other mechanism. The other is an elevation of the amount of error-prone repair activity present in the cells. Ames has managed to optimize things for a particular lesion going through a series of steps that give rise to mutation. Again, it is sort of a correlation between the coupling of repair and mutagenesis, but it is even stronger in this plasmid case than in the case of the cellular system. It turns out that all these plasmid-mediated effects (and there are a number of them; it is also a slight spontaneous mutator, it increases the re-activation of mutagenesis of UV-irradiated phage, and a variety of things) are dependent on $recA$ and $lexA$ (Walker, 1977). These are the two control functions that seem to be involved in control and regulation of the error-prone repair system. I have just recently found that it does not seem to be at all dependent on the $umuC$ locus (Walker, 1979). At this point, the most reasonable inter-pretation is that $umuC$ is a mutation in an operon that is involved in the production of some component that actually physically participates in error-prone repair. This has not been proved, but if it is true, pKM101 may well be carrying a component that actually physically participates in the process of error-prone repair.

Other evidence links repair and mutagenesis, as I have found by going through and isolating mutants of pKM101 looking for a loss of ability to enhance mutagenesis. I have found a number of such mutants, and Figure 5 shows typical data. Again, the number of revertants is a function of the amount of mutagen (Walker, 1978a).

Figure 6 shows what happens when you examine those pKM101 mutants for the ability to protect the cells against killing by UV. The figure gives the results obtained with strain hisG46 with and without the plasmid, with a mutant that completely knocks out mutagenesis, and with one that gives sort of intermediate mutagenic effects. So far I have not been able to uncouple them, either by their dependence on a chromosomal gene in the host or by mutating the plasmid.

Figure 7 shows an interesting effect. One reason why pKM101 is so particularly effective may simply be due to the more or less historical accident that the system was developed in Salmonella (Ames had been studying the histidine operon in Salmonella for a long time). If you look

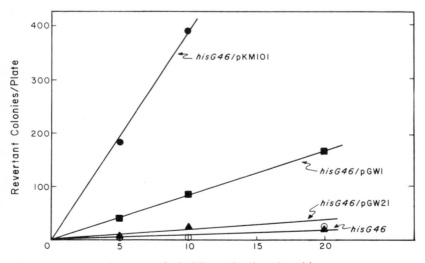

FIGURE 5
Effect of pKM101 and pKM101 mutants on the reversion of the missense mutation hisG46 by 4-nitroquinoline-1-oxide. Reversion was measured on petri plates and spontaneous revertants have been subtracted. Strain hisG46 (O), hisG46/pKM101 (●), hisG46/pGW1 (■), hisG46/pGW21 (▲).

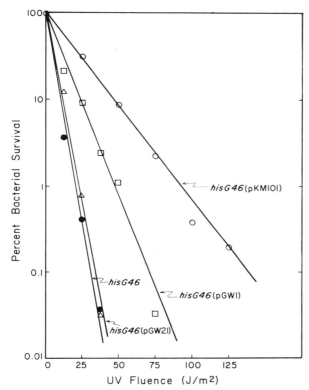

FIGURE 6
Effect of pKM101 and pKM101 mutants on the survival of
strain hisG46 after exposure to UV irradiation; hisG46 (●),
TA92 (O), GW203 (□), GW274 (Δ).

at Weigle-reactivation in Salmonella, this inducible phage
reactivation is very small compared to the amount of
reactivation that you see in E. coli. The most one sees is
a two- to fourfold reactivation in Salmonella, but it is
relatively easy to get 100-fold or more in E. coli (Walker,
1978b). When you introduce pKM101 into the strain,
however, you get some increase in the recovery of the
phage even in the nonirradiated host. Then the amount of
reactivation you get goes up quite dramatically.

There is an interesting point about this sort of thing.
Normally, UV damage to phage is not mutagenic in a
nonirradiated host. You have to induce the error-prone
repair system in order for the UV damage in the phage to
be mutagenic. Yet, in the presence of the plasmid, even in
the nonirradiated host in this condition, you find that
damage to the phage becomes quite mutagenic.

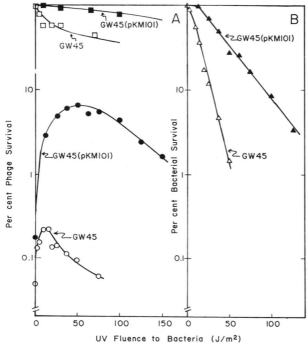

FIGURE 7
Effect of pKM101 on Weigle-reactivation of phage P22.
(A) Survival of UV-irradiated (300 J/m²) P22 on GW45 (O)
and TA92 (●).   Survival of nonirradiated P22 on GW45 (□)
and TA92 (■).   (B) Survival of the bacterial strains GW45
(Δ) and TA92 (▲) after UV irradiation.

Table 1 lists some mutation frequencies of UV-
irradiated phage P22 as a function of the UV dose given the
host (Walker, 1978b).   The essential point is that the
mutation frequency of the irradiated phage is not substantially different from that of the nonirradiated phage if
there is no plasmid present in the host.   If there is plasmid
present, you get about a 20-fold increase in the amount of
mutagenesis even in the nonirradiated host.   Irradiating it
further, you can get an even larger increase in mutagenesis
in the phage. So the plasmid may be making the cell behave
as if it were partly constitutive for this error-prone repair
process.   It can be turned on even more by damaging the
host, but it is already partway there as far as being able
to process damage in a fashion that gives rise to mutation.
One thing is quite different from the cellular system.
Figure 8A (Walker, 1979) (which depicts basically a repeat

TABLE 1
Effect of pKM101 on Frequency of Clear-plaque Mutants of P22

Bacterial strain	UV to P22 (J/m²)	UV to bacteria (J/m²)	P22 survival (%)	Reactivation factor	Clear-plaque mutants among survivors (%)[a]	Induced mutation factor
GW45	0	0	100		0.033	
GW45	250	0	0.085	1	0.049	1
GW45	250	2.5	0.13	1.5	0.080	1.6
GW45	250	5	0.13	1.6	0.075	1.5
GW45	250	13	0.10	1.2	0.064	1.3
GW45(pKM101)	0	0	100		0.036	
GW45(pKM101)	250	0	0.87	1	0.96	1
GW45(pKM101)	250	6	3.2	3.6	0.98	1.0
GW45(pKM101)	250	33	2.6	3.0	0.81	0.84
GW45(pKM101)	250	78	1.8	2.0	0.93	0.97
GW45(pKM101)	400	0	0.037	1	0.88	1
GW45(pKM101)	400	6	0.36	9.7	2.0	2.3
GW45(pKM101)	400	33	0.38	10	2.2	2.5
GW45(pKM101)	400	78	0.26	7.0	1.5	1.7

[a]For each entry for GW45, 45,000 to 80,000 plaques were screened for clear-plaque mutants. For each entry for GW45(pKM101), 25,000 to 75,000 plaques were screened.

of an experiment by Radman and his coworkers [Defais et al., 1976]) shows the effect of a period of postirradiation incubation in the Weigle-reactivation experiment in which the cells are incubated for some period of time before adsorption of the phage. It takes a few minutes to induce this error-prone repair system. If chloramphenicol is present during this period of preincubation, it is removed before addition of the phage. You find that, whereas in the absence of plasmid you see a continued induction of the ability to reactivate phage, when chloramphenicol is present there is a decay of this ability. When you put pKM101 into a strain and look at Weigle-reactivation, you get an apparent increase.

I expected that when I did the induction experiment in

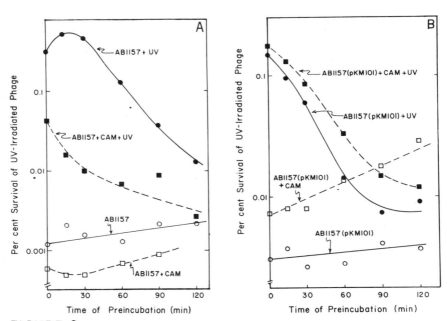

FIGURE 8
Effect of chloramphenicol on kinetics of Weigle-reactivation response in E. coli K-12 with and without pKM101. (A) Survival of UV-irradiated λ (320 J/m^2) in nonirradiated (O) and irradiated (39 J/m^2) (●) AB1157 not treated with chloramphenicol and in nonirradiated (□) and irradiated (50 J/m^2) (■) AB1157 treated with chloramphenicol (100 μg/ml). (B) Survival of UV-irradiated λ (385 J/m^2) in nonirradiated (O) and irradiated (45 J/m^2) (●) AB1157 (pKM101) not treated with chloramphenicol and in non-irradiated (□) and irradiated (58 J/m^2) (■) AB1157 (pKM101) treated with chloramphenicol.

a pKM101-containing strain, de novo protein synthesis would be required and that it would be very similar to the host system., The results of that experiment (shown in Figure 8B), however, really did not show any effect of chloramphenicol on the kinetics of the Weigle-reactivation response in the plasmid-containing strain.

In mammalian systems, if there is an analogous error-prone repair system of some sort, you probably do not want such an activity turned on all the time. It might increase the rate of spontaneous mutation. Here is an example of a case where you can turn on this activity by damaging the host, yet it does not seem to require de novo protein synthesis. Rather, instead of being an induction, it looks more like an activation of some preexisting protein. Often "error-prone" repair is equated with "inducible," at least in mammalian systems. This might just provide at least a caution to people thinking along those lines.

Lately, I have devoted a lot of energy to trying to figure out what the plasmid pKM101 does. We have it in minicells, which is an excellent background for looking at just the plasmid-encoded proteins. We have plasmid mutants, we have cloned derivatives of the plasmid, and we have insertions into the plasmid of translocatable elements that knock out its ability to increase mutagenesis. We are in the middle of sorting all this out.

A lot of the Ames system is very dependent on this plasmid and some of it still has not been straightened out. Ames kept making improvements every year, and finally the test reached the level where people were happy with it and it was critically evaluated. That does not necessarily represent the limit of what the test can do. The introduction of the _tif_ mutation, which causes constitutive expression of the error-prone repair system, at least in E. coli, increases the mutagenic rate quite considerably (Walker, 1977). One cloned derivative of pKM101 increases MMS mutagenesis fivefold more in E. coli than does pKM101 itself. With the current guideline situation you are not allowed to introduce recombinant DNA in Salmonella. So we have not been able to see whether this would help the tester strains or not.

In any case, just to close out here, I wanted to mention a couple of the other short-term tests in this context. Devoret and his coworkers have developed a test that looks at the induction of lambda by chemical agents (Moreau, Bailone, and Devoret, 1976; Moreau and Devoret, 1977). That test measures the induction of the system and finds chemicals that will induce the error-prone repair system, lambda, and all these coupled functions. So it is not specifically asking whether a compound is mutagenic or not, but rather whether it is the kind of compound that can turn on these $\underline{recA}^+$, $\underline{lexA}^+$-dependent error-prone repair systems. There are some indications that the error-prone repair system, once turned on, may be a sort of mutator gene that just randomly mutates and gives untargeted mutagenesis, so this may be a reasonable sort of system with which to work.

The biggest complaint I have with the current short-term tests is with what are termed repair tests, which do not directly measure mutagenesis. Normally, the kind of system used involves taking cells that are wild-type for DNA repair and comparing them with a strain that has a mutation affecting some aspect of DNA repair. The classical system that has been used takes a $\underline{polA}^+$ mutant and compares it with a polA mutant, so that you are comparing one cell that has polymerase I with one that lacks it (Slater, Anderson, and Rosenkranz, 1971). Polymerase I seems to participate in a number of repair systems. So far, the systems that have been suggested, published, and used are relatively unsophisticated. The polA test is most widely used and does not incorporate the removal of any of the other repair systems, which would certainly improve the sensitivity of the test. Also, there is nothing to permeabilize the cells; there is not a deep rough or an envA mutation--the things that would help larger molecules to get into the cell. Government agencies are spending a lot of money to evaluate two systems: the Ames test, which has taken a lot of genetic work to make it sensitive, and the polA mutant, which Eisenstadt, I, or any number of people could probably improve considerably as a testing vehicle with a few weeks of work.

DNA Repair

RICHARD SETLOW

Biology Department
Brookhaven National Laboratory

What is known about DNA repair in E. coli and most bacterial systems has already been discussed. The difficulty in extrapolating these data to mammalian systems is that the putative first enzyme in excision repair, the so-called "UV" endonuclease, really has not been isolated. So we have a profound conceptual difficulty that makes problems when we get to mammalian cells. Numbers will give an idea of the magnitude of the problem. In E. coli, there is good experimental evidence that UV-induced changes in DNA, called pyrimidine dimers, are the cause of much of the lethality and many mutations. The number of pyrimidine dimers per chromosome per mean lethal dose is shown in Table 1. For E. coli wild type, they are in the neighborhood of 3,000. Even though wild-type cells are very good at repairing such damage, they are ultimately affected by them. If you investigate mutants deficient in excision repair, so-called uvrA mutants, the numbers are around 50, so you can see that excision repair in itself results in about a 60-fold decrease in E. coli sensitivity. In a double mutant, recA uvrA, those numbers come down to about 1 dimer per bacterial chromosome.

The existence of numbers such as 50 rather than 1 for excision-deficient cells led to the search for other repair mechanisms described as postreplication repair. Even though wild-type cells are very proficient at repairing damage, they never can do it 100%. The important concepts are the kinetics of the processes of replication and repair and whether the replication is what has been termed error-free or error-prone. Obviously, if you blocked replication and permitted repair to take place, you would have a much happier state of affairs for a cell than if you let both go on and asked a cell to replicate past a lesion before it was repaired. In most systems the two processes

TABLE 1
Pyrimidine Dimers per *E. coli*
Chromosome at D_{37}

Genotype	Dimers
Wild-type	3,000
uvrA	50
recA	20
uvrA recA	~1

Data from Setlow and Setlow (1972).

go on at the same time. You do not say "here's an insult,
repair it, and then I'll think about replicating it." Those
are complications in E. coli.

The kinds of excision repair systems known at present
are given in Table 2. Most of the information comes from
data both in E. coli and in mammalian cells. My colleague
James Regan and I (1974) categorized excision repair into
two types. One type is called long patch, where a region
of DNA of the order of 100 nucleotides is removed and
replaced, even though the initial damage itself might only
have been 1 or 3 nucleotides. It appears that the system
cannot quite accommodate cutting out small pieces--as if it
gets ahead of itself. This long-patch type of repair follows
UV damage and many other bulky types of damage, presumably those caused by the polycyclic aromatic hydrocarbons, such as N-acetoxyacetylaminofluorene, nitroquino-
line oxide, and many other compounds. The second
category is short patch--on the order of 1-10 nucleotides.
It is characterized by its existence in cells that are exposed
to X-rays or some alkylating agents. Presumably, an
alkylating agent can lead to a depurination that can be
repaired by a simple break and rejoining.

A short time ago I heard of a third kind of excision

TABLE 2
Excision Repair Systems

Patch size	Damaging agents
Long (~100 nucleotides)	UV and its mimetics
Short (1–10 nucleotides)	ionizing radiation, apurinic sites, etc.
Zero (0 nucleotides)	dealkylation of O-6 alkyl guanine

repair that applies to alkylation damage. It is felt that the major damaging alkylation product (not the principal numerical product, but the major alkylation product) is O-6 alkyl guanine (the major product numerically is N-7 alkyl guanine, but the N-7 seems to have very few biological consequences compared with the O-6). At a recent meeting Pegg (1978b) described evidence that there is an enzyme in rat liver that removes the alkyl group from the O-6 and gives back guanine (see also Pegg, 1978a). This repair does not affect the polynucleotide. You would not detect this repair by any easy physical test unless you happened to have a specific marker on that methyl group, and most people do not do that. It might be detected in a muta- genesis test. I call this repair a zero patch; zero nucleo- tides are removed and replaced, and it seems to be docu- mented for the O-6 alkyl guanine.

In the other tests, long- and short-patch repair can be detected by various biochemical or biophysical means that look at changes in the parental DNA, such as the incorporation of nucleotides by repair replication or unscheduled synthesis. The big advances in this area have come from the recognition that there are mutants that are sensitive to various environmental agents. Of course, the point of all this is that the sensitivity of an organism to such an agent (chemical or physical) in the environment depends not only on what the agent is, but also on whether the cells can repair the damages. You can see that there can be big differences in the effectiveness of various agents; these differences are also reflected in the mutageni- city of various compounds. At a given dose, the uvrA mutant would be mutagenized much more than wild type.

The extension of these ideas to mammalian cells comes from the recognition that there are human mutants that are deficient in repair. James Cleaver (1968) had the bright idea to look at human mutants that got skin cancer at early ages--so-called xeroderma pigmentosum (XP) individuals. Such individuals, diagnosed clinically, have 100% cumulative incidence of skin cancer by the age of 10 or 12. They are characterized by the fact that their cells are deficient in one or more DNA repair mechanism. Veronica Maher (Maher and McCormick, 1976) and her collaborators have shown that XP cells are also mutagenized very readily by UV and that the cells themselves are also sensitive to UV. XP happens to be a very peculiar case in that we know a great deal about the disease and we know the etiologic agent-- sunlight--very clearly. We know that the individuals are deficient in repair; their cells are mutagenized to a high rate in culture, and there is a high incidence of skin cancer. The concentration of homozygotes in the population is of the order of 1 in 10^5; the heterozygotes in the population are estimated to be in the neighborhood of 1 in 100. The homozygotes are very sensitive; the heterozygotes, as far as has been determined epidemiologically, are close to normal. They do not seem to be at much greater risk than normal individuals.

It is of interest that xeroderma pigmentosum cells in culture are sensitive not only to UV, but also to many other agents. They are both mutagenized by and are more sensitive (killed) to these other agents. As far as the clinical disease is concerned, however, UV swamps out any other environmental agent that might affect such individuals.

Finding UV-repair defects among XP individuals has stimulated the search for other human genetic diseases in which there is a high propensity for cancer, and several have been found (Setlow, 1978). Ataxia-telangiectasia (AT) is also associated with a high cancer incidence; it is estimated that the cumulative incidence of cancers (most of which may be lymphatic) among such individuals may amount to 10%. The etiologic agent is not known; we just know that they are a high-cancer-risk population. What is known is that cells of such individuals, and the individuals themselves are very much more sensitive to X-rays, i.e., maybe fivefold. The idea to look at X-ray sensitivity came about because some AT individuals had very severe reactions to X-ray cancer therapy. Although the cells and the individuals are sensitive to X-rays, that does not mean that their cancer arises from ionizing radiation in the environment. There are a number of chemicals to which cells from these individuals are sensitive--alkylating agents, MNNG, and MMS, for example. But whether the people are sensitive to these agents is another matter. The interesting thing here is that the concentration of homozygotes is of the same order as found for XP--about 1 in 10^5--and they are also high risk.

The heterozygotes have been subjected to an epidemiological analysis by Swift and coworkers (1976), and among the heterozygote population they find a higher risk for cancer than in the normal population. Let me give you some examples from their data. Heterozygotes less than 45 years of age have a fivefold greater risk of cancer death than the average population, so they are a high-risk group.

EHRENBERG: Cancer of which sites?

SETLOW: Of several sites, if I remember.

The epidemiology was all done on mortality records. The biggest change is in young individuals. For the total population up to age 75, which is the highest age looked at, cancer mortality was 50% higher than the normal population. It appears that AT heterozygosity is shifting the incidence curve to lower ages.

The molecular nature of AT is not clear. AT cells in culture are very sensitive to X-rays. Approximately one-half the cell strains looked at are defective in repair of one form or another. One-half of them seem to be proficient in repair, which indicates extreme heterogeneity (that these arise for different reasons) or we are not looking at the right kind of repair. Whether it is a repair that involves zero patch, and no one has looked at it, or whether they do not perform repair is just not clear. So, when I say "defective in repair," you have to remember that this is based on an experiment, and maybe people have done the wrong experiment.

But all the cells are sensitive (in terms of killing) to X-rays. We just do not know why. They are all also sensitive to alkylating agents.

There is a syndrome called Fanconi's anemia in which, according to Swift (1971), the heterozygotes are also at higher risk than the average population. The homozygotes die from numerous hematological abnormalities as well as face a high risk of leukemia. The heterozygotes in this population have been estimated by Swift to account for 5% of all leukemia deaths. They are present in the general population to the extent of 1 in 100, and therefore 5% is a fivefold excess over average.

As far as we know, the deficiency in this case is in a kind of a repair that is quite different from long-, short-, or zero-patch repair. It seems to be a deficiency in the repair of cross-links, something that joins two DNA strands together. So cross-linking agents such as mitomycin C, psoralen plus light, and so on affect such cells much more than they affect normal cells, and the cross-links persist for longer periods of time. The etiologic agent for the high incidence of cancer, however, is not known.

BREWEN: Are they also defective in repairing protein-DNA cross-links?

SETLOW: I have not seen anything on that.

The environmental agents, if any, involved in ataxia-telangiectasia or Fanconi's anemia are not known. Luckily for us, the etiologic agent of xeroderma pigmentosum is known, and that is why we have a lot of background information on it.

In summary, mammalian cells that lack repair systems are more sensitive to a number of agents. There is a correlation, but not a superb one, between such deficiencies and increased cancer, although for AT and Fanconi's anemia we do not know what the environmental agents are. Incidentally, the models that most people like to use for human cells in culture are rodent cells, and rodent cells in culture are all (at least as far as UV is concerned) in the class of xeroderma pigmentosum--deficient in one way or another in excision repair. So even though they are easy to grow, they are not necessarily a good quantitative model.

WATSON: Is that because of their thick skin?

SETLOW: No, these are cells in culture.

RAY: And that does not apply to primary cultures, I would gather.

SETLOW: It applies to primary cultures if they are taken from mice after birth.

BREWEN: Mouse embryos are deficient?

SETLOW: Not if you get cells from very young embryos. It appears that in the rodent system the UV excision repair system is really there genetically; it gets turned off at some time, maybe because the animals realize they have a thick skin and do not need it. It is there, but it is turned off some time during late gestation.

RAY: When you say that, are you speaking about epithelial cells as a comparison between rodents and humans, or are you talking about all cells including specific organs such as the liver?

SETLOW: In the rodent system, epithelial cells and fibroblasts have been studied. With regard to human cells, most of the work has been done with fibroblasts. I know that normal human epithelial cells are proficient in excision repair. There were some early experiments done to look at the ability of the skin of XP individuals to do unscheduled synthesis after UV--experiments that would not be permitted nowadays. Such experiments presumably showed that epithelial cells are deficient, so there does not seem to be any tissue dependence for repair of UV damage. People have not looked carefully at the tissue dependence for repair of damage caused by many other agents, such as alkylating agents.

FLAMM: Lieberman and his colleagues (Ambacher, Elliott, and Lieberman, 1977) have done some of that work. Many of the mouse species they looked at were not competent with respect to UV repair in somatic cells.

The were competent with respect to both long-patch and short-patch repair with the whole series of chemicals, in certain instances exceeding human cells in their ability to repair damage induced by certain types of chemicals.

SETLOW: The problem with chemicals, as with the alkylating agents, is that you are not really sure what product to study. You want to look at the deleterious product, and in the case of alkylating agents the major product is relatively nondeleterious, so you can look at that. You are not sure what its biological significance is. But you are right, it is not clear what goes on in rodent versus human cells except for UV.

I want to present some NIH data (Table 3) on xeroderma pigmentosum to emphasize what a dramatic difference there is between normal people and XP individuals. This is an analysis by Jay Robbins and his collaborators (1974); it indicates the fact that multiple tumors develop. The table also illustrates that XP individuals have a high incidence of malignant melanoma. Basal and squamous-cell carcinomas are relatively innocuous cancers to deal with, but that is not true of malignant melanoma. It is a serious disease in the white population and seems to be increasing at the rate of 5% or 6% per year. The XP data implicate damage to DNA, if you want to put it that way, in malignant melanoma. Individuals who are defective in that repair have a prevalence of 50% in this sample, whereas the normal incidence in the general population is just a few in 100,000 per year.

In a fit of frenzy I at one time (Setlow, 1978) made a compilation showing the various chemicals that have been tested with XP, AT, and Fanconi's anemia cells (Table 4). I was making the point that cells deficient with one agent, which is how these cells are characterized in the first place, end up being deficient in repair with a large number

TABLE 3
Some Characteristics of 13 Individuals with
Xeroderma Pigmentosum

Percentage with skin tumors	100
Average age of first tumor, (yr)	10 ± 5
Tumors per individual	40 ± 30
Percentage with malignant melanoma	54

Data from Robbins et al. (1974).

TABLE 4
Damaging Agents or Products for Which Cells Are Repair-proficient
or Repair-deficient

Proficient	Deficient
Xeroderma pigmentosum	
Ionizing radiation	UV
strand breaks	dimers
anoxic	protein DNA links
4-NQO (minor compound)	strand breaks
NO-carbaryl	Ionizing radiation
NO-Me guanidine	anoxic
MNNG	4-NQO
MMS	AAF damage
MNU	ICR, 170
EMS	Aflatoxin
N-7 alkyl guanine	K-region epoxides
Proflavin + light	Br benzanthracene
Propane sultone	Br_2 Me benzanthracene
Mitomycin C	EMS
	O-6 alkyl guanine
	Psoralen + light
	Chlorpromazine + light
	BCNU
	HNO_2
	Decarbomyl mito C
Ataxia telangectasia	
Ionizing radiation	Ionizing radiation
strand breaks	chromosomes
endonuclease sites	survival
Mitomycin C	endonuclease sites
MMS	Actinomycin D
UV	Mitomycin C
AAF damage	MMS
Fanconi's anemia	
Decarbomyl mito C	Mitomycin C
MNNG	Psoralen + light
4-NQO	HN_2
MMS	DNA crosslinks
UV	Gamma rays

Cells are categorized on the basis of survival, host-cell reactivation, or chromosomal, biochemical, or biophysical measures of repair (a listing in both categories means that there are several products of an agent or that all cell lines are not the same) (Setlow, 1978).

of other agents, most of which have no obvious connection with UV. AT cells are also sensitive to a wide variety of agents and proficient with a large number. It seems as though these repair-proficient anomalies in mammalian cells--the clues to which are taken from bacteria, whose science is in a bad state--span a wide range of chemicals. Agents that damage DNA are bad, and conceivably there exist sensitive subsets of the population that one has to worry about--perhaps, for example, heterozygotes of AT or of Fanconi's anemia.

NEEL: Your estimates of heterozygote frequencies are based on the assumption that the entity is genetically homogeneous. As we know, there are now about eight subgroups or eight complementation groups for XP, two at least for AT, and MacPaterson, at a recent symposium (1977), said he got tired of doing that kind of work. These are independent loci, and that fact could double these heterozygote frequencies. Earlier in this conference there was a question about mutable strains of people and these would be candidates.

SETLOW: These are mutable as cells. There was some question at a conference we attended as to whether fibroblasts of AT were mutable or not; some people said no, and I just was not wide awake enough to say "to what agents?" I do not know whether they really tested the right agent or the wrong agent.

RAY: The work you and others have done showing that the intrinsic or inherent repair capability of the same kind of cell taken from a variety of species can differ has been very interesting--the difference between human and rodent cells, for example. Has anyone any knowledge at this point about the inherent or intrinsic repair capability for organs with a very low mitotic index, such as the liver and bladder, compared with organs with a very high mitotic index, such as the villi of the intestines, hair follicles, and certain parts of the reticuloendothelial system? I have wondered whether this is known; has anyone looked at this?

EISENSTADT: Have liver and brain been compared with respect to repairing out of nitroso . . .?

RAY: Liver and brain?

EISENSTADT: Yes.

SETLOW: Yes in so far as repairing some kinds of alkylation. This is part of the evidence that leads to the circular kind of argument that we get into. Whichever was the sensitive tissue--brain in this case--did not remove O-6 alkyl guanines as readily as liver and so this is some evidence that O-6 alkyl guanine is bad.

BREWEN: But what about the data of Strauss and collaborators (Scudiero et al., 1976) on leukocytes?

SETLOW: The data show that when leukocytes with a relatively low repair rate are stimulated to divide they have an increased repair rate.

BREWEN: For UV damage, but they do repair X-ray damage without stimulation.

SETLOW: Confluent cells are just as good for UV or a number of the chemical damages as growing cells, but, again, that is the same cell.

RAY: I guess the question at the back of that is whether or not some of this inherent or intrinsic repair capability could indeed be related to sensitivity or resistance to carcinogenic agents in those particular organs.

SETLOW: People attempted to guess at the lethal product or the mutagenic product, such as O-6 versus N-7 alkyl guanine, and determined that the O-6 in brain lasts for a long time, whereas it does not last for a long time in liver.   Therefore, the rate of repair is important.   But obviously the rate of repair has to be related to the rate of proliferation in that tissue.

RAY: That is why I asked about mitotic index in the first place.

SETLOW: I cannot really answer that.   For X-ray damage, almost all kinds of cells repair at reasonable rates. Let me add one point that came up in the previous presentation: the ability of cells to reactivate or to have some sort of inducible activity.   In mammalian cells, there is a viral system that also has been used in the same sort of way.   This is a system in which an irradiated virus shows a higher survival if it is plated on irradiated cells--or cells treated with a number of chemical carcinogens.   There is reactivation of UV-irradiated viruses for a number of chemical types of damage to mammalian cells.   It is not as dramatic as in bacteria.   That is probably the best evidence for an induced repair system.

WALKER: It is probably worth mentioning that with XP, too, if you look for more than one biochemical effect, the different complementation groups seem to be lacking more than one activity.   It is as though they were lacking some regulatory . . .

SETLOW: They lack one, they lack the other. It is a rather complex system. There are in the neighborhood of six to eight complementation groups. We do not have that number in E. coli where we cannot even analyze three, so to speak. We do not know what the defect is in E. coli--whether it is uvrA, B, or C. It seems that in xeroderma pigmentosum it could be A through H.

EHRENBERG: With reference to dose-response curves, very often people believe, at least on the quasi-scientific level, that if you have a repair system, there must be a threshold of the effects. That is, at very low doses the repair might be error-free and complete. I have seen an investigation quoted where the repair of O-6 alkylation had been determined with regard to dose response down to very low doses. I do not know who did that, but it was certainly a study in the United States.

SETLOW: I think Pegg (1978a) may have done that. It is true that if you go down to very low dose rates or doses (which is what we are exposed to, not acute rates as in all these experiments), you would expect much more efficacious repair. But in the case of UV, I would argue that this is a simplistic point of view for the following reason. Even though we all talk about pyrimidine dimers as being the big thing, they are not the only thing. There may be a number of other products that are not repaired as effectively. Even when you go to low dose, there are still other products. For example, just to put this in perspective, I put down the number of pyrimidine dimers per chromosome per mean lethal dose. For XP cells, for the whole chromosome set, this number is about 10^5.
        There are lots and lots of products, most of which are ignored--after all, these are distributed among 40-odd chromosomes. This really means that there are appreciable numbers of other products about whose biochemical characteristics we know little--for example, DNA-protein cross-links. Unfortunately, we only measure the ones we know something about and can measure easily. Some might be at the level of 10, which you really would not detect by the means we have; they might not be effectively repaired. There is no way of my getting at that problem with mammalian cells.

LEE: May I make a comment about repair in germ-cell stages? I will consider this in historical order. Rejoining of chromosomes is at least one method that would require repair--mechanism unknown and prob-

ably rather complex. But 30 years ago Muller showed
from the kinetics of rejoining in mature sperm that
chromosomes do not undergo rejoining until after the
egg is fertilized. This process of chromosome rejoining is apparently turned off at the midspermatid
phase. The latest spermatid and mature spermatozoa
do not have the capability of chromosome rejoining,
whereas the early stages do.

About four years ago Sega did work on unscheduled DNA synthesis. In this case, synthesis
occurred normally, of course, by premeiotic replication. In the presence of a variety of mutagens,
including alkylating agents, X-rays, and so forth, the
unscheduled synthesis continued after meiosis until
about midspermatid stage and then it shut off. In
more recent work, Sega (1978) compares the stage of
unscheduled DNA synthesis and the stage of maximum
sensitivity of the germ-cell stage to dominant lethal
formation. The patterns are quite different for
different mutagens.

In the case of EMS, for example, the maximum
sensitivity for dominant lethality occurs 7 to 9 days
after treatment of the mouse, whereas the unscheduled
synthesis does not appear until a few days later.
They do not coincide. In fact, the beginning of the
scheduled synthesis is the end of the mutation-detec-
tion system in that germ-cell stage. The other
mutagens, however, have quite different patterns, so
even with the four or five different systems we
studied, there is not a consistent pattern between the
time of germ-cell stage sensitivity and the time of
unscheduled DNA synthesis.

A third type of experiment that may be related to
repair would be to measure the loss of the labeled
group on the DNA. An abstract by Janca (1977) is all
there is in the published literature. Unpublished work
on Drosophila has shown a loss of the labeled group in
the early germ-cell stages. From a midspermatid stage
only to mature spermatozoa, there is an accumulation
of the alkyl group, and loss from the sperm stored in
the female is at a rate that corresponds to the
published rates of hydrolysis, with no indication of
any enzymatic loss at all.

After fertilization, Janca has been able to
determine two points. He has a level of labeling in
the mature sperm, and he has the level 15 minutes
later. He has not been able to get a point between
those two. But there is a drop of some 40% to 50% of
the alkylation in that short period of time. The rate

would require many times that of hydrolysis. Apparently there is a change in the loss of the labeled alkyl group upon fertilization. It appears that in the germ-cell stage (in these two metozoans and humans), each individual is a result of a cell that passed through stages where the repair systems were shut off and stages where they functioned. At early cleavage, apparently there is replication of DNA and a repair system going. An error-prone system at that point would be predicted.

NEEL: May I suggest that you have failed to quote what might be the most spectacular example of all repair mechanisms in humans--the well-known failure to recover induced mutations from late eggs in irradiated female mice.

LEE: That is in the mouse, not in humans.

NEEL: No, but we do not yet have that kind of evidence.

LEE: I think there is some question as to whether the mouse ovary is reflective of the human female ovary. Grant Brewen would be better able to discuss that than I. Yes, I have limited my discussion here to the male, but certainly there is a very rapid change in the female system there; exactly which model we should use for humans, perhaps Brewen will discuss.

ABRAHAMSON: In the Drosophila female, repair goes on from oogonial stages up to stage-14 oocytes. You have stage 7, and between stages 7 and 14 there is about an 8-hour period. So somewhere in there you lose repair. Dean Parker showed that, and we did also (Parker and McCrone, 1958; Parker and Hammond, 1958; Abrahamson, 1961). The stage-14 oocyte does not repair again until after fertilization, which is a stimulating process. Grant, do you want to discuss the female?

BREWEN: Actually, I was going to talk about the female in my little presentation. But I will make this one point. The stage in the mouse oocyte that has 100% repair is stage 1; stage 2, the true dyctyate oocyte, does not exist in humans or for that matter in very many mammals.

PERSON: I want to criticize your phrase "100% repair." That is 0% survival.

BREWEN: Well, not quite, it is 0.1%. I was quoting Bill Russell when I said 100% repair (see review by Searle, 1974).

ABRAHAMSON: Its LD50 dose is 9 R and its LD99.9 dose
is 50 rad X-rays.   His lowest dose experiment was at
50 rad for the female for that stage, and it is true he
got zero mutation.

BREWEN: Fifty rad is the only dose for which there are
any data, because at any higher doses there are no
surviving oocytes.

EHRENBERG: Does the similarity between bacteria and
humans in various respects indicated here make it
possible to determine which test is applicable to risk in
humans?   The bacterial systems are made more and
more quantitatively sensitive simply to detect mutagenesis.   But such changes could increase the
difficulty of quantitation of risk.   For instance, great
increases in postreplication repair through these
plasmids would be abnormal but very practical for
detection.

WALKER: In terms of carcinogenesis, Ames has been looking at this correlation between carcinogenic potency
and mutagenic potency, having gone through the
world's cancer literature of the last 50 years or so
where there were test data that satisfied criteria set
up ahead of time.   He found a correlation (about which
he is not yet willing to say much) between carcinogenic potency and mutagenic potency covering a
six-order-of-magnitude scale (Ames and Hooper, 1978;
Meselson and Russell, 1978).   In that system he put in
things designed to pick up more and more of the
known carcinogens.   This he used as a yardstick for
calibrating the system as he went along.   What he
ended up with seems to be not a bad predictor of
potency, even though all he was looking for initially
was a yes/no response.   How that relates to mutagenicity, I don't know.

VALCOVIC: I would only add that this is for a relatively
small number of points on that curve, though.   A lot
of carcinogens are not on there.   It is a highly
selected sample.

FLAMM: Sure.   No one is saying that they biased it to
come out that way.   It is just that it has not covered
the whole universe of carcinogens because the data
have not been sufficient to meet those criteria.   Once
you have removed the nitrosamines and the nitro
compounds that are in the middle--one being too high
and the other being too low--you are left with points
just at either end.   It says essentially that things like
chloroform and chlorinated alkenes and alkanes are

very weak carcinogens, whereas things like aflatoxin
are very potent.

WALKER: Isn't it the other way around? There is a huge
cluster in the middle and then there are a couple of
things at each end.

FLAMM: Except if you remove the things that are producing problems--for instance, nitrosamines are not
registering as strongly for carcinogenicity as they do
in animals, whereas nitro compounds are registering as
too potent. But there are a lot of nitro compounds
and nitrosamines there because there are adequate
carcinogenicity data on them. I think what we really
need are people to do carcinogenicity experiments in
ways that will generate some useful information on the
potency in various animals.

Cytogenetic Studies and Risk Assessment for Chemicals and Ionizing Radiation

J. GRANT BREWEN

Biology Division
Oak Ridge National Laboratory

This discussion of the role of structural chromosome aberrations will ignore the numerical chromosome alterations that result from nondisjunction and polyploidy. An attempt will be made to restrict the comments to an objective evaluation of the data. This is particularly important because the analysis of chromosome aberrations often becomes very subjective. Since I assume that there may be a few who may lose their way amidst the cytogeneticist's jargon that I tend to slip into, I would like to define a few terms.

Cytogenetics, in my opinion, is just beginning to come out of the dark ages. I say that because we do not understand very many, if any, of the basic mechanisms involved in the formation of structural chromosome aberrations. So when I define the aberrations, I talk about chromosomes as if they were a piece of string.

Published light microscope photographs of chromosomes as they appear at metaphase of mitosis show two arms, called chromatids. The one thing that is very important in evaluating cytogenetic data is the structural unit of that chromosome involved in the aberration. In the normal proliferative cell cycle, there are four stages: G_1, S, G_2, and mitosis. We can subdivide these into three major components in terms of the level of the chromosome at which the aberration takes place or is formed. During G_1 the chromosome behaves as if it were a single unit; in other words, any damage produced during this stage of the cell cycle involves both chromatids. If you will imagine for one moment that we have what I call an interchange or a translocation involving two chromosomes as depicted in Figure 1, you will see either a dicentric--a chromosome with two centromeres--or a reciprocal translocation. It is important to bear in mind that dicentrics are almost always

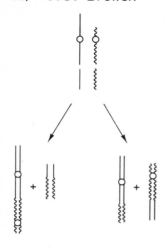

DICENTRIC   RECIPROCAL
                     TRANSLOCATION

FIGURE 1
Diagrammatic representation of the formation of chromosome-type interchanges.

lethal at the cellular level, so of course they are lethal at the organism level. There is a loss of genetic material. Furthermore, the two centromeres generate difficulties at cell division. Reciprocal translocations are not cell-lethal and they are heritable; hence, the translocation test that Flamm discussed.

On the other hand, if structural damage is produced during the S or G_2 portion of the cell cycle, the structural unit involved is the single chromatid. The equivalent aberration types, or exchanges, take on a different appearance. There is a phenomenon known as sister chromatid attraction. The two chromatids of the same chromosome are attracted to each other. If the chromosomes are wiggly and straight, as depicted in Figure 1, the sister chromatid attraction results in the configurations diagrammed in Figure 2. When that cell divides, four segregation products can be generated. One of them is a normal cell; that is, the nonexchange chromatids segregate together. Another is a translocation-bearing cell; that is, translocation is balanced, in the sense that the two exchange chromatids are recovered in the same cell. And last, another segregation pattern will create two duplication-deficient cells.

Let us assume for simplicity that each event occurs at equal frequency if we treat a population of dividing cells with X-rays. It is obvious that the reciprocal translocation

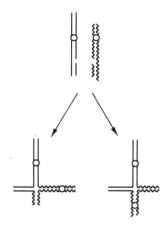

CHROMATID   CHROMATID
DICENTRIC   RECIPROCAL TRANSLOCATION

FIGURE 2

Diagrammatic representation of the formation of chromatid-type interchanges.

produced in G_1 will be recovered in every daughter cell. But in S and G_2 it will be recovered only in one of four daughter cells. It is important to remember that when I talk about chromatid-type damage, I am talking about one event, and when I talk about chromosome-type damage, I am talking about the other event. The probability of recovering these two events in the subsequent generations is different by a factor of 4.

This also applies to deletions. If we produce a deletion at the chromosome level, all daughter cells will carry a deleted chromosome. On the other hand, if the deletion is produced at the chromatid level, one of the daughter cells will carry a deleted chromosome; the other one will not and will live--it is viable.

Why does one even study chromosome aberrations? From the inception of studies on mutagenesis in <u>Drosophila</u> to today, it has been fairly obvious that structural chromosome aberrations constitute a major, if not <u>the</u> major, component of the genetic damage produced by practically any mutagenic insult in higher eukaryotic systems. In fact, Liane Russell (1971) has shown by complementation tests and also by testing the homozygosity or homozygous lethality that at least 50% of all the specific-locus mutations induced in oocytes and postmeiotic male cells are small chromosomal deficiencies.

I am going to assume here that the basic mechanism for producing a deficiency of that size is the same as that

for producing one large enough to be seen in a microscope.
Given that assumption, it is possible to discuss visible light
microscope work and correlate it, at least in the mouse, to
a proportion of specific-locus mutations. However, this has
to be done in a realistic fashion. We have to accept the
fact that most of what is seen in a light microscope are in
fact lethal events. I would venture to guess that 99.9% of
the simple deletions seen in a light microscope are lethals at
the cellular level.

What do we know about chromosome aberrations? Four
pieces of data have been generated over the past 10 years
that elucidate somewhat the molecular mechanism of aberration formation in higher cells. The first piece of evidence
was generated by Evans and Scott (1964, 1969). They
showed that if a normally proliferating cellular system was
treated with alkylating agents, no structural damage was
observed until approximately 6-8 hours later. All the
damage observed was of the chromatid type. The next
experiment was to apply [^{3}H]thymidine. They found that
the appearance of chromosome aberrations coincided with the
appearance of cells that incorporated the isotope. So they
identified the sensitive stage as being the S stage, or the
time of replicative DNA synthesis. This was done for
maleic hydrazide and nitrogen mustard. From that we
generalize that all alkylating agents operate mechanistically
the same way. They require an intervening round of DNA
replication to convert the lesion that is put into the
chromatin into an actual structural aberration.

The second piece of evidence comes from an experiment
I did with Jim Peacock about 10 years ago (Brewen and
Peacock, 1969). This experiment was quite simple-minded.
We simply labeled cells with [^{3}H]thymidine. On the basis of
the observation of the semiconservative replication and
segregation of the chromosomal subunits demonstrated by
Taylor, Woods, and Hughes (1957), we asked, "If a
particular type of aberration is produced, how are these
segregating subunits associated end to end?" Figure 3
summarizes the experimental rationale. If the molecular
target was DNA, the two strands of the duplex of each
chromatid would be restricted in their end-to-end association. If DNA was not involved, the end-to-end association
would be expected to be random. We could then induce
polyploidy and recover these as dicentric chromosomes. If
there was a restriction in the way that the strands of the
DNA duplex associated end to end, we would expect to get
either all of one or all of the other autoradiographic pattern
depicted in Figure 3. If there was no restriction, the two
patterns would be expected to occur in equal frequency.

When we analyzed the autoradiograms, we found that
99% of the chromosomes so generated had a label segregation

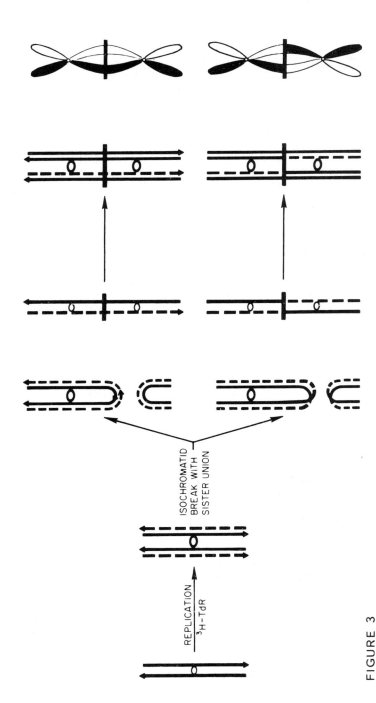

FIGURE 3

Diagrammatic representation of the alternate types of end-to-end association of the segregating chromosomal subunits. For simplicity, the subunits are represented as the helices of a single DNA molecule. The dotted line indicates the presence of [³H]thymidine and the solid chromosome regions indicate the presence of a label. (Reprinted, with permission, from Brewen and Peacock, 1969.)

101

pattern, which we interpreted as meaning that there was a restriction in the end-to-end association in aberration formation because of the physiochemical properties of DNA, and that therefore DNA was probably the principal target in the formation of this aberration.

The third bit of evidence comes from an experiment of Griggs and Bender (1973), in which they utilized an amphibian cell line that was capable of performing photo-reactivation. They synchronized, plated, and UV-irradiated cells in G_1. This was done in duplicate, and they then photoreactivated one population but not the other. They collected cells at the subsequent mitosis and found that in the absence of photoreactivation, there was an extremely high frequency of chromatid-type aberrations--aberrations that were formed as the cell passed through replicative DNA synthesis. They argued that since photoreactivation removed specifically pyrimidine dimers, the pyrimidine dimer in the template strand caused a gap in the nascent strand which was subsequently translated into structural damage.

The confirmation of that observation by Sasaki (1973) constitutes a fourth bit of evidence. He took peripheral leukocytes from xeroderma pigmentosum (XP) and normal patients and treated them with 4-nitroquinoline-oxide (4NQO) and UV. Leukocytes from XP patients cannot excise the pyrimidine dimers, or the lesions put into the DNA by 4NQO. The interval between treatment and the onset of DNA replication in these cells is approximately 24 hours. Sasaki found that the normal cells had in fact repaired the lesions and the chromosomes were normal, whereas in the XP cells, where there would not be any excision-type repair, there were massive amounts of chromosome damage.

These four pieces of evidence indicate two things: DNA is the principal target, and more importantly, certainly, for alkylating agents and for UV, an intervening round of DNA replication is necessary to produce some effect. Keeping this in mind, how can we use this information in making either qualitative or quantitative risk estimates for humans or for mice? For a long time, the method of measuring the mutagenic capacity of a chemical was the dominant-lethal test. One intriguing fact is that if you look at the spectrum of dominant-lethal effects in terms of stage sensitivity, curves like those shown in Figure 4 (Generoso and Russell, 1969; Brewen et al., 1975; Ehling, 1977) are generated. When one samples cells that were spermatogonial at the time of treatment, one very rarely, if ever, recovers dominant lethals, heritable translocations, or specific-locus mutations (Ehling, 1971; Cattanach, 1975).

The dogma in mammalian mutagenesis is that the spermatogonial cell is the cell of importance because it sits

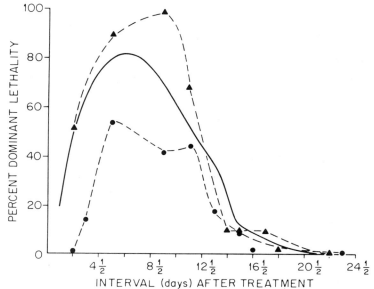

FIGURE 4

Yield of dominant lethals, with time, after injection of male mice with either EMS or MMS. The solid line is a generalized representation of the 300 mg/kg EMS data of Generoso and Russell (1969). The dotted lines are frequencies of embryos carrying at least one lethal chromosome aberration (Brewen et al., 1975).

there for the entire reproductive lifetime of the male and can accumulate damage. With chemical mutagens, the difference in sensitivity between the postmeiotic stages and the spermatogonial cells is measured not in orders of magnitude, but in infinity, because no lethal effects are recovered from spermatogonia. So it is zero as compared with 50% or 100%. On the other hand, if you do the experiment by going directly to the animal, removing the testes, and making cytological preparations, there is abundant chromosome damage in the differentiating spermatogonia. Why aren't they ever recovered? If you did an experiment with X-rays and with a chemical, you would find that X-rays produce cytologically observable damage in spermatogonia equivalent to that produced by an appropriate dose of a chemical mutagen; with X-rays, however, dominant lethals are recovered, but with a chemical mutagen they are not.

Let us imagine that we have in the testes a spermatogonial stem cell, which is what we are really interested in. It is going through a normal proliferative cell cycle as a

G_1, as an S, as a G_2; it then goes through mitosis and begins a new cycle.   Observations made on somatic cells have shown that cells in the act of replicating DNA are extremely sensitive to most of the alkylating agents tested. Remember that most chromosome damage is lethal at the cellular level.   That means that if I treat a cell in S and produce a reciprocal translocation of the chromatid type, I have one chance in four of ever recovering it, because of segregation.   But if into that same cell I introduce three or four deletions, for example, I ensure that it will die.   That is precisely what happens.   The cells are sensitive; they are hit with a massive dose of a compound; they are killed. The G_1 and G_2 cells are not affected; they survive, producing normal cells that go through the spermiogenic cycle, and the chromosomal damage is not recovered.

If the same experiment is done with bone marrow cells, precisely the same effect is found.   At the higher concentrations, however, it is possible to recover the S-phase cells.   In [^{3}H]thymidine tagging experiments (Luippold, Gooch, and Brewen, 1978), it was seen that bone marrow cells that were replicating their DNA were recovered and found to contain aberrations.   In the spermatogonia, at very high doses, the S-stage cells never reached mitosis; they suffered interphase death.   So that is the first question--and answer.   We have an explanation for why you do not recover this sort of typical effect when spermatogonial cells are treated with these mutagens.

There are exceptions to this generalization in that some chemicals are truly radiomimetic.   That is, they produce chromosome aberrations at all stages of the cell cycle.   Examples of these are 8-ethoxy- and methoxy-caffeine, cytosine arabinoside, streptonigrin, phleomycin, and bleomycin.   Polyfunctional alkylating agents such as thio-TEPA and triethylenemelamine (TEM) appear to be mildly radiomimetic but do require replicative DNA synthesis to produce a maximal effect.

The experiments on normal human leukocytes, described by Luippold, Gooch, and Brewen (1978) demonstrate this.   If we treat cells in what we call G_0 (prior to PHA stimulation), we detect a low level of chromatid-type damage; we also detect a low but significant level of chromosome-type damage--in other words, chromosome-type aberrations that must have been produced prior to replicative DNA synthesis.   If we stimulate the cells and treat them shortly after stimulation, we detect more chromatid-type damage but not any more of the chromosome type (Table 1).

If the cells are treated just before they enter the replicative part of the cell cycle, the level of damage is increased by a factor of 3.   The way I would interpret these data is that if there is sufficient time for the cell to

TABLE 1
Frequencies of Chromosomal Aberrations Observed in Human Leukocytes after
Treating Different Stages of the Cell Cycle with 1×10^{-5} TEM

Cell stage treated	No. of cells scored	Chromatid deletions (%)	Chromatid exchanges (%)	Iso deletions (%)	Rings plus dicentrics (%)	Anchromatic lesions (%)
G_0	300	4.0	0.7	11.0	3.3	5.0
Early G_1	300	11.3	6.3	22.0	5.3	8.0
Late G_1,[a]	300	37.3	38.0	61.0	5.3	19.7
G_1 control	300	2.7	0.0	0.7	0.3	1.3
S^b	300	18.7	7.3	37.7	0.0	19.0
S control	300	2.7	0.0	3.7	0.0	0.3
G_2,[a]	300	8.0	0.0	2.7	0.3	3.3

Data from Brewen (1977).
[a]Unlabeled cells only.
[b]Labeled cells only.

handle the lesion prior to the DNA replication, only a low level of damage is observed. On the other hand, if the cell is treated just prior to DNA synthesis, there is insufficient time for repair and a maximal effect is observed.

To prove that this is not a fluke, we have treated cells in G_2 and have gotten very little effect. But one thing about these data that bothers me is that when we treat cells while they are replicating the DNA, we get a lower effect than when we treat just prior to S. I think this is an artifact of excessive killing; we are recovering cells that for some unknown reason did not quite get the dose.

We can do the same experiment in mouse germ cells. Here we want to look at the effect of TEM on primary spermatocytes. Generoso et al. (1977) published a paper that showed that if you treat primary spermatocytes with X-rays or TEM during pachytene, you can recover equivalent amounts of dominant lethality in the next generation. The X-ray dose was about 400 R and the TEM dose was about 2 mg/kg. If you analyze the first meiotic division of the primary spermatocyte, you see a large amount of damage after X-rays but a negligible level of damage after TEM. In other words, these aberrations had not been formed in the primary spermatocyte following TEM treatment. But they had appeared in the zygote, because dominant lethals and heritable translocations are recovered.

We went back and did the experiment again in a slightly different way with longer time intervals between treatment and meiosis (Luippold, Gooch, and Brewen, 1978). With only a 6-day interval there is no effect, with 9 days no effect, with 11 days no effect, but with 12 days a significant level of damage appeared, and with 13 days there was a highly significant level of damage. Concomitant with that, we are now recovering cells that were in the premeiotic S phase for the spermiogenic cycle (Table 2). In other words, there is a correlation between the level of chromosome damage and DNA synthesis.

If most chemicals require replicative DNA synthesis to produce structural aberrations, why do we obtain dominant lethality when postmeiotic stages are treated? There is no replicative DNA synthesis after the early primary spermatocyte stage, but dominant lethality and heritable translocations can be induced throughout that long period of spermiogenesis. In fact, the most sensitive male germ-cell stages appear to be the spermatid and spermatozoan stages. In addition to this, Generoso and colleagues (Generoso and Russell, 1969; Generoso, Huff, and Stout, 1971) have demonstrated that dominant lethals can be induced in oocytes in which the last replicative DNA synthesis occurred in oogonial stages prior to birth. In the last few years, a new technique has been applied to the study of this problem. It consists of treating the parents of choice, mating the animals, removing the fertilized oocytes, and culturing them to the first zygotic cleavage division (Payne and Jones, 1975). At this time, the paternal and maternal chromosomes can be analyzed for structural chromosome damage.

TABLE 2
Frequency of Labeled Diplotene-Diakinesis Figures and Chromosome Aberrations at Various Intervals following Treatment of Primary Spermatocytes with 1.0 mg/kg TEM and [³H]dThd (Controls)

Time interval (days)	Treatment	No. of cells scored	Chromatid plus isochromatid deletions (%)	Chromatid exchanges (%)	Labeled figures (%)
6	[³H]dThd	200	0.0	0.0	0.0
6	TEM	400	0.0	0.0	0.0
9	[³H]dThd	200	0.0	0.0	0.0
9	TEM	400	0.25 ± 0.25	0.0	0.0
11	[³H]dThd	100	0.0	0.0	0.0
11	TEM	200	0.5 ± 0.5	0.0	0.0
12	[³H]dThd	100	0.5 ± 0.5	0.0	28.5
12	TEM	400	12.8 ± 1.8	0.5 ± 0.4	84.5
13	[³H]dThd	100	0.5 ± 0.5	0.0	70.5
13	TEM	150	68.7 ± 6.8	0.0	95.7

Data from Brewen (1977).

    To date, two compounds have been studied in some
detail using this technique. We have studied the effect of
methyl methanesulfonate (MMS) on both the postmeiotic male
germ-cell stages and the maturing oocytes (Brewen et al.,
1975; Brewen and Payne, 1976). In addition, we have
studied the effect of TEM on oocytes (Brewen and Payne,
1978). Matter and Jaeger (1975) have studied the effects
of TEM on postmeiotic male germ cells. The results of our
study of MMS effects on the male are summarized in Figure
4. The data are expressed as percent dominant lethals and
correspond to the frequency of first-cleavage embryos that
had at least one lethal chromosome aberration in the
paternal genome. For the sake of comparison, the dominant-lethal data of Generoso and Russell (1969) for EMS are
also summarized. These latter data were used because EMS
gives the same stage-sensitivity pattern as MMS, and the
data were more complete than any published for MMS. The
aberrations observed consisted principally of chromatid-type
deletions and exchanges with the odd chromosome-type
exchange. The data show an excellent correspondence in
stage sensitivity for both chromosome aberrations and
dominant lethality (Figure 4). Also, the preponderance of
chromatid aberrations suggests that the aberrations were
formed during pronuclear DNA synthesis in the zygote.
The studies of Matter and Jaeger on TEM effects did not
include an analysis of stage sensitivity, but their data did
show that the amount of dominant lethality observed could
be accounted for by the number of embryos carrying
chromosome aberrations.
    Experiments similar to those done on the male germ
cells have also been done on oocytes. In this instance,
however, it is possible to analyze oocytes at metaphase I,
after treatment with the chemical and, in a parallel group of
animals, analyze the chromosomes at the first cleavage
division after an intervening round of DNA synthesis. The
data from experiments with MMS and TEM are summarized in
Tables 3, 4, and 5. The data show that both compounds
produce very few, if any, structural chromosome aberrations in the meiotic oocytes, but a considerable number are
observed in the maternal genome of the first-cleavage
zygote. Furthermore, the majority of cytogenetic damage is
restricted to those oocytes that were ovulated within the
first week after treatment. This pattern is the converse of
that seen for ionizing radiation, where the more-mature
oocyte stages are the least sensitive except for those only a
few hours from ovulation. As in the case of the male
studies, the predominant aberrations observed were
chromatid-type.
    Two facts emerge from these experiments. One is a
confirmation of observations made earlier in dominant-lethal

TABLE 3
Chromosome Aberration Yields at the First Cleavage Mitosis after Treatment of Dictyate Oocytes with MMS

Dose (mg/kg)	Interval (days)	No. of cells scored	No. of cells with aberrations						Expected lethality (%)
			0	1	2	3	>3	shattered	
Control	—	100	100	0	0	0	0	0	0
50	2.5	75	70[a]	2	2	0	0	1	8.0[a]
50	6.5	50	47	3	0	0	0	0	6.0
50	10.5	50	49	1	0	0	0	0	2.0
50	14.5	50	50	0	0	0	0	0	0
100	0.5	50	40	4	0	0	0	6	20.0
100	1.5	50	43	3	1	0	1	2	14.0
100	2.5	50	40	5	1	1	0	3	20.0
100	6.5	50	43[a]	5	0	0	1	1	16.0[a]
100	10.5	50	47	3	0	0	0	0	6.0
100	14.5	50	50	0	0	0	0	0	0

Data from Brewen and Payne (1976).
[a]Includes a triploid zygote.

studies that the most important male germ-cell stages in terms of risk are the postmeiotic stages. The second is that due to the delayed effect of many chemicals, in the sense that they produce chromatid-type aberrations in the early embryo, it is conceivable that mosaics can be produced in mammals as in Drosophila. Further research is needed to elucidate this possibility. At the moment, it appears difficult to make quantitative risk estimates for

TABLE 4
Chromosome Aberration Yields in Metaphase-I Oocytes following a 100-mg/kg Dose of MMS

Interval (days)	No. of cells scored	No. of deletions	No. of exchanges
Control	200	0	0
0.5	100	1	0
2.5	100	0	0
14.5	100	0	0

Data from Brewen and Payne (1976).

TABLE 5

Frequency of Chromatid Aberrations Observed in Metaphase-I Oocytes and Female Pronuclear Chromosomes following Treatment of Female Mice with Either 0.8 or 1.6 mg/kg TEM

Dose (mg/kg)	Interval (days)	Metaphase I			First-cleavage zygotes			
		no. of cells scored	deletions (% ± S.E.)	exchanges (% ± S.E.)	no. of cells scored	deletions[a] (% ± S.E.)	exchanges[a] (% ± S.E.)	cells with multiples[b] (%)
0	0.5	200	0.5 ± 0.5	0.0	50	0.0	0.0	0.0
0	4.5	—	—	—	50	2.0 ± 2.0	0.0	0.0
0.8	0.5	150	0.7 ± 0.7	0.0	75	47.9 ± 8.1	26.8 ± 6.1	5.3
0.8	2.5	125	0.0	0.0	50	16.0 ± 5.7	4.0 ± 2.8	2.0
0.8	4.5	100	3.0 ± 1.7	0.0	50	4.0 ± 2.8	2.0 ± 2.0	0.0
1.6	0.5	150	2.0 ± 1.2	0.7 ± 0.7	75	193.1 ± 25.8	105.4 ± 16.9	61.3
1.6	2.5	145	1.4 ± 1.0	0.0	50	44.9 ± 9.6	16.0 ± 5.7	2.0
1.6	4.5	110	2.7 ± 1.6	1.8 ± 1.3	90	11.1 ± 3.5	1.1 ± 1.1	2.2
1.6	6.5	125	1.6 ± 1.1	0.0	50	8.2 ± 4.1	12.2 ± 5.0	4.0
1.6	10.5	125	0.8 ± 0.8	0.0	75	13.5 ± 4.2	1.4 ± 1.4	1.4

Data from Brewen (1977).

[a]These frequencies are based on total number of cells less those with multiple aberrations that could not be quantitated.

[b]These represent cells that had too much damage to be analyzed quantitatively.

chemicals based on the cytogenetic data; as I have tried to show, the mere existence of a chromosome aberration in a particular cell after exposure to a chemical mutagen does not necessarily mean such events will be recovered in the next generation.

Chromosome aberrations have been useful, however, in improving and modifying the risk estimates for ionizing radiation. The aberration type that has been studied in greatest detail is the reciprocal translocation. This is principally because it is heritable and thus qualifies as a true genetic effect. The most extensive work has been done in the mouse. The experiments consist of irradiating the testes, waiting an appropriate length of time, and then analyzing the diplotene-diakinesis figures for the presence of translocations. The translocations are readily seen because they result in multivalent configurations. Several dose-response curves have been generated for acute X- and gamma-irradiations (Leonard and DeKnudt, 1967; Searle et al., 1971; Preston and Brewen, 1973). The results have all been very similar in that the yield increases approximately linearly with dose up to 600 R and then decreases with increasingly higher doses. When the data are fit to the model $Y = bD$, the coefficient ranges from $2.0\text{-}2.5 \times 10^{-4}$ translocations/cell/R. A reduction in the dose rate, or an increase in the length of time taken to administer a dose, results in a decrease in yield. This reduction reaches a minimum at 1.3×10^{-5} translocations/cell/R at a dose rate of 1×10^{-3}/rad/minute (Searle et al., 1968; Pomerantseva, Vilkina, and Svanov, 1975; Searle et al., 1976). In a study performed on marmosets, with two dose points for humans, we (Brewen, Preston, and Gengozian, 1975) found that the rate of induction of translocations was 7.7×10^{-4} translocations/cell/ R for acute X-irradiation (Figure 5). This value is three to four times higher than those found in the mouse. If we assume that the dose-rate effect is the same in all three species, we would predict a translocation yield in humans of about 4×10^{-5} translocations/cell/R at very low dose rates.

All of these translocations have been analyzed at meiosis of the primary spermatocyte. Thus, those frequencies must be corrected by 1/8-1/4 to arrive at an expected recovery rate in the next generation. This gives values of $1\text{-}2 \times 10^{-4}$ translocations/offspring/R with acute exposures and $0.5\text{-}1.0 \times 10^{-5}$ translocations/offspring/R with chronic exposures.

Based on the data of Jacobs, Frackiewicz, and Law (1972), the spontaneous rate of all newly formed balanced reciprocal translocations, including Robertsonian, is about $2\text{-}3 \times 10^{-4}$/gamete/generation. This value is undoubtedly

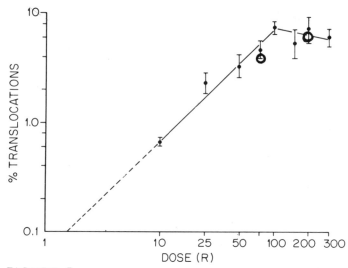

FIGURE 5

Log/log plot of the frequency of translocations in marmoset testes after various acute X-ray doses. The open symbols are observations for humans (Brewen and Preston, 1978).

an underestimate. These are old data, accumulated before we had the refined banding techniques. I would say, as a human cytogeneticist of sorts, that at that time the accuracy obtained by somatic-cell analysis was 25-33%. In other words, we were missing anywhere from 75-67% of all the translocations. If they were in the balanced form, with no phenotypic problems, no clinical manifestations--these are done on newborns--they were not picked up. Neel indicated earlier that the frequency of observed chromosomal abnormalities is increasing as a result of refined techniques. A lot of that is because banding now allows us to detect many more of them. The true spontaneous yield could be anywhere from 8 to 12 × 10^{-4}. If this corrected spontaneous rate is then divided by the induced rate, doubling doses of 4-12 R and 80-240 R are obtained for acute and chronic human exposures, respectively. These values are close to those obtained for specific-locus mutations.

BAUM: Doesn't it bother you that you apparently have a linear function rather than a quadratic function as this is a two-event process?

BREWEN: It did at first. When we first started doing our

own work on mouse translocations, I was convinced that if we analyzed the data in a log/log plot, the slope would be greater than one. We have the data now, but the interpretation is very complicated. It is a function of cells going through sensitive and resistant phases of the cell cycle (Cattanach and Mosely, 1974; Preston and Brewen, 1976). At higher and higher doses, you kill off more and more of your sensitive cells. You recover proportionately fewer translocations. In fact, I understand (the data are not published) that in an experiment where the male was irradiated with a reasonably high dose that killed off all of the sensitive cells, leaving only a small population of semisynchronous resistant cells, a dose-response curve done 24 hours later resulted in a large two-track component. We are trying to do that experiment ourselves right now. All of this indicates that the linear dose-response curve is an artifact of these subpopulations.

With X-rays, we have the old issue of stage sensitivity. When I was in graduate school, Hsu, Dewey, and Humphrey (1962) published a paper describing stage sensitivity. For years a great dialogue raged between Stanley Revell and the rest of the cytogenetic (or radiation biology) community on the shape of the dose-response curve for simple deletions. He insisted that it was a quadratic, and everybody else agreed with Carl Sax that it was a linear dose-response curve. Stage sensitivity played a vital role in that issue, as it does in oocyte sensitivity to ionizing radiation.

We took up the problem of risk assessment in the female. One of the problems that came up was in Russell's original work on specific-locus-mutation induction in oocytes at two dose levels, namely 50 and 400 R (Russell, 1972a). In the male, the curve was linear--these are purported point mutations, so they should increase linearly with dose. In the female they did not. In other words, the mutation rate/locus/rad at 400 R was considerably higher than it was at 50 R. It was not a true quadratic.

To explain these data, you could say it is principally a two-track process resembling that for chromosome aberrations, or that a repair system operating in the oocyte is very efficient at low doses but becomes less efficient at higher doses because it is being inhibited or saturated. That is what Russell suggested (1972b). That means, then, that if you have repair influenced by the total dose, and conceivably by dose rate, then you might get very low effects for chronic irradiations.

In fact, this was observed when the experiments were done in the female. Exposures protracted over several weeks gave a very low mutation yield that approximated zero (Carter, 1958; Russell, 1963, 1972a). There was some debate about that. This got me involved in the question of oocyte sensitivity. One of the things that puzzled me was that if you looked at the data on dominant-lethal induction in oocytes, there was a great heterogeneity depending on when the female was mated (Russell and Russell, 1956). We began looking at structural damage to the chromosomes as a function of oocyte maturation. Female mice were irradiated and induced to ovulate at various times after irradiation. The chromosomes of the metaphase-I oocytes were analyzed for structural aberrations; the results are plotted in Figure 6. The sensitivity increases until about 9 days prior to ovulation and remains relatively constant until sterility sets in. By sterility, I mean it is impossible to recover enough oocytes to do a cytogenetic analysis. That does not mean that those females are sterile and that they will never have any more offspring. But we cannot recover enough eggs to do cytogenetics. The cytogenetic data show a two- to threefold difference in the oocyte sensitivity when week one is compared with subsequent intervals.

When the specific-locus data were generated, at 50 R they came from offspring conceived from weeks one through six; at 200 R, from weeks one through six; and at 400 R, from week one (Russell, 1977). The dose-response curve was quadratic from 50-200 R and linear from 200-400 R.

A striking thing in these data is that the time pattern of sensitivity to specific-locus-mutation induction is exactly

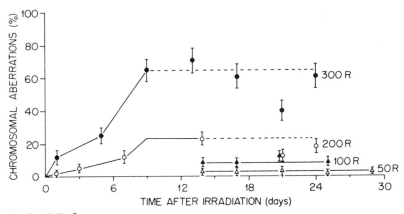

FIGURE 6
Yield of total chromatid aberrations at various times and doses after irradiation of mouse oocytes (Brewen, 1977).

the same as that for cytogenetic damage. In other words, for conceptions that occurred prior to day seven the specific-locus-mutation rate is approximately one-third to one-half as high as it is for conceptions that occurred from day seven through week six (Russell, 1977).

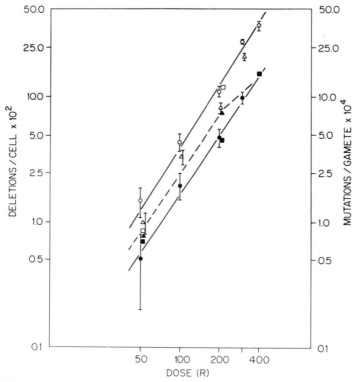

FIGURE 7

Log/log plot of both the present cytogenetic data and the specific-locus data of Russell (1972a, 1977). The lower solid line is an eye fit of the data obtained from the less-sensitive oocytes ovulated during the first week after irradiation. (●, deletions; ■, specific-locus mutations.) The upper solid line is an eye fit of the data obtained from oocytes ovulated during days 9½ to 24½ in the case of the deletions (O) and weeks two to six in the case of specific-locus mutations (□). The dashed line is an eye fit of the pooled data from days 1½ to 24½ for deletions (Δ) and weeks one to six for specific-locus mutations (▲), except at doses above 200 R where the line is drawn to fit only the first-week data. Standard errors are indicated for the deletion data.

Both the cytogenetic and specific-locus data have been analyzed as a function of stage sensitivity. That is, the data from days two through seven were analyzed separately, as were the data from weeks two to seven. This analysis is presented in Figure 7.

Remember there are only specific-locus data from conceptions that occurred in the first week at 400 Rad. So I do not have a 400 Rad data point for the cytogenetics but I do have one for 300 Rad. The week-one data for both end points have a slope of 1.7, as do the week-two to week-six data. When they are pooled, the slope from 50-200 Rad is 1.7 but then approaches 1 from 200 Rad on up. In other words, it would be very easy to say that there is less and less efficient repair as the dose increases, and that at 200 Rad the repair competence of the oocyte system is saturated. Now all the mutational events, which are being formed as a linear function of dose, are recovered. If the data are broken down into the various stages of differing sensitivity, specific-locus mutations and cytologically scored deletions, in fact, follow the same dose-response kinetics. If the specific-locus data are fit to $y = a + cD^2$, the P values are all in excess of 0.6; in fact, some of them are 0.95.

There is one point I want to make which relates to risk assessment. I think these experiments support Russell's (1977) contention that the chronic effects would be dramatically low, because if this is the mechanism, then with protracted exposure the probability of getting two independent events occurring simultaneously is very low, and you would not expect many mutations or many chromosome aberrations.

I think there is hope for cytogenetics in risk estimation. I am not sure whether the story with chemicals will ever be as clear as with ionizing radiation, because we are burdened with the problem of extreme stage sensitivity. We have looked at effects in the female, and we see that in oocytes there is no effect, but in the embryo there is a tremendous effect. We will have to try these experiments across species to see whether some of the rules and regulations that I have outlined here concerning chemical effects in somatic cells really apply to germ cells. I am not sure they do.

Radiation-induced Cancer

JOHN W. BAUM

Safety and Environmental Protection Division
Brookhaven National Laboratory

I have been asked to summarize the animal and human data base on radiation carcinogenesis and to touch briefly on mathematical models that may relate to mutagenesis and carcinogenesis and may therefore be useful in extrapolating from moderate doses to effects one might find at very low doses. My review will employ a number of illustrations taken from the recent literature, especially from the recent reviews of the National Academy of Sciences committee (NAS, 1972) and the United Nations scientific committees (UNSCEAR, 1962, 1972, 1977).

The first three figures show dose-effect relations for skin cancers in rats (Figure 1), bone cancers in mice (Figure 2), and kidney tumors in rats (Figure 3). These data are used to illustrate two points. First, resistive tissues (requiring kilorads for significant tumor induction) tend to have sigmoid dose-effect relations; second, more densely ionizing radiations (such as alpha particles) are usually more effective than X or gamma radiations in inducing tumors. The shapes of these and similar curves for bone cancers in humans (see data later on radium dial painters) caused many people concerned with radiation protection in the 1940s and 1950s to think that there might be a "threshold" dose below which no cancers would be produced.

Other data, such as shown in Figure 4 for leukemia induction in mice, in Figure 5 for thyroid tumor induction in rats, and in Figure 6 for mammary neoplasms in Sprague-Dawley rats, suggest that the more sensitive tissues may respond even at very low doses, and the slope of the dose-response curve at low doses may be nearly linear. In fact, the data for 0.43 MeV neutrons (Shellabarger, 1974) shown in Figure 6 show a dose response with a $D^{0.4}$ relation. This function is a curve that, on linear paper,

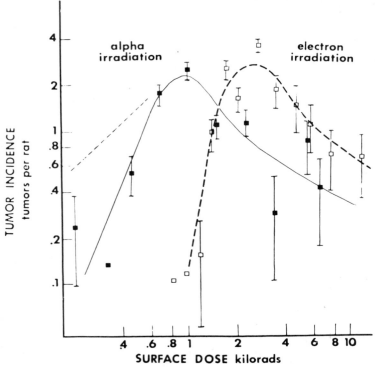

FIGURE 1

Log-log plot of the cumulative tumor incidence at 76 weeks versus surface dose for alpha and electron irradiation. The dotted line at the left represents a linear dose-response relationship. (Reprinted, with permission, from Burns et al., 1968.)

rises more steeply at low doses than at higher doses and is therefore in contrast to the earlier sigmoid-type curves.

Figure 4 illustrates a difference frequently observed between chronic and acute exposures for sparsely ionizing radiations such as X and gamma radiations. The effect for chronic exposure is often less than that for acute exposure. This generality has exceptions, and, unfortunately, for whole-body exposures, the exceptions may dominate the dose-effect relation for humans at low doses.

Figure 5 shows results for radiation-induced thyroid tumors in Long-Evans rats. The thyroid is a moderately sensitive organ in both animals and humans. The dose response is perhaps linear at very low doses; it peaks and then comes down again. An important concept in modern radiation protection standards as suggested by the ICRP (1977) is detriment. Detriment considers both the prob-

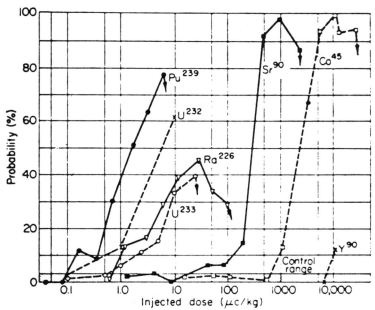

FIGURE 2
Average probability of dying with a malignant bone tumor as a function of isotope dose in mice. (Reprinted, with permission, from Finkel, 1959.)

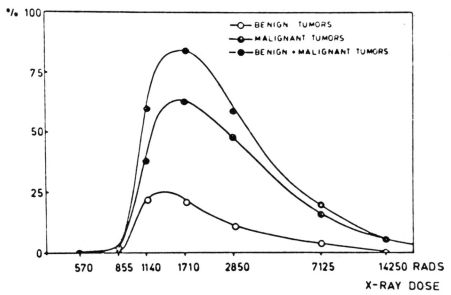

FIGURE 3
Percent of rats with kidney tumors as a function of X-ray doses. (Reprinted, with permission, from Maldague, 1969.)

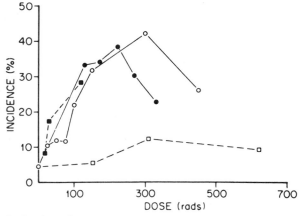

FIGURE 4
Myeloid leukemia in male mice. (O) Single exposure; (□) daily exposures. Open symbols denote results with gamma rays and X-rays; solid symbols denote neutrons. (Reprinted, with permission, from Upton, Randolph, and Conklin, 1970.)

ability of inducing an effect and the severity of that effect. This important concept should also be considered in the chemical area. For example, there may be more thyroid tumors induced in animals and humans than other types,

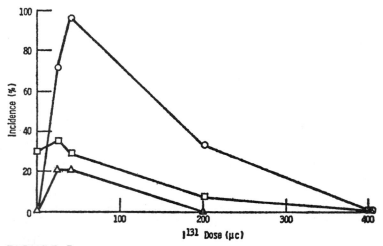

FIGURE 5
Incidence of thyroid tumors in male Long-Evans rats given injections of various doses of [131]I. (O) Follicular adenoma; (□) alveolar carcinoma; (Δ) papillary and follicular carcinoma. (Reprinted, with permission, from UNSCEAR, 1962.)

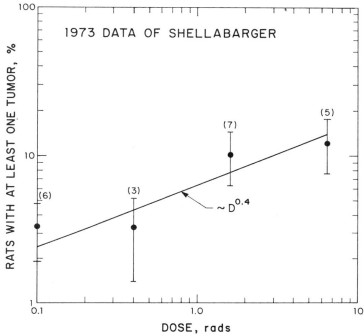

FIGURE 6
Mammary tumors in rats; 0.43 MeV neutrons, 210 days post-irradiation. (Reprinted, with permission, from Shellabarger, 1974.)

but thyroid surgery is usually successful and the mortality rate for thyroid cancer is much less than that for other cancers.   So reduced mortality is integrated into the consideration of risk from this insult.   It is given a mortality weighting factor of about 0.1 in the human risk-estimate scheme.

Figure 7 shows Vogel and Zaldivar's (1969) results for mammary induced tumors in rats.   The lower set of data is for the control group; vertical data lines reflect animals that developed a mammary tumor.   The height of the line is proportional to the number of animals that were first found to have mammary tumors on that day; a short line, for example, represents one animal, and the tallest line represents four animals.   About 50% of these animals develop mammary tumors naturally if they live long enough. In the control group, there is some spread in occurrence time, but the spread in occurrence time is changed markedly even at as small a dose as 5 rad.   We start seeing tumors very early in the irradiated animals.   In general, when the dose is higher, the percent incidence increases. So both promotion and induction are occurring.

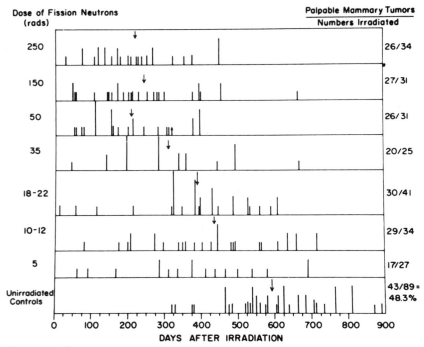

FIGURE 7
First appearance of mammary neoplasia in irradiated female Sprague-Dawley rats. (Reprinted, with permission, from Vogel and Zaldivar, 1969.)

I have been asked to look at these data in terms of models. Unfortunately, I think the term model means different things to different people. I shall refer to mathematical models that tie data together. These data can be considered in terms of the old somatic mutation theory or model of carcinogenesis, now more properly called multiple-event model. It may be that a somatic mutation, or perhaps just a gene alteration (turning off or turning on of a gene), is involved.

The natural incidence rates for these tumors (see Figure 8) increase very steeply, as a fifth power of time (not dose). This implies, in the multiple-event model, that five events are required to complete the initiation process for cancer induction in these animals. In an analysis of Vogel's data (Baum, 1976), this simple model did not fit the data well unless I assumed that two events occurred simultaneously along the track of a proton recoil, produced in this case by neutron irradiation. The dose-effect curve in this system is interesting; the response follows a power function that has an exponent less than 1.

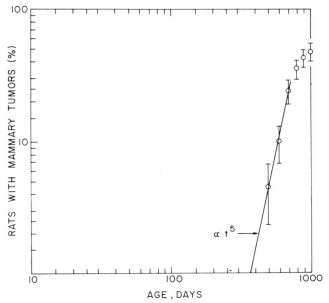

FIGURE 8
Percentage of rats with mammary tumors of natural incidence after passage of time. (Reprinted, with permission, from Vogel and Zalidvar, 1969).

Figure 9 illustrates the steps in the model in which one assumes that events occur naturally at a constant rate and that there are six different classes of cells. Initially, all cells in the animal are in class 0. As these events (mutations or whatever) occur, some of the cells in the animal move to progressively higher classes until finally one cell is in class 5; that presumably completes the initiation process. Then, during the promotion phase, the animal's initiated cell is stimulated to divide, and the tumor becomes apparent in a short time.

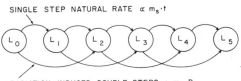

FIGURE 9
Steps in the multiple-event model of carcinogenesis. (Reprinted, with permission, from Baum, 1976.)

Normally, one would assume that radiation would induce one of these steps and simply add to its natural occurrence. But in this particular experiment, it looked as though the radiation-induced steps occurred two at a time. This was unique.

This model is very interesting because it possibly applies to a broad spectrum of insults. In other words, radiation, chemicals, and natural processes of all sorts could be operating to cause these steps. So this model eventually may help to tie radiation, chemicals, and natural processes together in one overall scheme.

The data of Shellabarger shown in Figure 6 illustrated a power-function dose-effect relation with exponent less than 1 (the slope of the dose-effect line is 0.4). Part of the explanation for this is that the data were obtained at 210 days postirradiation; therefore, one sees a distortion of what would be seen if the animals were followed to the end of their lives. The model predicts that, following the animal to the end of life, the dose response ought to be a linear function of dose. Cutting the experiment short distorts the apparent dose response and switches this power function to a lower value. For example, if one started with a power function that was quadratic, it could switch toward linear. In this case, it is even less than power 1. This is of great interest for extrapolation. The curve on a linear plot looks like that shown in Figure 10. Extrapolating from the last point on the upper curve back toward zero, one underestimates the risk.

This is frequently done in human epidemiological studies. One often looks at the population over some period of time--10 or 20 years--and does not necessarily follow it to the end of its normal life span. Thus, one can get a distortion. In fact, in the early Japanese data (discussed later) that sort of thing was observed.

Figure 10 shows tumor penetrance for Drosophila, an animal that is not very frequently looked at in terms of tumor induction. These data are for melanotic tumors (there is some question as to whether they are a legitimate type of tumor). When one strain was crossed with another, the offspring were even less sensitive than either of the two parents. Genetic factors obviously are important and are also extremely complex. In general, the more sensitive strains may have more nearly linear responses. In a mixed population of these three strains, the sensitive population would dominate the dose response at low doses.

The human population is highly heterogeneous. Suppose some people are 100 times more sensitive than others, then Figure 11 illustrates the kind of thing that can happen. If a small subfraction of the population has a D_0 or an induction dose of 1 rad (that is, 63% of that subpopu-

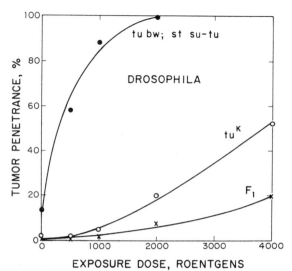

FIGURE 10
Tumor penetrance for <u>Drosophila</u>. (Reprinted, with permission, from Burnet and Sang, 1964.)

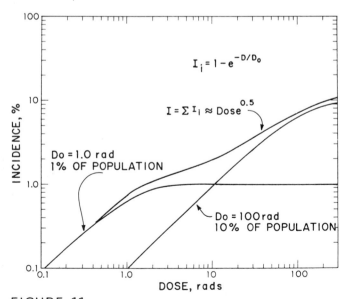

FIGURE 11
Dose response for hypothetical heterogeneous population.
(Reprinted, with permission, from Baum, 1973.)

lation would be induced to have cancer with a dose of, hypothetically, 1 rad), that subpopulation would tend to saturate at a very small dose of a few rads. One hundred percent of that population would have been affected. If there is another subpopulation--say, 10% of the total--that has a D_0 of 100 rads, it will add to the total picture in the manner shown. The composite of these two populations would then sum to give the top line in Figure 11. Because of the statistical uncertainties in the data, a line with a slope of about one half would probably be fit to the data; it would have a power function of one half. Thus, population heterogeneity can also drive these dose-response curves toward a power function less than the inherent underlying power functions of the subpopulations.

There is another peculiarity of some dose-response data. In some male mice, leukemia induction increased approximately linearly with dose while pulmonary tumors decreased. Looking only at pulmonary tumors, one might have concluded radiation was good for these animals. This complexity of the overall picture has not received much attention. Should we be concentrating on sensitive systems that are early measurable, or is it the total picture that is

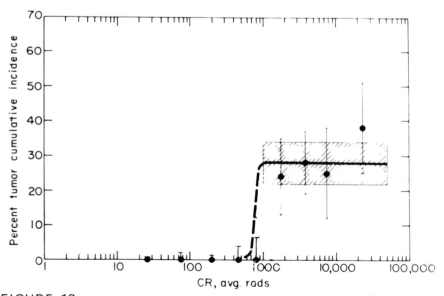

FIGURE 12

Observed tumor cumulative incidence or occurrence in "epi-demiologically suitable" cases. The shaded region corresponds to the mean occurrence p = 0.28 ± 0.06 between 1,000 and 50,000 CR. (Reprinted, with permission, from Evans, Keane, and Shanahan, 1972.)

important?   Similar   decreases   are   found   for   particular
tumors in RF females and males of another strain of mice
when irradiated with either X-rays or neutrons.

I will now turn to a brief review of human data.   The
early data of Robley Evans at MIT (Evans, Keane, and
Shanahan, 1972) again illustrate that bone tumors are not
readily   induced   (see   Figure   12).   There   is   a   quasi-
threshold type of response.   As more and more data has
accumulated, the Argonne group (Rowland et al., 1971) has
calculated a somewhat different dose response for radium
dial painters (see Figure 13).   The curve has a quadratic
component and a cell-killing type of function.   This would
be somewhat different from the threshold assumption in that
even at low doses there is a finite response.

Another very important set of human data (shown in
Figure 14) involves British spondylitic patients who were
treated for arthritic conditions of the spine.   The response
for leukemia is approximately linear, but quadratic functions
could perhaps also be fit within the 90% confidence interval
lines.

Important   human   information   also   comes   from   the
offspring of mothers who were irradiated with diagnostic
X-rays while the child was in utero.   Data from England

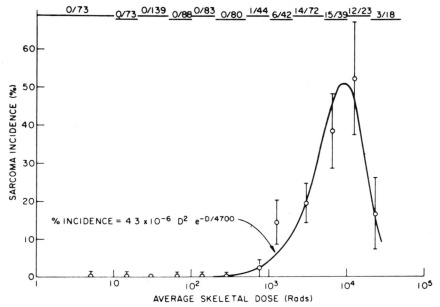

FIGURE 13
Semilogarithmic plot of percent incidence of sarcomas as a
function of initial radium burden.   (Reprinted, with permission, from Rowland et al., 1971).

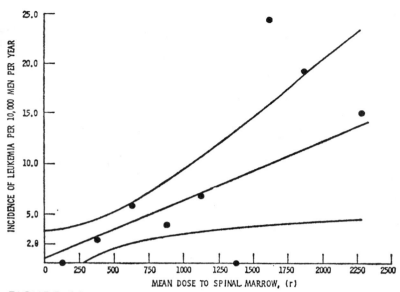

FIGURE 14
Incidence of leukemia in relation to mean spinal marrow dose
of therapeutic irradiation. The regression line was obtained
after weighting the rates according to their reliability and
is given by $Y = 0.00586X + 0.38$; the 95% probability limits
of the value of Y for each value of X are shown by the
curved lines. (Reprinted, with permission, from UNSCEAR,
1962.)

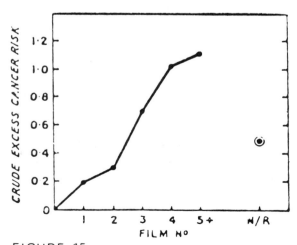

FIGURE 15
Crude dose-response curve. Crude excess cancer risk as a
proportion of the normal risk (N/R = no record). (Reprinted, with permission, from Stewart and Kneale, 1970.)

128

(Stewart and Kneale, 1970) (see Figure 15) again show approximately linear dose response. The apparent excess induction in these children is about ten times greater than would have been expected from previous human data. These data have many uncertainties and are fairly controversial. Shore and others (Shore, Robertson, and Bateman, 1973) in the United States have broken the data down into different epochs--different periods of time during which the data were gathered. Their results are shown in Figure 16. They point out that the slope of the dose-response curve changed with the period during which the data were accumulated. In the last period, from 1960 to 1965, the response seems to be parallel to the axis and implies no response.

Why would the response be changing in this way if it were a true dose-effect relationship? Perhaps there is a problem with dosimetry or with the accuracy of recording

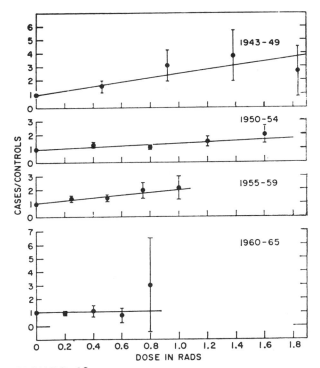

FIGURE 16
Linear least-square fits for case/control ratios as functions of radiation dose for the four epochs. The zero dose points were excluded in the curve-fitting. (Reprinted, with permission, from Shore, Robertson, and Bateman, 1973.)

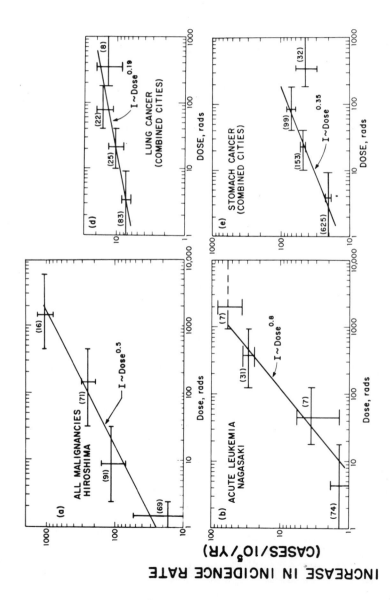

INCREASE IN INCIDENCE RATE (CASES/10³/YR)

(a) ALL MALIGNANCIES HIROSHIMA — I~Dose^0.5 — Dose, rads

(b) ACUTE LEUKEMIA NAGASAKI — I~Dose^0.8 — Dose, rads

(d) LUNG CANCER (COMBINED CITIES) — I~Dose^0.19 — DOSE, rads

(e) STOMACH CANCER (COMBINED CITIES) — I~Dose^0.35 — DOSE, rads

130

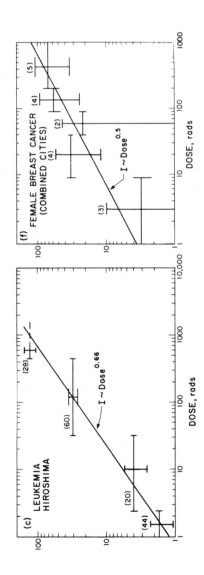

FIGURE 17

Cancer data for Hiroshima and Nagasaki victims. (Reprinted, with permission, from Baum, 1973.)

the number of films taken. A second problem is that these
data yield a much higher incidence per unit dose than was
observed in fetuses exposed in the Japanese populations at
Hiroshima 'and Nagasaki.   Nonetheless, the most recent
United Nations report (UNSCEAR, 1977) on the subject
indicates that the data are being accepted as probably
correct.

For all malignancies in Hiroshima and for Japanese
women with breast cancers, the dose response was about a
one-half power function in early analyses (Baum, 1973) (see
Figure 17). This was surprising; it had not been pointed
out previously in human data. As time goes on, the slope
of that curve is gradually changing--it is about 0.7
now--and, eventually, according to that multiple-event
model, we would expect it to be linear when the population
has completed its life span. Other female breast cancer
data (shown in Figure 18) are approximately linear as a
function of the number of fluoroscopies.

There are several sets of radium 224 data like those
shown in Figure 19. It is interesting that children are a
little more sensitive than adults. These data have also
been analyzed in terms of protraction. The excess inci-

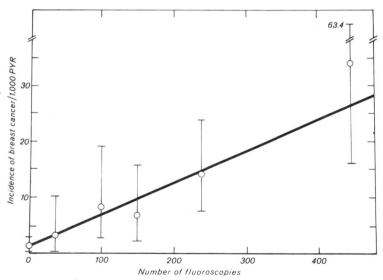

FIGURE 18
Incidence of breast cancer per 10^3 PYR (1966 data) against
the number of fluoroscopies received. The error bars
represent 90% confidence intervals, and the line is the
best-fitting, weighted, least-squares regression line.
(Reprinted, with permission, from NAS, 1972.)

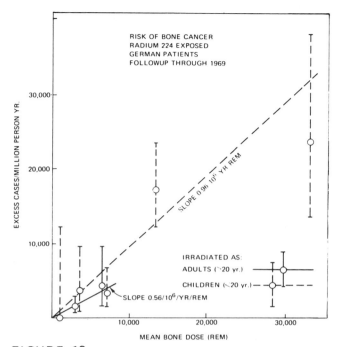

FIGURE 19
Dose-response data for bone cancer in German patients
given radium 224 therapeutically. Open circles and dashed
error bars: patients given doses as children (under 20
years of age); closed circles and solid error bars: patients
given doses as adults (over 20). (Reprinted, with permission, from NAS, 1972, after Spiess and Mays, 1970.)

dence is about five times greater for those patients who
were dosed in a protracted manner rather than acutely.
Contrary to what we would have expected, protraction was
more--not less--hazardous.
    Radiation protection standards are an important
reference point because the system is developed to a much
greater extent than for any other agent. In the current
system of ICRP recommendations (ICRP, 1977), three basic
questions have to be considered. First, one must justify
the exposure. Second, there should be a net benefit (the
benefits must outweigh the detriments). Third, the dose
should not exceed the annual limit. It is usually fairly
obvious that an operation is beneficial. If an operation is
beneficial, then one must optimize in terms of cost effectiveness. This is done by considering the cost per unit
reduction in risk. One does not have to analyze benefits
further once it has been shown that the operation has a net

benefit.   One does have to ask how much it costs to reduce
the risk.   Units on cost and also on risk are needed.   So,
in radiation, for example, one talks about dollars per human
rem.   The Nuclear Regulatory Commission has suggested in
some of its guides that one use a value of $1,000 per human
rem.   As soon as one is willing to do that, one can go to
the engineering analysis and design work needed to answer
questions such as the one raised here concerning ethylene
oxide.   How much exposure should we permit?   It becomes a
question of the cost of the damage that is going to result--
the risk--versus the cost of reducing that risk.

EISENSTADT: I am not sure I understand what you are
     saying about benefit; you are not arguing that you do
     not want to quantify the benefits?

BAUM: No, but usually the net benefit is large and is not
     dealt with in much detail.   If there is a net benefit,
     then the thing that should be quantified is the cost of
     reducing the risk.   We do not want to permit people to
     get radiation exposure from wearing radioactive jewelry
     when that has a rather trivial benefit and we can
     substitute some other thing for the radium to give the
     same effect.   X-rays, for example, are obviously bene-
     ficial in medical practice, but how beneficial?   It is
     almost impossible to measure the benefits.   But we do
     not have to.   We can ask, "If a person is going to get
     a certain dose from this X-ray, how much does it cost
     to reduce that dose a small amount?"   We can compare
     that cost to the risk costs and minimize the total.   Say
     that the exposure we are going to give is 10 millirems.
     That is a risk of about $10 based on the units we dis-
     cussed, so we ought to be willing to spend up to $10
     to reduce that exposure.   Of course, we should
     consider the total reduction summed over a long period
     of time, the number of people examined, and all such
     related factors to arrive at the long-term cost effec-
     tiveness.
          It becomes fairly clear that in medical practice,
     by very small expenditures of money, we could very
     much improve the cost effectiveness.   In the design of
     nuclear power plants, the question may be whether to
     put up a higher stack or to install a better filtration
     system.   We sum the dose that is going to be received
     by all the people in the environment.   We multiply the
     human rems by $1,000 and get some measure of the
     insult in dollars.   This gives an idea of how much we
     ought to be willing to spend in order to reduce that
     insult.

Low-dose and Species-to-Species Extrapolation for Chemically Induced Carcinogenesis

DAVID HOEL

Biometry Branch
National Institute of Environmental Health Sciences

In this presentation I will attempt to review the statistical procedures that are currently used for estimating a low-dose carcinogenic effect in humans from data obtained in animal-based studies.

To extrapolate outside the experimental range to the low environmental levels to which humans are commonly exposed, one must have both actual experimental data and some mathematical formulation relating response to dose. For chemical carcinogenesis, animal data are typically derived from long-term studies (such as those generated under the NCI Bioassay Program) in which lifetime total cancer incidence is observed for various groups of animals exposed to different levels or doses of the chemical of interest. Often in radiation experiments (but rarely with chemical exposures) there may even be sufficient data to study the relationship between age and cumulative cancer incidence at several dose levels.

The mathematical models commonly used to depict the relationship between response and dose generally fall into one of two categories. Either they focus on a dichotomous response, such as the presence or absence of some speci-fied condition, or they attempt to relate the distribution of the time until occurrence of a given event (e.g., tumor onset or death) to dose level. Examples of dichotomous-response models include the one-hit and probit formulations. The most frequently employed time-to-occurrence models are the log-normal (Blum, 1959; Druckrey, 1967) and Weibull (Chand and Hoel, 1974; Peto and Lee, 1973). The latter distributions are related to the use of the probit and extreme-value distributions, respectively, for dichotomous responses.

Interest in the probit grew out of an early attempt by Mantel and Bryan (1961) to develop a conservative upper bound for the unknown underlying dose-response curve, which they assumed to be convex in the low-dose region. They selected the probit for their model because it seemed to provide a reasonable fit to many of the experimental data sets they had encountered (and not because of any mechanistic arguments supporting its usage). Mantel and Bryan adopted a fixed slope of 1 in order to generate a shallow (conservative) dose response and then estimated the upper bound of the low-dose response using the observed data.

Although the probit and many related curves, such as the logistic, will all tend to provide similar fits to the observed data in the experimental dose range, they can generate risk estimates (for a specified dose) that differ by as much as three orders of magnitude when extrapolating to incidence rates in the 10^{-6} to 10^{-8} range. As a result, it is important to develop a rational basis for selecting among competing extrapolation models. In an attempt to address this issue, the more recent low-dose extrapolation research efforts have emphasized the ability of the proposed model to reflect underlying biological mechanisms that might logically be involved in the process of tumor formation.

The series of papers that have been published on the multistage model of carcinogenesis constitute an important advance in this area. Under the multistage model it is assumed that the cancer originates as a "malignant" cell that is initiated by a series of somaticlike mutations occurring in finite steps. It is also assumed that each mutational stage can be depicted as a Poisson process in which the transition rate is approximately linear in dose rate. Then the lifetime probability of tumor onset can be expressed approximately as

$$P(d) = 1 - \exp \{- (q_0 + q_1 d + \ldots + q_k d^k)\},$$

where $q_i \geq 0$ for all i, and k corresponds to the number of transitions or mutational stages.

Statisticians at the NIEHS, in conjunction with co-workers at other institutions, have developed a sophisticated computer algorithm for fitting the multistage model to laboratory data which does not require the value of k to be specified in advance. The types of fits obtained when this algorithm is applied to actual laboratory data are illustrated in Figure 1, which summarizes the results of an analysis of animal cancer-screening data for vinyl chloride, chloroform, DDT, dimethylnitrosamine, and dieldrin performed by Guess, Crump, and Peto (1977). In each of the data sets depicted in Figure 1, curve C corresponds to the maximum-likelihood estimate of excess risk based on the observed data. Curve A is the asymptotic upper one-sided 97.5%

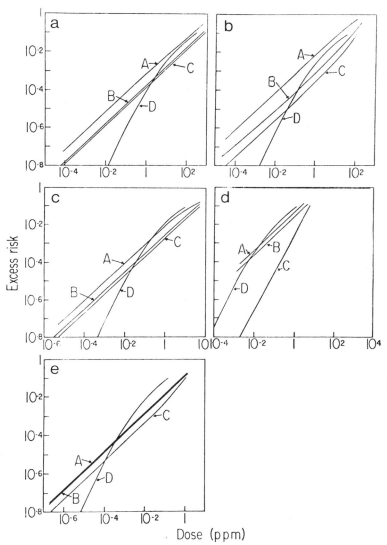

FIGURE 1

Results of analysis of animal screening data for vinyl chloride, chloroform, DDT, dimethylnitrosamine, and dieldrin. In each of the data sets, curve C corresponds to the best-fitted estimate of excess risk, curves A and B represent two different estimated upper bounds to C, and curve D is the corresponding Mantel-Bryan upper bound for the given data set. (Reprinted, with permission, from Guess, Crump, and Peto, 1977.)

137

confidence limit on excess risk at each dose. Curve B is
the third highest of 100 estimated values of excess risk,
based on 100 computer simulations. Curve D represents the
one-sided upper 97.5% confidence limit on excess risk
computed using the Mantel-Bryan procedure. An
interesting feature of curve D (which has been used by a
number of regulatory groups to predict low-dose risk) is
that although it is initially conservative (i.e., in the
intermediate dose range), the tail of the Mantel-Bryan or
probit procedure goes to zero very rapidly, faster than
other dose-response models. Thus, in the low-dose region,
you will, in fact, be underestimating risk with the Mantel-
Bryan procedure relative to most other models.

An important point to notice in each set of curves
depicted in Figure 1 is that the upper confidence curve
(curve A) is always approximately linear in the low-dose
region. This approximate linearity holds even when the
maximum-likelihood estimate of excess risk (curve C) does
not contain an (estimated) linear component, as is illustrated by the dimethylnitrosamine data. Although the linear
component of the true dose-response curve may be so small
that it has no appreciable effect on the maximum-likelihood
estimate in the experimental dose range, one always has to
allow for the possibility of its existence. As a result, it
becomes the dominant term in the upper confidence limit
when one extrapolates down several orders of magnitude to
the low-dose region. Thus, there may be a very pro-
nounced difference between the best estimate of the
underlying dose-response curve and the corresponding confidence bound on this estimate for any given data set.
This type of discrepancy may be encountered with compounds for which the multistage model is not necessarily
applicable--that is, in instances where there is no good
evidence for direct carcinogenicity. For example, if you
attempt to fit the saccharin data, you will find that there is
no apparent linear term, although the data are not very
adequate. The same result holds for much of the animal
data on chlordane.

Table 1 displays the maximum-likelihood fits and the
extrapolation estimates for two separate sets of simulated
data from a hypothetical megamouse experiment. The data
for experiment 2 are almost identical to those for experiment
1, differing for only 11 of the 8,000 test animals--a difference that could easily arise by chance if both sets were
generated from the same underlying dose-response curve.
Yet this apparently trivial difference in responses is
sufficient to cause the best fit to the experiment-2 data to
include a modest linear component, whereas the corresponding fit for the data from experiment 1 has no linear term.
Therefore, when one considers excess risks of the magni-

TABLE 1

Hypothetical Data Illustrating Extreme Sensitivity of Best-estimate Extrapolation to Minute Changes in Data When Background Is Present and True Curve Is Flat

Data

	Response	
Dose[a]	exp. 1	exp. 2
0	103	100
2	99	99
15	100	105
30	109	112
35	131	131
40	187	187
45	305	305
50	506	506

Best-estimate Dose-Response Curves

Exp. 1 $P(d) = 1 - \exp[-(0.105 + 1.1 \times 10^{-15}d^7 + 1.5 \times 10^{-14}d^8)]$

Exp. 2 $P(d) = 1 - \exp[-(0.106 + 1.6 \times 10^{-4}d^1 + 1.2 \times 10^{-14}d^8 + 7.2 \times 10^{-17}d^9)]$

Low-dose Extrapolations

Increased risk	Dose	
$P(d) - P(0)$	exp. 1	exp. 2
10^{-8}	5.40	7.20×10^{-5}
10^{-7}	7.20	7.20×10^{-4}
10^{-6}	9.60	7.20×10^{-3}
10^{-5}	12.80	7.20×10^{-2}
10^{-4}	17.09	0.72
10^{-3}	22.78	7.20

Data from Guess and Crump (1978)
[a]Number of animals tested was in each case 1,000.

tude of 10^{-6} to 10^{-8}, the extrapolated doses for the two experiments can differ by as much as five orders of magnitude. So it appears that even with experiments on the megamouse scale, it is very unlikely that an investigator will be able to establish the nonexistence of a linear component in the data or avoid the relatively conservative estimates associated with linearity in the low-dose region.

ZIPSER: That is just what you expect intuitively if you are trying to predict the frequency of one in a hundred million on the basis of statistical observations in which each sample has a thousand. Any kind of statistical fluctuation of one tumor is going to throw you off by three orders of magnitude.

Figure 2 provides some additional quantitative insight into the conservatism of the linearity assumption in the low-dose region. The figure depicts a hypothetical (unknown) dose-response curve for which a linear bound has been estimated based on the observed tumor incidence at dose d_E and the known background rate. Suppose that one wished to estimate the true dose d_A associated with some specified risk l_A by the corresponding "linear" dose d_L. If

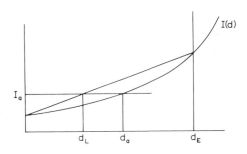

$$I_a - I(0) \simeq I'(0) d_a$$
$$1 + p \simeq I(d_E) / I(0)$$

$$R(p, k) \equiv \frac{d_a}{d_L} \lesssim \frac{p}{k[(1+p)^{1/k} - 1]}$$

R		P	
	0.1	1.0	10
k 2	1.02	1.21	2.16
5	1.04	1.35	3.25
∞	1.05	1.44	4.17

FIGURE 2
Hypothetical dose-response curve and the corresponding linear upper bound estimated from the observed incidence at experimental dose d_E. The accompanying table (Crump et al., 1976) displays upper bounds on the ratio of the actual dose corresponding to a given level of risk to the estimated linear dose for a variety of experimental conditions.

1 + p   denotes the increase in risk relative to background corresponding to exposure at dose d_E--that is, if

$$1 + p = I(d_E) / I(0),$$

then it can be shown that the ratio of d_A to d_L is bounded by a function p and k, the number of mutational transitions in the underlying multistage model. Typical values for this ratio (Crump et al., 1976) are also depicted in Figure 2. If, for example, d_E were a doubling dose (i.e., if p = 1), and if one were willing to assume a two-stage carcinogenic process, then the ratio of d_A to d_L would be bounded by 1.21. If an infinite number of stages were assumed, then the ratio would be bounded by 1.44.

ABRAHAMSON: Does that mean you are overestimating the risk by 20-44%?

HOEL: Yes.   And although that is a fairly reasonable margin of error, it does demonstrate the importance of background.   The background risks at each transitional stage in the carcinogenic process have been incorporated into the model, and the manner in which corrections are made for background can have a significant effect on the estimated risk.   In the Mantel-Bryan procedure, the correction for background is made in an independent sense using Abbott's formula (i.e., background is removed and the remaining probability of tumor is distributed proportionally among the animals still at risk).   Alternatively, background can be regarded as additive on the log scale.   The treatment of background is quite important if it is mechanistically an additive-type process, as is assumed with the multistage model.

RAY: When you say background, are you talking about tumors at a given site and then, with dose, you get an increase in tumors of the same type, same target organ?   Obviously, other tumors are taken care of differently.

HOEL: We are assuming that we are focusing on a specific tumor type.

Some mention was made of susceptibility, but not much work has been done in this area.   Recently, we have investigated a few topics that we hope will have some bearing on this question of susceptibility.   For example, suppose that an individual has an age-specific cancer-incidence rate of the form $c\lambda(t)$, where c represents some sort of susceptibility factor for the individual in question. Then the probability that this individual will develop a tumor by time t is of the form

$$P_c(t) = 1 - \exp\{-c\Delta(t)\},$$

where

$$\Delta(t) = \int_0^t \lambda(t)\,dt.$$

Averaging over the entire population yields an incidence rate of

$$h(t) = P'(t) / [1 - P(t)],$$

where

$$P(t) = \int P_c(t)\,dG(c),$$

and $G(c)$ represents the distribution of susceptibility in the population. It can be shown that $h(t)$ is bounded by $\lambda(t)\cdot\mu_G$, where $\mu_G = \int c\,dG(c)$ is the mean susceptibility. Under mild regularity conditions, it can also be shown that $h(t)$ will tend to zero. These theoretical results have a number of practical implications. First, it appears that if you impose this type of susceptibility mixing on the underlying probability structure, you are not going to be able to take a single-stage mechanism and make it look like a multistage one. (This was one of our initial questions when we began this research.) Second, under this modified model you can cause the age-specific incidence rate to decrease in time. This finding may at least partially explain the reported (e.g., HEW, 1970) decline in age-specific, white male lung cancer death rates in the most elderly age groups.

All of this discussion has been focused on low-dose extrapolation. However, greater quantitative errors in risk assessment are probably associated with species scale-up than with the dose-response models. There has not been much work on this subject. We know of approximately 25 compounds or chemicals that are human carcinogens. These compounds--with the possible exception of arsenic and benzene--also tend to be carcinogenic in one or more animal species. In his report on the health hazards of chemical pesticides, Meselson (NAS, 1975) reviewed several of the known human carcinogens and concluded that there were sufficient human dose data for the six compounds cited in Table 2 to make a quantitative comparison of animal and human risk on a dose-rate basis. In calculating his relative risk estimates, Meselson appears to have compared the ratio of lifetime tumor incidence to total accumulated dose (ex-

TABLE 2
Summary of Relative Risks Most-sensitive Animal Species

Compound	Animal model	Total dose per body weight	Average daily dose rate mg/kg	Average daily dose rate mg/surface area
Benzidine[a,b]	rat: mammary	2.0	17.7[c]	2.7[c]
Chlornapha- zine[a,b]	mouse: lung	5.0	7.0[c]	2.0
DES[d]	mouse: cervix and vagina	<41.2	<1.2	<16.6
Aflatoxin B₁[b]	rat: liver	14.6	2.4[c]	2.7
Vinyl chloride	mouse: lung	291.7	8.3	117.5
	rat: liver	52.5	1.5	9.8
Cigarette smoke	mouse: lung	3.6	9.7[c]	1.4

[a]Animals observed for less than half their normal life spans.
[b]Animal risk estimates averaged over more than one dose level.
[c]Denotes an excess human risk.
[d]Human and animal risk may not be directly comparable because humans were exposed in utero and mice received a single postnatal injection.

pressed in mg/kg) for humans with the corresponding ratio for the most sensitive animal species tested. He obtained values similar to those shown in Table 2 and concluded that for benzidine, chlornaphazine, and cigarette smoke, the animal and human risks were quite similar. For aflatoxin B₁, vinyl chloride, and DES, the animal risk exceeded the corresponding human risk; that is, higher risks would be predicted for humans on the basis of the animal data than were actually observed.

In making these types of comparisons, the first issue that should be addressed is the question of the most appropriate dosage unit. For example, if dosage is expressed in terms of average daily dose rate over an expected lifetime instead of total accumulated dose rate (thereby taking animal and human relative life spans into account), the risk estimates given in the second column of Table 2 are generated. These estimates suggest that humans often tend to be at about the same or even greater risk than the corresponding test animal. Expressing the lifetime average daily dosage in surface area units rather than kilograms of body weight appears to bring the animal and human data into even closer agreement. However, these conclusions need to be qualified for a variety of reasons. Some of the tumor-induction rates observed in the various animal experiments may have been sufficiently large

to cause the linear approximation to the presumed underlying multistage model to be inadequate. Furthermore, the
animal incidence data for both chlornaphazine and benzidine
were obtained from animals that were observed for less than
half of their normal life expectancy. Correcting the
observed incidence rates associated with these two compounds for incomplete follow-up would certainly increase the
estimated animal risk. Depending on the specific nature of
the correction, better overall agreement between animal and
human risk estimates might be attained by expressing
dosage on the basis of body weight rather than surface
area. In any event, the data summarized in Table 2 should
illustrate the importance of the units in which the dose rate
is expressed in the estimation of relative human risk.

INFANTE: For vinyl chloride, what is the site you are
        looking at in humans? I thought these were site-
        specific cancers. It seems that one always over-
        estimates when looking at animal versus human data.
        In one epidemiological study, where we had quite a
        significant excess of liver cancers, three angiosarcomas
        in that population could not be counted just because
        they were misdiagnosed. The pathologist did not read
        the data right. When these were confirmed, we still
        could not include them in the analysis. That is just a
        very blatant example.

HOEL: We are reviewing all of the data that formed the
    basis of the calculations reported in Table 2.

We are focusing a great deal of attention on vinyl
chloride, attempting to obtain our own animal data, as well
as reexamining all of the epidemiological data available to
us. In reexamining the industrial cohort data from which
most of the human risk estimates are derived, it is important to remember that industrial exposures are generally
limited to only a fraction of an individual's total life span.
Thus, the manner in which cumulative tumor incidence is
adjusted to reflect this lack of lifetime-exposure data can
significantly alter the risk estimates of interest. For
example, consider a hypothetical cohort of workers exposed
to some specified chemical at a daily dose rate d for a
period of t years. If their observed lifetime tumor-incidence rate is denoted by I, then the corresponding
estimated cumulative incidence rate resulting from a
continuous lifetime exposure at rate d would be $I \times (70/t)$,
ignoring latency and assuming a simple proportionality
between dose and incidence. On the other hand, if you
adopt a cumulative Weibull hazard function in which risk is
proportional to duration of exposure raised to the power k
(where k corresponds to the number of required transitions

TABLE 3
Values of $(70/t)^{k-1}$

k	t				
	10	15	20	25	30
4	343	101.6	42.9	22.0	12.7
5	2401	474.3	150.1	61.5	29.6
6	16807	2213.3	525.2	172.1	69.2

in the presumed underlying multistage model), then the estimated cumulative tumor-incidence rate would be given by $I \times (70/t)^k$ Thus, if cancer risk is not linearly related to the length of exposure, assumption of such a simple proportionality could result in a lifetime tumor-incidence rate that is underestimated by a factor of $(70/t)^{k-1}$ Table 3 displays values of the amount by which incidence rate might be underestimated in typical industrial settings. For instance, if a group of workers were exposed for 20 years to a chemical that required five transition stages to produce a malignant tumor, and if a linear adjustment were made for nonlifetime exposure, then the cumulative incidence rate could be underestimated by a factor of 150. Of course, all of these calculations are very simplistic. They do not take into account such issues as repair mechanisms, synergistic and/or antagonistic effects resulting from exposure to multiple risk factors, differences in the effective dose at the site of action, and the administered dose, and a variety of other issues related to pharmacokinetics (e.g., Gehring's work at Dow). However, they do give some indication of the care that has to be exercised in assessing human data.

Estimating Radiation-induced Genetic Disease Burdens

SEYMOUR ABRAHAMSON

Department of Zoology
University of Wisconsin

The following brief description of the methodology employed by the BEIR committee in developing their risk estimates for genetic effects of radiation is presented in the hope that some of these approaches might also be applicable to chemical mutagens. First, let me update the category of genetic diseases and their current incidence levels based on recent data developed by Trimble and Doughty (1974) from the medical records of a British Columbian population. Because this population was limited to children up to the age of 10, it is necessary to adjust the figures to include diseases of late onset. The data of Jacobs, Melville, and Ratcliffe (1974) were used for the chromosomal diseases. The generally agreed upon incidences are displayed in Table 1.

To assess the influence of radiation in a meaningful way, it is important to develop a method for converting induced-mutation-rate data into a form that describes how many more cases of these various types of diseases will be introduced. Knowing the number of new mutants introduced into a population by, say, 1 rem of exposure does not provide an appropriate assessment of the harm. There-

TABLE 1
Incidence of Genetic Disorders

Type of disease	Current incidence per million liveborn
Autosomal dominants	10,000
X-linked recessives	400
Irregularly inherited	90,000
Chromosomal abnormalities	
unbalanced rearrangements	500
monosomies and trisomies	4,000

fore, the BEIR committee employed a <u>relative-mutation-risk</u> procedure, a value that is the inverse of the doubling dose--the amount of irradiation required to double the current incidence of mutationally maintained disease assuming the population is continuously exposed to that level of radiation until a new equilibrium is reached. This will become clearer with the following example.

Assume the average human gene mutation rate is 0.5×10^{-5}-0.5×10^{-6} (A) and the average induced gene mutation rate per rem of exposure for both sexes in mice is 0.35-0.5×10^{-7} (B), then the doubling dose is A/B = 10-140 rem (BEIR computed a doubling dose of 20-200 based on somewhat different induced mutation rates in mice) and the relative mutation risk per rem is B/A = 0.1-0.007.

For the dominantly determined diseases, we assumed the equilibrium time was five generations. The relative mutation risk per rem would therefore be $10,000 \times 0.007$ (or $\times 0.1$) or 70-$1,000$ additional diseases/10^6. In the first generation there would be one-fifth as many--that is, 14-200. Essentially the same calculation can be applied to the X-linked diseases, except that the equilibrium time is taken to be six generations: $400 \times (0.007$-$0.1) \times 1/6 =$ <1-6 first-generation cases.

For irregularly inherited diseases (which constitute the great bulk of the diseases), there were two other uncertainties to be considered. The first, and still the most uncertain assumption, was the mutational component of these diseases. It was agreed that the mutation component probably did not exceed 0.5 nor was it lower than 0.05.

The second assumption was that these mutations had a ten-generation equilibrium time and that 1/10 of the effect would be expressed in the first generation. The calculation for this category (per rem of exposure) was $90,000$ $(0.007$-$0.1) \times (0.05$-$0.5) \times (0.1) = 3$-450 newly induced cases per million liveborn.

In the interests of brevity, I will not attempt to detail here the somewhat more complex analysis required to estimate the frequency of chromosomally abnormal births from the induced frequency of chromosome aberrations observed in mouse gametes. Since the publication of the BEIR report, we have available better data on induced frequencies in human and marmoset spermatogonia (Brewen, Preston, and Gengozian, 1975; Brewen and Preston, 1978) and on aberrations induced in mouse oocytes (Brewen and Payne, 1976, 1978; Uchida and Freeman, 1977). Let me suggest that the newly induced cases of unbalanced translocations probably range between 3-40 and 1-25 for numerical disorders (monosomies and trisomies). These values encompass the limits derived by different risk-estimating groups.

For the total of all effects, the approximate value is 40-720 new cases, and the "best" estimate is probably the geometric mean of this range. That number is 170 cases per rem per million liveborn.

All of these values are sensitive to such procedures as the method of calculation of doubling dose and particularly to the estimated mutational component for the irregularly inherited diseases. Small changes here could easily halve or double the final estimates.

Finally, I think that where reasonable estimates for the induction of a given class of damage (mutation or chromosome aberration) can be demonstrated for a given "dose" of specific mutagen, it should be possible to introduce these values into the specific category to which they relate.

DISCUSSION

ZIPSER: I am confused about something. At a certain dose (and I do not know what it is) of whatever, either genetic defects appear or cancer is present. All people get cancer if they live long enough. A certain percentage of the population is genetically predisposed. So it seems to me that the place on the curve where we should deal with additional doses is the place where the people are. It may not be exactly determinable, but it is not the low dose--certainly not for carcinogens. I do not see the rationale that is going on here.

ABRAHAMSON: What rationale don't you see? I am missing your point.

RAY: The point is: What would an additional dose do if you can guess where you are on that curve? You are not at the bottom of it.

ABRAHAMSON: In almost all the experiments that are done, the mouse is an indicator of mutation rate. We are going to estimate what the risk is or what the mutation rate is by extrapolating from something in the range of a 50- to 300-R exposure.

ZIPSER: This is very much greater than the background.

ABRAHAMSON: That is right. The human background we are talking about is in the range of 5 rem per 30 years. Humans get a 100 millirem per year background--at a very low dose rate.

ZIPSER: But it is not a tremendous difference between the lowest dose you are looking at in the background, even for radiation.

ABRAHAMSON: If you are talking about 5 rem received over 30 years.

ZIPSER: Nothing is observed where we just double the background doses.

ABRAHAMSON: There has been no experiment done in the mouse which results in adequate data for a dose of less than 50 R in the female or less than 300 R in the male (there is one exception to this, but the statement is basically correct). It is necessary to extrapolate from those doses and correct them for the influence of dose rate.

RAY: This is for genetic effects?

ABRAHAMSON: For genetic effects in which the end point being scored is primarily the specific-locus-mutation rate. In the mouse germ-cell system, as well, you have end points such as reciprocal translocations or deletions or dicentrics, as Grant Brewen described. I do not recall what the lowest dose was for trans-missible gross chromosomal changes.

BREWEN: Ten rad.

ZIPSER: Is that a lifetime dose or what?

ABRAHAMSON: The doubling dose is just another way of saying the dose that will be required to double the current incidence of genetic disease when given over enough generations. If the current value is 94,000 cases and you gave the doubling dose for enough generations, you would no longer see 94,000; you would see, roughly, 180,000 cases. Is that reasonably clear? Once you get those sets of numbers, you apply them into these estimates.

RAY: Again, what is the assumed doubling dose?

ABRAHAMSON: The dose that will double the spontaneous incidence of mutation or current incidence of disease; it is the same thing whether you look at first genera-tion or equilibrium time. The dose that the BEIR report gives is roughly 20-200 rem. Neel has looked at the Hiroshima and Nagasaki data. Would you suggest that the doubling dose is in the range of 100-1000 rems for humans based on your end points?

NEEL: We would say that for acute it is not less than, say, 30, and then make some kind of adjustment for the chronic, depending on how you want to adjust. There is one other magnificent uncertainty there that I have mentioned. You are using the UNSCEAR data, and I developed an argument that the recessive component in human disease, the null traits that are surfacing all over medical genetics now, may be much, much greater than the dominant component.

ABRAHAMSON: Which number do you want me to put in there?

NEEL: If I work with the estimate, you see how easily those figures are overdone!

ABRAHAMSON: I am very flexible.

NEEL: That is one of the things that bothers me about this whole numbers game; how flexible some people are. I said there were 5,000 critical proteins that might be subject to null mutants and result in disease if they are absent. Using Drosophila data from Mukai and Cockerham (1977) on the ratio of electrophoretic to null variants, I came up with a figure that, at conception, nulls would be 10%--the same figure you have for the multifactorial. The big catch is that we do not know how many of those nulls make it to birth; it may be like chromosome aberrations, where we know we are losing nearly 90%; that is a tremendous unknown right now.

ABRAHAMSON: But the equilibrium time must be so damn long for the most part that the first-generation effect, which we are usually interested in, would be extremely low, wouldn't it?

NEEL: It is a square-root function, of course; if there are enough of them there, it gets very tricky. It is less than the dominants, we will agree on that.

ABRAHAMSON: We are generally talking about dominants somewhere in the range of 20-200 or 50-500, depending on the exact number you are looking at in the first-generation effect.

NEEL: The average handicap is between 20-40% for the dominants that you work with in human genetics. You get your equilibrium times as a function of that. So that is about right.

ABRAHAMSON: We all agree that there is considerable uncertainty. Right now, the largest value of uncertainty and the largest contribution come from the complexly inherited traits. We do not know what the mutational component is; we have never really studied it. The BEIR committee report said the mutational component or contribution that would go up proportionally with increasing dose would be somewhere between 5% and 50%; that is the outside limit. There is no reason to change those limits now as there is no further information on them.

BAUM: Is that recessive number actually uncertain by a factor of 100?

ABRAHAMSON: That is what Neel says.

NEEL: In the last 5 to 10 years in medical genetics, individual, rare entities that collectively add up to quite a bit have literally begun to come out of the woodwork. Technically, you would have to call them recessives. There is a heterozygote effect, but the homozygote exhibits the phenotypic disease that we deal with in medicine. They are beginning to add up to a much greater impact than we realized. I think the UNSCEAR figures just did not recognize this.

ABRAHAMSON: Obviously, the British Columbia figures did not indicate that great a recessive effect (Trimble and Doughty, 1974). Something in this range was also found when the British Columbian children were looked at over a 10-15-year period.

SUTTON: Trimble and Doughty, using their technique, did not find the number of dominants that many other studies predict.

ABRAHAMSON: They found too few dominants. We all agree that they probably underestimated the dominants because they looked at children up to the age of 10, and many dominants have late onset of development, so the estimate was really close to 1,000. Before he died, Trimble had planned to bring it up to a value of 10,000, after talking to a lot of human geneticists who said he missed about 90%.

NEEL: You see how bad those figures are. Trimble had 1,000 in the dominant category, whereas the Northern Ireland study had 3% (30,000). The Northern Ireland study was very high in dominants and Trimble was very low, and when he was confronted with these facts, he then backed away from them. I do not take that British Columbia study too seriously, Seymour.

RAY: Are you calling the heterozygote state normal phenotype?

NEEL: The terms dominant and recessive are increasingly losing their meaning. We still use them because we have to; but for the biochemical traits (and damn near everything in genetics is ultimately biochemical), increasingly you can detect in the heterozygote the abnormality associated with the abnormal gene. So true recessiveness--I don't think we would argue about

this--is increasingly rare as we begin to get at the
molecular basis of disease.

ABRAHAMSON: In fact, in <u>Drosophila</u> there was never an
indication of much true recessiveness;   all recessive
mutants have some kind of heterozygous effect in
Muller's kinds of studies.   There would be about a 2%
detriment in the heterozygous condition.

To answer Zipser's question, if I just estimate
what the risk is for 1 rem of radiation, you can now
ask what it will be for 5 rem of radiation.   That is
what the background level would for a 30-year period.
You can ask what each additional rem will give you in
terms of human exposure relative to such things as
nuclear power plants, medical X-rays, or what have
you.   You can plug that in and come up with some
level of risk.

RAY: What you are saying then, correct me if I am wrong,
is that 1 rem of radiation will produce (including
first-generation effect, which you calculated to be 2%)
an equilibrium-time effect of 10% to 14%.   You add
10-14% to these rates per 10^{-6} lifetimes.   Is that what
you do per rem?

ABRAHAMSON: Or you can say that since we have always
been exposed to background radiation, approximately
10% (or maybe 20-30%) of these 100,000 cases might be
due to background.

EHRENBERG: May I make one comment on Neel's estimate
of the lower limit of the doubling dose in the Hiroshima
and Nagasaki material?   Could one really use the
doubling dose as a measure here, considering the
difference between laboratory animals and humans with
respect to the pressure from all the chemical mutagens
in food and in environment?   One would expect, a
priori, that the doubling dose would be higher in
humans.

ABRAHAMSON: I would expect the doubling dose to be
lower, but maybe I am misinterpreting something.

NEEL: Our estimate did not apply to chemicals at all.

EHRENBERG: Of the spontaneous mutations resulting from
unknown causes, a small fraction are due to background radiation.   Considering other unknown causes,
there are many more chemical mutagens in the human
environment than there are in the environment of
laboratory animals.   You would therefore expect, a
priori, that the spontaneous mutation frequency would
be higher in humans than in laboratory animals; you
have a higher pressure of mutagens.

NEEL: I understand what you are saying. Humans have a long life span and their germ cells are exposed to the chemical mutagens to a much greater extent than are the germ cells of the animals.

ABRAHAMSON: Although it is true that our spontaneous incidence of human mutation has a lot of variable associated with it, we do find that the spontaneous mutation rate per locus for almost every organism we look at is in the range of 10^{-6}. The spontaneous mutation rate per locus for <u>Drosophila</u> is about 3×10^{-6}; for the mouse it is about 7×10^{-6}; and for humans it is in the range of 10×10^{-6}. They all cluster pretty close to each other.

NEEL: I guess I would say the uncertainties are tremendous. So far, spontaneous mutation rates in any animal, even <u>Drosophila</u>, have measured only a small portion of the total spectrum.

ABRAHAMSON: We have looked at 13 loci in <u>Drosophila</u>, 7 loci in the mouse, and about 25 loci in humans.

NEEL: The estimate you are using for humans, for instance, is based entirely on dominant mutations. We have agreed how atypical the dominants may be. We are only now in a position to make good mutation-rate estimates. We will not have to make these extrapolations in another few years.

ABRAHAMSON: I do not know whether we are going to do much better. I do not know whether you are going to change these values by a factor of 2.

NEEL: I think you will agree that, up until recently, for humans we have had to work with traits on a gross phenotypic level, and we do not trust those rates. Even in <u>Drosophila</u> we have worked on a pretty gross phenotypic level. We are only now becoming able to get down to a more biochemical level and measure mutation rates as they affect protein. So I think spontaneous rates in higher eukaryotes are up for grabs.

SUTTON: But in human hemophilia we do know something about the protein. We know that virtually all cases of hemophilia produce a cross-reacting protein, so it does involve a chemical change in that protein, and the mutation rates, however bad, are in the same range as the others.

NEEL: They are higher than what was quoted; they are 2×10^{-5}/locus/generation.

RAY: Just one comment. You take an induced mutation rate increase of 10-14%, and the chemical producing that is equivalent to the effect of 1 rem of radiation, right?

ABRAHAMSON: That is one way to go. Another way would be to take any interval of this. You can look at the concentration of chemical that humans would be exposed to which would give a certain increase in dominants, in chromosome rearrangements, and what have you, and at least limit it to that with which your observation is dealing. I think this is an important point; we know that a given dose of X-rays is going to produce both chromosome aberrations at a given frequency in germ-cell stages and also various levels of "gene mutation." With chemicals, that may not be the case. The range of induction frequency relative to gene-mutation frequency may be orders of magnitude apart. Do you not agree with that?

LEE: It may go from zero to a very large number.

ABRAHAMSON: So you have to be much more careful with your extrapolations for chemicals; if you are extrapolating for the induction of translocation, you cannot say what the mutation rate will be for a gene mutational system. If you are using sex-linked recessive lethals or specific-locus-mutation induction with a chemical, you cannot then predict what it is going to do in terms of chromosome aberration, because we do not have any real knowledge of the spectrum from one to the other at this stage.

NEEL: But there is another problem. Your lowest point on the mouse curve is 50 R of acute radiation. We just had an erudite presentation of curve-fitting and the problems of extrapolation.

ABRAHAMSON: The extrapolations for both the male and the female mouse are done on the basis of chronic exposures, not on the basis of acute exposures.

NEEL: But a 2-week dose at 300 R (1 R every 67 minutes) would still be acute for humans.

ABRAHAMSON: In the male, Russell (Russell and Kelly, 1976) employed dose rates of 0.001 R per minute and he has recently employed 0.0007 R per minute to obtain an exposure of 300 R.

BREWEN: You can no longer demonstrate statistically a significant decrease in the mutation yield.

NEEL: But you are still extrapolating down to where a

slight shift in your curve can change your end result by a factor of 10, if I followed the argument here. When you get down to exposures as low as the human exposure, 5 R over 30 years, your extrapolation does not have to be very far off to change your estimate by a factor of 10.

ABRAHAMSON: But I guess I am prepared to make that overestimate.   If there is something strange about a very, very chronic exposure in which one ionization track passes through a cell every 72 hours versus one track through a cell every 8 hours and there is a different . . .

NEEL: It is not just the chronic, it is the error in your curve, every point has a factor of uncertainty about it.

ABRAHAMSON: Right.   You put that into your weight and linear regression analysis, and that gives you an upper limit.

NEEL: You usually run one straight line, I think.   But you do not commonly state the uncertainty; that is, the standard error of that prediction.

BREWEN: Of course you do.   It is at least 100%.

NEEL: Only a factor of 2.   I do not think that is what we heard about some of the extrapolations in curve-fitting.

ABRAHAMSON: They did not have the data base that we have.

NEEL: Of course, that is the difference.   They were able to simulate the data base, so they knew the true situation.

BREWEN: We have one real dose point.

NEEL: You have one low-dose point and you do not want to be bothered by any more.

VALCOVIC: No, he said real dose.

ABRAHAMSON: I do not understand Neel's point.

NEEL: My point is that I would expect that the uncertainty in the extrapolation, given the standard error of the curve-fitting and the fact that you are extrapolating way off in humans the observed doses...

ABRAHAMSON: Not doses, dose rates.

Risk Assessment of Ethylene Oxide and Other Compounds

LARS EHRENBERG

Wallenberg Laboratory
Stockholm University

The principles we use for risk assessment of mutagenic and carcinogenic compounds can be illustrated by using ethylene oxide as a model compound. One reason for choosing this compound as a model is its occurrence as the single or predominant mutagen/carcinogen in certain environments such as sterilization plants.

Tests in various systems, ranging from bacteria to mammals, tell us that ethylene oxide is mutagenic. Cancer tests, although negative,[1] are considered inconclusive. A quantitation of the risk to individuals or to populations at given exposure doses or collective exposure doses, respectively, of ethylene oxide comprises a number of experimental and computational operations.

From a toxicological point of view, these steps are partly unconventional, as is also the scientific background. The unconventionality consists mainly in the utilization in the evaluation of one compound, such as ethylene oxide, of data for other compounds. These compounds are: (1) other epoxides, (2) other 2-hydroxyalkylating agents, (3) other alkylating agents, and (4) compounds giving rise through metabolism or chemical reaction to ethylene oxide or any of the compounds in 1-3.

---

[1]Note added in proof: H. Dunkelberg (personal communication) has recently demonstrated tumors in mice at the site of subcutaneous injection of ethylene oxide.

The original data presented in this paper were obtained in projects supported by the Swedish Natural Science Research Council and the Swedish Work Environmental Fund.

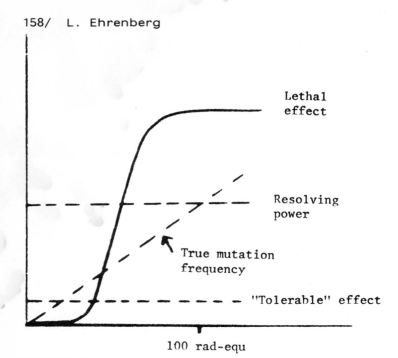

FIGURE 1
Hypothetical curve: True mutation frequency versus dose, illustrating how lethality (solid line) could prevent detection of a nonacceptable risk (lower horizontal line) in a test with the resolving power shown by the upper horizontal line.

The toxicological judgment of reaction products of ethylene oxide is a conventional requirement.

QUANTITATIVE ANALYSIS OF DATA

There are three main reasons why the quantitative analysis of existing data is needed:

1. to make quantitative risk assessments for man from positive biological tests,
2. to get a measure of the resolving power of biological tests, and
3. to clarify the question of whether a negative test excludes a nonacceptable risk.

The last point is related to the question of whether designations of chemicals as carcinogens and noncarcino-

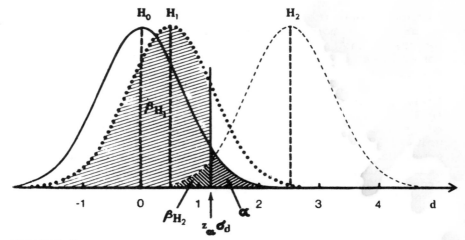

FIGURE 2
Illustration of type-I (α) and type-II (β) errors. Sampling distributions of differences d between test and control samples. H_0: null hypothesis; H_1 and H_2: counterhypotheses that give a large and a small β error, respectively, when H_0 is rejected at α = 0.05. (Reprinted, with permission, from Ehrenberg, 1977.)

gens, or mutagens and nonmutagens (cf. McCann et al., 1975a), are correct. This problem is illustrated in Figure 1, which shows how a nontolerable mutagenic potency of a compound may remain undetected because its lethal action (in other cases it could be its solubility) prevents testing with a sufficiently high safety margin. Statistically, the question of whether a negative test excludes a nonacceptable risk is answered by calculating the probability (type-II or β error) that the null hypothesis, H_0, is false. Figure 2 illustrates the sampling distributions of the difference d = 0 (H_0) between test and control samples and of two hypothetical differences, e.g., corresponding to a maximum tolerable response. Rejecting H_0 at the 5% level (α = 0.05), H_0 will be falsely accepted in some 70% of the cases if H_1 is true (β = 0.70) but only in some 3% of the cases if H_2 is true. Only in the latter case is β small enough (0.03) to permit a negative test to be considered reliable.

USE OF RADIATION RISK AS A STANDARD IN THE EVALUATION OF GENETIC RISKS OF CHEMICALS

Ionizing radiation is the only environmental factor that has been subjected to quantitative risk estimates. We have

suggested that the risk philosophy developed for radiations
be used as a model for stochastic effects of chemicals, and
we are trying to go one step further by investigating the
possibilities of applying the unit of radiation risk as a
general unit of chemical risk by establishing the "rad-
equivalence" of a unit dose of a chemical (see Ehrenberg,
1974; Ehrenberg and Osterman-Golkar, 1977; Ehrenberg,
1979).   Our concept of rad-equivalence is based on dose
and reaction rates and is therefore different from the "rec"
unit of Committee 17 (1975), which cannot be used for
generalized risk estimates.   There are three important
generalizations that can be made and these favor our approach. These generalizations, which will be discussed in
detail below, are:

1.   the linearity (at low doses) of dose-response
      curves,
2.   the finding that mutation frequency is determined
      by the number of alkylations of certain centers of
      DNA, and
3.   the finding that the number of such alkylations
      per unit amount of DNA that is associated with
      the same response as 1 rad of γ-radiation is the
      same in bacteria, plants, and mammals.

Dose-Response (Risk) Relationships
of Stochastic Effects at Low Doses
of Radiations and Chemicals

In discussions of genetic risks from chemical pollutants, low
doses or low dose rates are of primary importance. Most
investigators of dose-response curves for mutations induced
by radiations or chemicals agree that these curves are
linear through a broad range of doses, or at least at low
doses. Table 1 summarizes a few studies of this kind.
Three of these cases are illustrated in Figures 3 through 5:
the now classical linear dose response of X-ray-induced
recessive lethal mutations in Drosophila, already established
in the 1930s (Figure 3); the linear-square dose response of
somatic mutations in Tradescantia stamen hairs, a very
sensitive system investigated down to 0.25 rad X-rays and
0.01 rad 0.43 MeV neutrons (Figure 4); and the linear
component at low doses even of a typical SH-inhibitor such
as chloroacetone (Figure 5).   Figure 4 also shows the
decrease in mutation frequency often encountered at the
higher doses in experiments with radiations as well as with
chemicals (for ethyl methanesulfonate, cf. Turtóczky and
Ehrenberg, 1969).

TABLE 1
Linearity of Dose-Response Curves for Chemically or Radiation-Induced Mutations

System, effect	Mutator	Dose response	Figure	Reference
Drosophila, recessive lethals	X-rays	linear	3	Timoféeff-Ressovsky and Zimmer (1947)
E. coli Sd-4, mutation to streptomycin independence	ethyl methanesulfonate	linear at low doses, exponential at higher doses		Hussain and Ehrenberg (unpublished data); Turtöczky and Ehrenberg (1969)
E. coli, same as above	diepoxybutane	same as above		same as above
E. coli, same as above	ethylene oxide	linear		Ehrenberg and Hussain (1979)
Tradescantia, somatic mutations in stamen hairs	X-rays; neutrons	X-rays: linear-square, with linearity predominant at low doses; neutrons: linear	4	Sparrow, Underbrink, and Rossi (1972)
E. coli Sd-4	chloroacetone	linear at low doses, exponential at higher doses	5	Hussain and Ehrenberg (unpublished data)
Barley, waxy mutations in pollen grains	ethylene oxide in air, treatment during meiosis	linear below 200 ppm for 24 h, exponential at higher doses		Lindgren (1971)

161

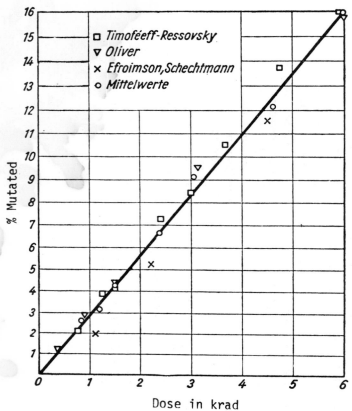

FIGURE 3
Dose response of X-linked recessive lethal mutations in
Drosophila. Data from early investigations. (Reprinted,
with permission, from Timoféeff-Ressovsky and Zimmer,
1947.)

The shape of dose-response curves for induced cancer
has been the subject of much debate, especially with regard
to the existence of a safe threshold dose. It has been
generally accepted, however, that human data for radiation-
induced cancers are best-fitted to linear curves down to low
doses, as can be illustrated by the leukemia incidence in
A-bomb survivors at Hiroshima (United Nations Scientific
Committee, UNSCEAR, 1972).

In some experiments, a threshold dose may have been
falsely inferred from a curve where the detection level was
so high that zeros were obtained at low doses (Figure 6).
The old data in Bryan and Shimkin's now-classical tests

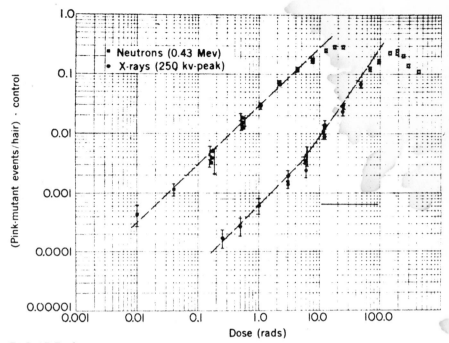

FIGURE 4
Dose-response curves for somatic mutations induced in
<u>Tradescantia</u> stamen hairs by neutrons and X-rays.
(Reprinted, with permission, from Sparrow, Underbrink,
and Rossi, 1972.)

(1943) with benzo(a)pyrene, dibenzanthrazene, and methylcholanthrene were presented as fractions of animals with
tumors (linear scale) versus log dose, giving the image of a
declining effectiveness at low doses. However, if you apply
the equation for a one-hit effect (Figure 7) and present the
fraction of unaffected animals in log scale, you get a
negative linear function of dose. Figure 8 shows the
Bryan-Shimkin data for methylcholanthrene plotted in this
way. Figure 9 shows the corresponding data from a study
on female sex-organ cancer after treatment of rats with a
directly alkylating agent, ethylnitrosourea (Ivankovic,
1969). Within the limits of error, these data are consistent
with a one-hit effect. The only data we have on a tested
epoxide are those obtained by Shimkin et al. (1966) on the
frequency of lung adenomas induced in A/Jackson mice by
diepoxybutane (Figure 10). A theoretical curve through
the highest point and through the control point (a general
control for that material) has been introduced into the

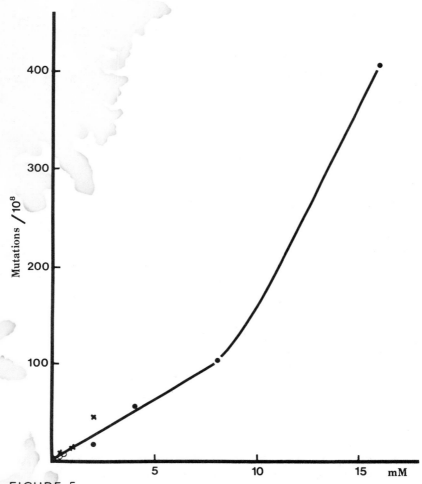

FIGURE 5

Dose-response curve for mutation to streptomycin indepen-dence in E. coli Sd-4 induced by chloroacetone in 1-hour treatments of stationary-phase bacteria at 37°C. (O, X, ●). Experiments on different occasions (Hussain, unpub-lished data).

figure. The data fit well to the theoretical one-hit curve. There is no reason to assume that the curves shown in Figures 8 through 10 are not linear.

Dose-response data for chemically induced cancer in man are very limited. If log (fraction of subjects without bladder tumors) in workers exposed to aromatic amines (Williams, 1963) is plotted against number of years of expo-

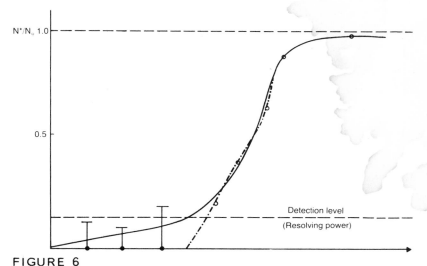

FIGURE 6
Hypothetical true dose-response curve (solid line) where
the linear component is not detected because of insufficient
resolving power. (N_o) Number of tested animals; (N^*)
number of animals with tumors; (—·—) false conclusion of
safe threshold.

sure, which is the only measure of dose possible, then,
according to the expressions in Figure 7, agreement rather
than disagreement with a one-hit curve is obtained.

Certain deviations from linearity have been recorded.
The drop in the response at high doses, of the type shown
in Figure 4, is of limited interest in the context of risks
associated with occupational exposures and exposures in the
outer environment. It should be remembered, however,
that linear extrapolation from observed points in this part
of the curve may lead to underestimates of the risk. This
has probably been done in estimates of cancer risks from
ionizing radiation (Brown, 1976; Ehrenberg, 1978).

$$N^*/N_o = 1 - e^{-kD}$$

$$N/N_o = 1 - N^*/N_o = e^{-kD}$$

$$\ln N/N_o = -kD$$

FIGURE 7
Basic expressions for dose dependence of one-hit effects.
Symbols are as described in the legend to Figure 6.

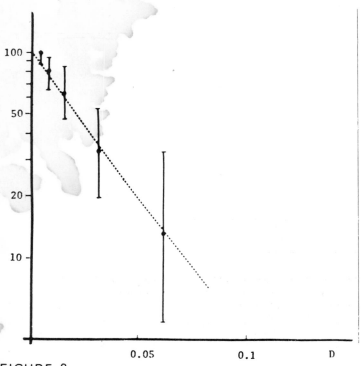

FIGURE 8
Dose response of tumors induced by methylcholanthrene. Fraction of unaffected animals (N/N$_o$) in log scale versus dose (D); 80% confidence intervals. (Reprinted, with permission, from Bryan and Shimkin, 1943.)

Of greater importance is the fact that in some investigations a positive deviation from linearity has been obtained at very low doses or dose rates. For example, a supralinear "hump" has been demonstrated for waxy mutations induced at doses of ^{90}Sr + ^{90}Y β-radiation below 0.1 rad per day during meiotic stages of barley (Figure 11; Ehrenberg and Eriksson, 1966 and papers cited therein). Similar dose-response curves have been described for mammary carcinomas induced in rats by neutrons (Figure 12; Shellabarger et al., 1974) and possibly also by γ-radiation (Rossi and Kellerer, 1972).

It is less clear whether dose-response curves for effects of ethylene oxide exhibit similar humps. One experiment with the waxy system in barley shows a tendency in this direction (Figure 13). It is very difficult, however, to get significance for such an effect. Embree's

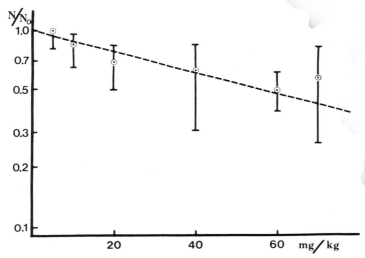

FIGURE 9
Dose response of tumors in female sex organs in pregnant
BD-IX rats treated with ethylnitrosourea. Fraction of
unaffected animals (N/N_o) versus dose in log/linear scale;
80% confidence intervals. (Reprinted, with permission, from
Ivankovic, 1969.)

(1976) data for micronuclei in the rat point in the same
direction (Figure 14).

The importance of this problem for risk estimates is
exemplified by Mary Lyon's (Lyon et al., 1972) challenge of
the practice employed by UNSCEAR (1972, 1977) and other
evaluating bodies of dividing by three the frequencies of
specific-locus mutations obtained in mice at high dose rates
in order to arrive at a figure valid for very low dose rates.
She and her colleagues showed that the curve of mutation
frequency per rad plotted against log (dose rate) is most
likely to be U-shaped. The rise in mutation frequency at
very low dose rates was not significant, but the idea of
Lyon et al. is supported by significant deviations of the
same kind in careful experiments with bacteria (Figure 15).
A likely explanation, although far from proved, might be
found in the induction of enzymes for "error-free" repair
(Hussain and Ehrenberg, unpublished data). The shape of
dose-response curves at low doses or dose rates for
chemically induced mutations is being investigated. Data
for ethylene oxide do not point unambiguously in either
direction.

A higher effectiveness at low doses has also been

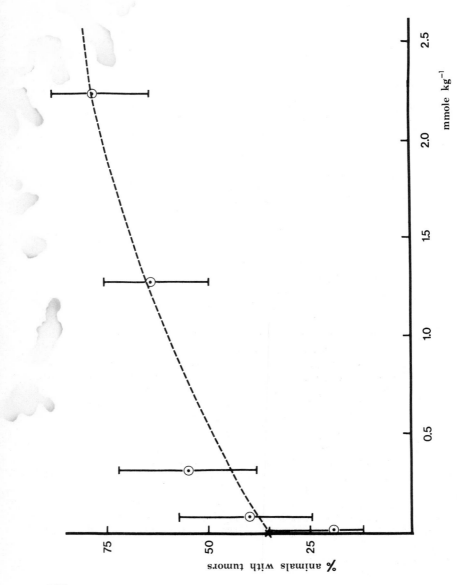

% animals with tumors

mmole kg^{-1}

FIGURE 10

168

observed in studies of the tumorigenic capacity of certain chemicals, such as benzo(a)pyrene (Hieger, 1959; Yanysheva, 1971). This effect might be due to a destruction of activating enzymes at higher intakes of the precarcinogen.

Generally, effects on activating and deactivating enzymes are expected to change the ratio of tissue dose to exposure dose, and mutation and tumor frequencies could still be a linear function of tissue dose. In contrast, induction and destruction of repair systems would cause true deviations from linearity. If the dose-response curves for γ-radiation and a chemical mutagen have the same shape (e.g., of the type shown in Figure 15), the rad-equivalence of the chemical risk could be retained, but at low doses a higher risk coefficient would have to be used for both agents.

Mathematical models have been proposed (with little support from biological theory) which suggest very low or zero cancer risks at low doses, e.g., Mantel and Bryan's (1961) linear relationship probit (cancer incidence) vs. log (dose) and Cornfield's (1977) "thresholded" one-hit curve, respectively. As illustrated in Figure 16, tumor frequencies are for the most part too uncertain for a decision to be made between such models and the hypothesis of linearity. Cornfield's threshold is ascribed to a hypothetical deactivation system that is fully effective at lower doses or in in-vivo concentrations. For ethylene oxide, the proportionality of tissue dose and exposure dose (Ehrenberg et al., 1974) permits the rejection of Cornfield's model at least down to doses as low as one-thousandth of the weekly dose received in work at the TLV, 50 ppm, which is still the present permissible weekly exposure dose in the United States.

We will always be able to find some dose below which experiments become practically impossible. We may con-

---

FIGURE 10
Percent of animals (A/J mice) with pulmonary tumors 39 weeks after 12 thrice-weekly intraperitoneal injections of L-diepoxybutane presented as a function of total amount injected. (·) Experimental points with 80% confidence intervals; (X) general control value; (---) theoretical one-hit curve,

response = $[1 - e^{-(aC_o + b)}] \times 100\%$,

through control and highest dose points (35% and 78%, respectively); (C_o) total injected dose (more correctly, initial concentration); (a, b) constants. (Data from Shimkin et al., 1966.)

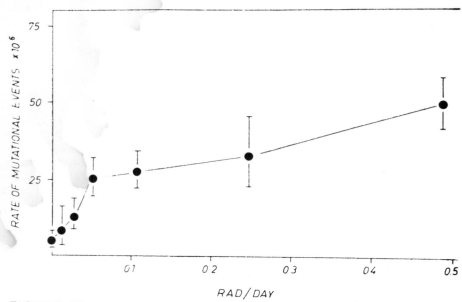

FIGURE 11
Relationship between induced frequency of waxy pollen grains and daily dose of ^{90}Sr + ^{90}Y γ-radiation; 90% confidence intervals are given. (Data from Ehrenberg and Eriksson, 1966.)

clude, however, that we have no data or theory that seriously sustains a general existence of safe thresholds of dose-response curves. In fact, available data are rather in agreement with linearity down to the very lowest doses. As illustrated in Figures 11 through 15, the curve may have a somewhat different slope at low doses, but such deviations seem to be of the order of a factor 3 or less. The reasoning of Crump et al. (1977) regarding the exposure of human populations to great numbers of cancer-initiating (and mutagenic) as well as cancer-promoting agents would also apply to repair-enzyme-inducing events, and this would tend to decrease the impact of deviations from linearity at low doses.

Relationship between Dose, Degree of Alkylation, and Mutagenic Effectiveness of Alkylating Agents

Mutagenic (and carcinogenic) chemicals are electrophilic agents or are converted to such by metabolic activation. The epoxidation of aromatic and aliphatic double bonds (e.g., ethene to ethylene oxide [Ehrenberg et al., 1977]) is one metabolic pathway that gives rise to electrophilic

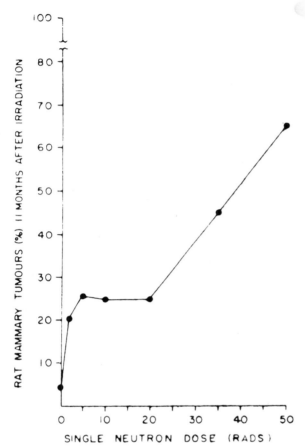

FIGURE 12
Neutron-induced mammary tumors in rats. (Reprinted, with
permission, from Shellabarger et al., 1974.)

compounds in vivo. To be able to compare the effects of
these compounds within or between test systems, it is
necessary to relate the effects to a defined dose.

The dose D in target cells, as a parallel to radiation
dose, may be defined as the time-integral of the concentration of the ultimate electrophilic compound (Ehrenberg et
al., 1974):

$$D = \int_t C(t)dt. \qquad (1)$$

Evidently, the radiobiological concept of dose rate (dD/dt)
corresponds to concentration (C).

Electrophilic agents, RX, react with nucleophilic com-

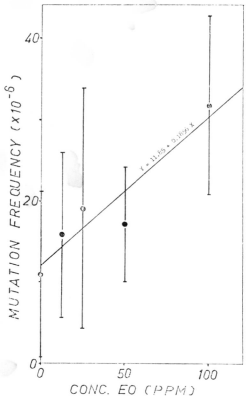

FIGURE 13
Frequency of pollen grains with waxy mutation (absence of amylose) following exposure for 24 hours of barley plants at meiotic stages to different concentrations of ethylene oxide in the air. (Reprinted, with permission, from Lindgren, 1971.)

pounds, Y^-, to give alkylated products, RY:

$$RX + Y^- \xrightarrow{k_{Y^-}} RY + X^-; \tag{2}$$

k_{Y^-} is the second-order rate constant for the reaction.

The rate of the reaction depends on both the structure of the alkylating agent, RX, and the nucleophilic strength of the compound Y^-. If the logarithms of rate constants k_{Y^-} are plotted as a function of the nucleophilic strengths, n, of compounds Y^-, a straight line is obtained for each alkylating agent (Figure 17). The slope of such a curve, the "substrate" constant s, expresses the dependence of the reaction rate on n. Using the equation for a straight

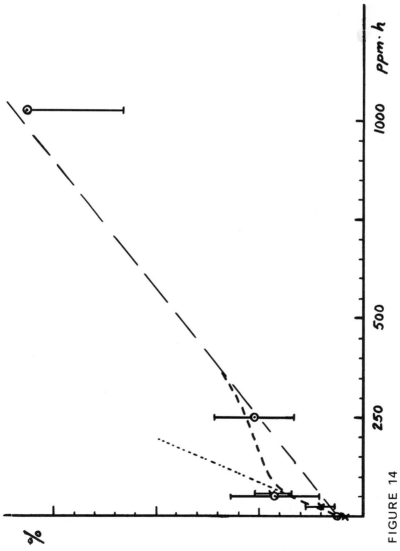

FIGURE 14

Frequency of polychromatic erythrocytes with micronuclei after exposure of rats to various doses (in ppm·h) of ethylene oxide. (Data from Embree, 1976; see also Ehrenberg and Hussain, 1979.)

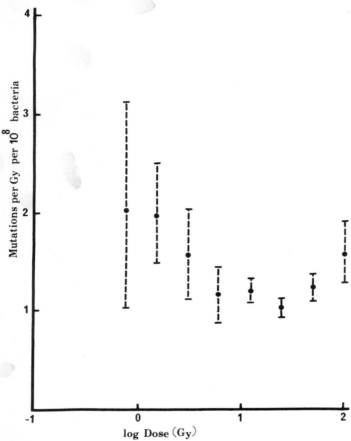

FIGURE 15
Frequencies per rad of reversion to streptomycin independence in E. coli Sd-4 exposed to γ-radiation; 80% confidence
intervals. (Pooling data from six experiments gives P<0.01
for a rise in the mutation frequency at low doses; data to
be published.)

line, the reactivity of an alkylating agent towards nucleophilic compounds of known strength may be calculated,
given, e.g., the reactivity with water (n = 0) and the
s-value (Swain and Scott, 1953; Osterman-Golkar, Ehrenberg, and Wachtmeister, 1970):

$$\log k_{Y_1} - \log k_{Y_2} = s \cdot (n_1 - n_2). \tag{3}$$

Compounds with a reactive oxygen, such as phosphate

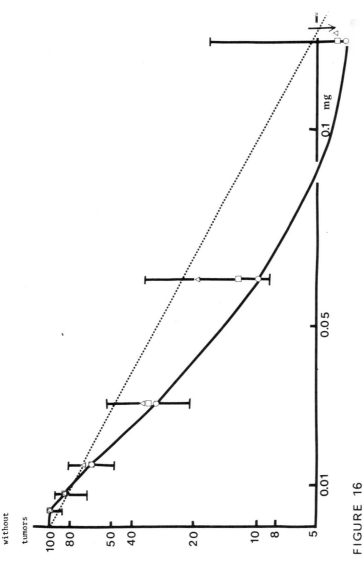

FIGURE 16

Log/linear presentation of fraction of animals without tumors in Bryan and Shimkin's (1943) study of 20-methylcholanthrene. The experimental points (Δ) are given with 80% confidence intervals and with the theoretical one-hit curve (···), as well as the points expected according to the models of Mantel and Bryan (1961) (□) and Cornfield (1977) (○, with curve as solid line).

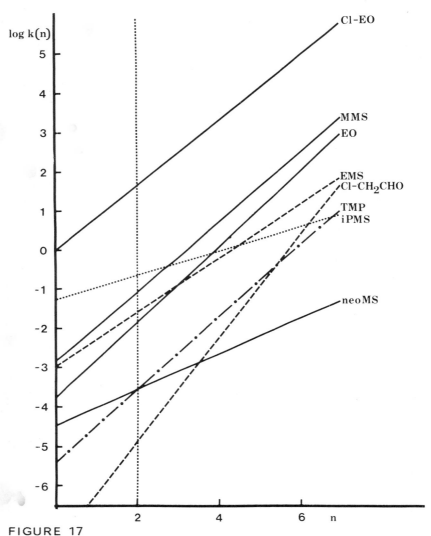

FIGURE 17

Dependence of reaction rates (at 37°C) on nucleophilic strength (n) (data from Osterman-Golkar, 1975). MMS = methyl methanesulfonate, EMS = ethyl methanesulfonate, iPMS = isopropyl methanesulfonate, neoMS = neopentyl methanesulfonate, EO = ethylene oxide, Cl-EO = chloro-ethylene oxide, Cl-CH₂CHO = chloroacetaldehyde, TMP = trimethyl phosphate. Alkylnitrosoureas (Veleminsky et al., 1970) and alkylnitronitrosoguanidines (Osterman-Golkar, 1974) generally have low s-values (low slopes).

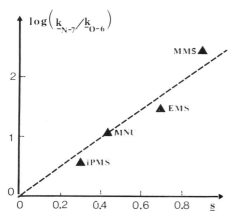

FIGURE 18
Ratio of relative extents of alkylation at the N-7 position of guanine in DNA to that at the O-6 position as a function of s. (Figure from Lawley, Orr, and Shah, 1971, 1972; corrected s-values introduced from Osterman-Golkar, 1975.)

groups, carboxylate groups, and oxygen atoms in nucleic acid bases, have low n-values (0-4); compounds with a reactive nitrogen have intermediate n-values (~3-5); and compounds with a reactive sulfur have high n-values (~5-7).

The rate of formation of the product RY (Equation 2) is given by the equation

$$d[RY]/dt = k_{Y^-} \cdot [RX] [Y^-], \tag{4}$$

and the degree of alkylation, $[RY]/[Y^-]$, of the nucleophilic compound may be calculated from the integrated equation

$$[RY]/[Y^-] = k_{Y^-} \cdot \int [RX]dt = k_{Y^-} \cdot D. \tag{5}$$

When a series of monofunctional alkylating agents were compared at equal dose, a proportionality was found between the mutagenic effectiveness in barley (Osterman-Golkar, Ehrenberg, and Wachtmeister, 1970) and micro-organisms (Turtóczky and Ehrenberg, 1969; Hussain and Ehrenberg, 1975; Osterman-Golkar and Wachtmeister, 1976) and the reaction rate at some low nucleophilicity, n~2 (cf. Figure 17). Since the product of rate constant times dose is equal to the degree of alkylation (Equation 5), the proportionality relationship observed means that a given number of alkylations per unit amount of certain nucleophilic centers, characterized by their nucleophilic strength

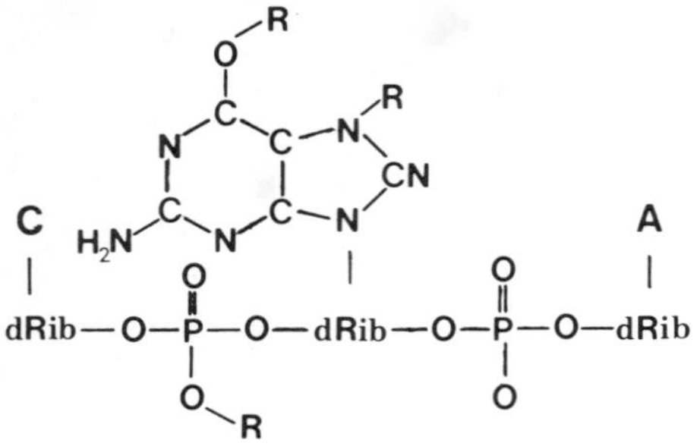

FIGURE 19
Some of the centers alkylated in DNA (R = alkyl).

n~2, give rise to the same mutation frequency irrespective of which alkylating agent is used.

The accuracy of the estimated n-value is still low, but it seems to exclude N-7 guanine, the most reactive center in DNA (n-value around 3.5), as the critical point. For the time being, the value n~2 should be understood as a mean value of a number of centers of low strength. It is, at present, not significantly different from, and may include, O-6 guanine, which, as inferred from the ratio of O-6 to N-7 alkylation, has an n-value of about 1.2 (Figure 18). The alkylation of certain other groups, e.g., the phosphate groups of the DNA chain (see Figure 19), might also have biological significance.

The observed proportionality

$$\text{mutation frequency} \propto [RY_{n=2}]/[Y^-_{n=2}] \tag{6}$$

permits the calculation of the degree of alkylation of the centers denoted $Y^-_{n=2}$ that is associated with the same response as the response to a unit dose of ionizing radiation. In the test systems used, the degree of alkylation 1×10^{-7} corresponded to 1 rad, with an uncertainty of a factor around 2:

$$1 \text{ rad} \longleftrightarrow [RY_{n=2}]/[Y^-_{n=2}] = 1 \times 10^{-7}. \tag{7}$$

Using the radiation risk as a standard (Ehrenberg, 1979; Ehrenberg and Osterman-Golkar, 1977), i.e., expressing the chemical risk in rad-equivalents, the following equation is obtained:

$$\text{risk} = D \cdot k_{n=2} \cdot 1 \times 10^7 \cdot \pi_i f_i \text{ rad-equ.} \tag{8}$$

A product of correction factors, $\pi_i f_i$, has to be introduced in order to correct for properties that modify the alkylation pattern or affect the biological response. These properties include steric effects (e.g., intercalation), charge distribution (which depends in part on solubility parameters), repair, etc. These factors may be worked out in suitable forward mutation systems.

Epoxides react with nucleophilic compounds to give products with an OH group in the β position:

$$Y^- + CH_2 \underbrace{\qquad}_{O} CH_2 + H_2O \longrightarrow CH_2 \underset{\underset{OH}{|}}{\qquad} CH_2 \qquad Y + OH^-. \quad (9)$$

The reactions are catalyzed by hydrogen ions. In estimates of risk connected with exposure to epoxides, the reaction products with water and chloride, glycols, and chlorohydrins have to be considered:

$$CH_2 \underbrace{\qquad}_{O} CH_2 + H_2O \xrightarrow{\ (H^+)\ } CH_2 \underset{\underset{OH}{|}}{\qquad} CH_2, \qquad (10)$$

$$CH_2 \underbrace{\qquad}_{O} CH_2 + Cl^- + H_2O \underset{(OH^-)}{\overset{(H^+)}{\rightleftharpoons}} CH_2 \underset{\underset{OH}{|}}{\qquad} CH_2 \qquad Cl + OH \qquad (11)$$

These products are formed especially in the stomach.

In several systems, ethylene chlorohydrin gives a mutation frequency higher than what would be expected from its very low reactivity (Ehrenberg and Hussain, 1979). One explanation is that at the slightly alkaline pH of cells, it is transformed to ethylene oxide (see Equation 11), which is three orders of magnitude more reactive. Even if only a small fraction of ethylene chlorohydrin is transformed to ethylene oxide, it would increase the mutagenic effectiveness.

Equation 8 is valid for forward mutation, but not for back mutation, in the test systems currently used. Table 2 shows a comparison of diepoxybutane and ethylene oxide in various systems recording forward and back mutation. In the forward mutation systems, E. coli Sd-4, Drosophila, barley, and Sch. pombe, a ratio of 16:100 was found for the mutagenic effectiveness per primary alkylation. A mean value of 30 may be used as a correction factor for difunctional epoxides. The killing effectiveness of diepoxybutane relative to that of ethylene oxide was approximately the same, indicating a genetic component in this effect.

In the back mutation systems, S. typhimurium His⁻ and N. crassa ad-3A, figures close to 1 were obtained for

TABLE 2
Relative Effectiveness of Diepoxybutane Compared with Ethylene Oxide in
Various Systems Recording Forward and Back Mutation

| System | Ethylene oxide | Diepoxybutane | | Triethylene melamine |
		mutation	killing	
Forward mutation				
E. coli Sd-4	1	16(10−25)	14	5,000
Drosophila	1	43	16	2,500
Barley, 22°C, chlorophyll mutations	1	~10[2a]	~10²	≥300
Barley, 3°C and 24°C, chlorophyll mutations	1	25−50		
Sch. pombe	1[b]	L~38 D~30 *meso* ~17	1×10²	
Back mutation				
S. typhimurium His⁻				
G46	1	1	30	17
TA1535	1	1.3	350	60
TA1535	1[c]	~0.5		
N. crassa ad-3A				
low doses	1	1−2	~1	
high doses	1	~0.3 (effectiveness) ~1 (efficiency)		

To illustrate the role of functionality, data for triethylene melamine are included, as
are data for the relative killing effectiveness of diepoxybutane.
Consult Ehrenberg and Hussain (1979) for references for data cited above.
[a]Earlier estimate referred to mutations per epoxy group.
[b]Propylene oxide has approximately 50−100% of the effectiveness of ethylene oxide
in this system.
[c]Glycidol is used as a reference.

the relative effectiveness of the two compounds. Thus,
these systems do not detect difunctionality. If you look at
the killing of these organisms, however, you have a factor
of 30 in G46 and a factor of 350 in the uvr-deficient strain
TA1535. The high sensitivity of the 1535 strain may result

conc. (M)

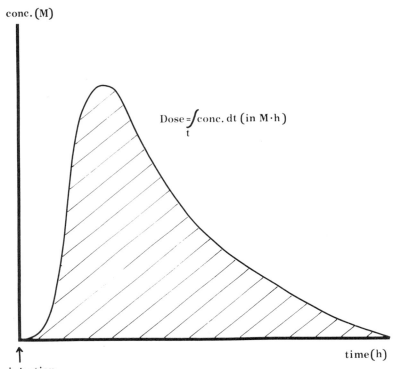

$$\text{Dose} = \int_t \text{conc. dt} \ (\text{in M·h})$$

time(h)

↑
injection
inhalation

FIGURE 20
Dose of a chemical in a target cell, defined here as the time
integral (shaded area, in M·h) of concentration (solid line);
see Equation 1.

from cross-linking of guanines in the DNA strand.   These
linked guanines bear a certain similarity to the thymine
dimers produced by UV (Ehrenberg and Hussain, 1979;
Lawley, Orr, and Shah, 1971, 1972).   As was shown in the
1960s (Haynes, 1964), there is a correlation between UV
sensitivity and sensitivity to difunctional alkylating agents.

IN VIVO DOSES OF CHEMICALS

Risk estimates for animals require knowledge of the in vivo
dose associated with the uptake of a certain amount of a
compound (Ehrenberg et al., 1974; Ehrenberg, 1974).
      The in vivo dose for a tissue is determined by the
rate of absorption, chemical and metabolic reactions,
distribution, transport, and excretion.   Independent of the
shape of the time-concentration curve (Figure 20), information on the tissue dose may be obtained from an analysis of

TABLE 3
Rate Constants for Reactions of Ethylene Oxide and Methyl Methanesulfonate with Some Biological Macromolecules at 37°C

Nucleophile	Ethylene oxide $k(l \cdot g^{-1} \cdot h^{-1})$	Methyl methanesulfonate $k(l \cdot g^{-1} \cdot h^{-1})$
Mouse hemoglobin (treatment of red cells)		
total	1.8×10^{-4}	1.2×10^{-3}
cysteine-S	0.5×10^{-4}	0.60×10^{-3}
histidine-N^{Im}-3	0.36×10^{-4}	0.12×10^{-3}
Mouse, protein in spleen cells (interphase fraction)	4.3×10^{-4}	
Mouse, protein isolated from spleen cells (interphase fraction)	2.9×10^{-4}	
Human hemoglobin (treatment of red cells)		
total	1×10^{-4}	
cysteine-S	0.05×10^{-4}[a]	
histidine-N^{Im}-3	0.14×10^{-4}[b]	
valine-α-NH_2	0.4×10^{-4}[c]	
DNA in mouse spleen cells (about 90% in Gua-N-7, corresponding to $k_{Gua-N-7} = 0.11 M^{-1} \cdot h^{-1}$)	1.0×10^{-4}	0.60×10^{-3}

Consult Ehrenberg and Hussain (1979) for references for data cited above.
[a]Unpublished data. Some uncertainty because of influence of oxygenation.
[b]Preliminary value.
[c]Unpublishd data.

the degree of alkylation of specific nucleophilic groups in cellular macromolecules, such as hemoglobin (Hb) and DNA (Ehrenberg et al., 1974; Osterman-Golkar et al., 1976, 1977). Hemoglobin has the advantage that it can also be obtained easily in large amounts from humans. Rate constants determined in vitro for reactions of ethylene oxide (and methyl methanesulfonate) with N-7 guanine in DNA and different nucleophilic centers in hemoglobin are given in Table 3. Using these rate constants and the degree of alkylation of the corresponding nucleophilic centers, the dose may be calculated according to Equation 5.

The rate of elimination of a compound from a tissue may be approximated by a first-order process. The dose may then be expressed as the initial concentration (or rather the total absorbed amount of the compound per unit

TABLE 4
Lethal Doses of Some Mono- and Difunctional Epoxides

	Mouse, i.p. in arachis oil		Inhalation during 4 h, rat			Other data		
	DL$_{50}$ mmoles/kg	rad-equ.	CL$_{50}$ ppm	uptake mmoles/kg	rad-equ.	CL$_{50}$ ppm	uptake mmoles/kg	rad-equ.
Ethylene oxide	(~5)[a]	(~150)[a]	6,000	42	(1,150)	835 (mouse) 1460 (rat)	9 10	(250) (280)
Propylene oxide	8.6	~250	4,000	28	(800)	1740 (mouse) 4000 (rat)	18 28	(500) (800)
Glycidol	4.1	~300						
Epichlorohydrin	2.3[b]	~250[c]	250	1.8	(~150)			
Diepoxybutane	0.29	~250[c]	(>125) ~175	1.2	(1,000)	90 (rat)	0.63	(500)
Diglycidyl ether	0.38							

Consult Ehrenberg and Hussain (1979) for references for data cited above.

Uptake from air estimated assuming that all material in the minute volume (1.0 l/kg in mouse, 0.66 l/kg in the rat) is absorbed. Tissue doses estimated assuming the rate of elimination to be the same in both species and for all compounds as for ethylene oxide in the mouse, $\lambda = 4.6$/h. The rad-equivalence was determined from 125 rad-equ. per mM $\cdot$ h of ethylene oxide.

[a] Intraperitoneal injection of saline solution; in our own experiments with mice and rats, the acute toxicity (with death on the following day) has sometimes amounted to lower values, 2.5–5 mM.

[b] Somewhat lower values (1.0–1.5 mmole/kg) have been reported.

[c] Correction factor f of Equation 8 set equal to 30 (for functionality).

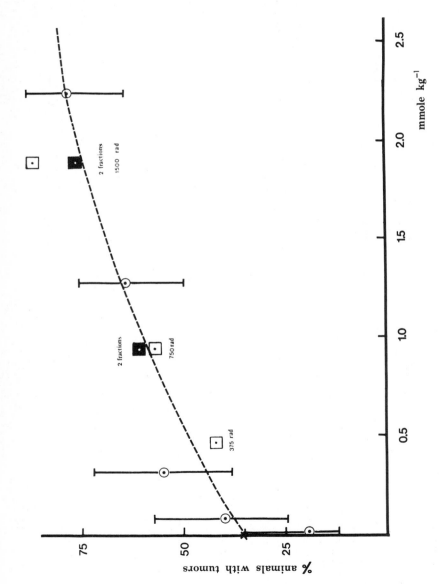

FIGURE 21

184

weight), C_o, times the average retention time in the tissue, $1/\lambda$ (λ is the rate constant for elimination):

$$D = C_o \cdot 1/\lambda. \tag{12}$$

Thus, if the rate constant λ is known, the dose D may be estimated.

The rate constant λ for ethylene oxide has been determined in mice (Ehrenberg et al., 1974; Osterman-Golkar et al., 1976). There is strong reason to believe that other epoxides, such as propylene oxide, glycidol, and epichlorohydrin, are eliminated at approximately the same rate (Ehrenberg and Hussain, 1979). This is indicated, for example, by the DL_{50} of the compounds. The doses of a series of epoxides, in mmole/kg body weight or ppm·h, giving 50% lethality are presented in Table 4. If we calculate the in vivo doses according to Equation 12, using λ = 4.6/h, and translate these doses to rad-equivalents (Equations 12, 5, and 8), values in reasonable agreement with the killing dose for radiation are obtained.

For diepoxybutane, a correction factor 30 (the factor for difunctionality evaluated from data on the relative mutagenic effectiveness [Table 2]) has been used in these calculations. If using the factor 30 we calculate the rad-equivalence of doses of diepoxybutane giving lung adenomas in mice (Shimkin et al., 1966; see Figure 10) and compare these data with Yuhas's (1976) data for frequencies of tumors induced by radiation, a good agreement between chemically induced and radiation-induced frequencies is obtained (Figure 21). Regrettably, the mouse strains were not the same, but as the two strains have the same control value, a tentative comparison of this kind seems permissible (see Ehrenberg and Hussain, 1979). Due to the large differences between mouse strains there is a need for good dose-response curves for the induction of cancer by both chemicals and radiation in the same animal strains.

Applying Equation 8 for some genetical end points in experiments with epoxides, the values found deviate throughout from expectation by less than a factor 2. These data comprise dominant lethal mutations (Embree, Lyon, and Hine, 1977) and micronuclei (Figure 14; Embree, 1975) in the rat, as well as Moutschen's (1961) study of chromosomal

---

FIGURE 21
Similar to Figure 10, with points for X-ray-induced tumors in RFM mice (Yuhas and Walker, 1973; Yuhas, 1976) in the scale of the rad-equivalence of diepoxybutane.

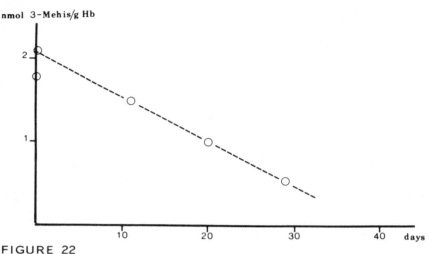

nmol 3-Mehis/g Hb

FIGURE 22
Amounts of 3-methylhistidine in hemoglobin recovered at different times after acute exposure (intraperitoneal injection of dimethylnitrosamine at 23.3 µmoles per kg body weight). The two points on the far left represent samples drawn after 1.5 hours and 5 hours. (Reprinted, with permission, from Osterman-Golkar et al., 1976.)

aberrations induced in the gonads by diepoxybutane. The consistency of these and other data with theory appears to be greater and more general than could be accounted for by coincidence.

It has been shown experimentally that alkylated products of hemoglobin obtained after treatment with ethylene oxide and methylating agents have a high stability in vivo (Osterman-Golkar, 1975; Osterman-Golkar et al., 1976; Segerbäck et al., 1978). Figure 22 shows the amounts of 3-methylhistidine recovered in hemoglobin at different times after acute exposure of mice to dimethyl-nitrosamine. The decrease with time, reaching the value zero after 40 days (the life-length of mouse red blood cells), demonstrates that red blood cells of different ages have been alkylated. This stability provides the basis for the use of alkylation of hemoglobin to integrate doses obtained during a long period of time.

At chronic exposure, the degree of hemoglobin alkylation is built up during one life-length (t_{er}) of the red cells, which is 126 days in man,

$$[RY]_{acc}/[Y^-] = a \cdot t (1 - t/2t_{er}),
\qquad (13)$$

and reaches a steady state after time $t=t_{er}$ at $a \cdot t_{er}/2$,

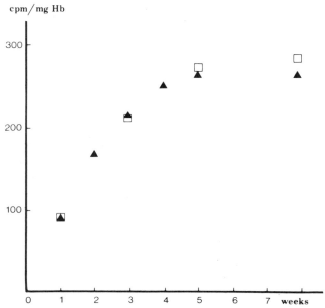

FIGURE 23
Accumulation of alkylated groups in hemoglobin after weekly intraperitoneal injections of [^{3}H]MMS. The mice were weighed before every treatment and received the same chemical dose, 15 mg MMS per kg body weight per injection. (□) Experimentally determined values; (▲) values calculated from Equation 13. (Reprinted, with permission, from Segerbäck et al., 1978.)

where a is the increment per unit time (Figure 23) (Osterman-Golkar, 1975; Segerbäck et al., 1978).

From measurements of the content of 3-hydroxyethyl-histidine in the hemoglobin of employees at an ethylene oxide sterilization plant where the exposure doses (in ppm·h per day) could be reconstructed with some reliability, the tissue dose, and hence the risk, per ppm·h could be estimated (Calleman et al., 1979). The most probable value for persons at "low physical activity" was estimated to 10 mrad-equivalents/ppm·h. At "medium physical activity", the alveolar ventilation, and hence the risk, would be approximately doubled.

CARCINOGENICITY OF ETHYLENE OXIDE

Several arguments can be put forward to sustain the suggestion that the two cancer tests with ethylene oxide so far published (see footnote 1) give false negatives.

TABLE 5
β-Error of Negative Cancer Tests with Ethylene Oxide Estimated on the Basis of Expectation from Positive Tests with Diepoxybutane

Compound	Test	Dose	Cancer	β, %
LD-Diepoxy-butane	Swiss mouse, skin application of acetone solution	$3 \times \sim3$ mg/wk = 0.105 mmole/wk	frequency found 6/30 = 0.2	—
Ethylene oxide	same as above	$3 \times \sim10$ mg/wk = 0.68 mmole/wk	expected (H_1) 0.043; found 0/30	30
LD-Diepoxy-butane	Sprague-Dawley rat, s.c.	1 mg/wk; total 2−3 mmoles/kg	10/50 = 0.2	—
Ethylene oxide	albino rat, s.c.	total 23 mmoles/kg during 94 days	expected (H_1) 0.07; found 0/12	≈40

Data from Ehrenberg and Hussain (1979).
$\beta = (1 - p_{H_1})^n$; p_{H_1} = expected frequency; n = number of animals.

Using data for the established carcinogen diepoxy-butane, the counterhypothesis (H_1, cf. Figure 2) for evaluating the β error of the negative tests with ethylene oxide could be formulated, taking into consideration the proportionality between dose and response as well as the correction factor f=30 for the difunctional agent (Ehrenberg

TABLE 6
Total Numbers of Tumors Induced in Female Wistar Rats by Ethyl Methanesulfonate and 2-Hydroxyethyl Methanesulfonate at Two Dose Levels

		Tumors in 20 rats	
	Dose, mmoles/kg	found	expected
CH$_2$H$_5$Ms	7.4	17 (6)[a]	—
	14.8	23 (6)	—
HOCH$_2$CH$_2$Ms	7.4	1 (6)	0.7
	14.8	3 (2)	1.4
Control	0	0	

Data from Miller and Miller, see Ehrenberg and Hussain (1979).
[a]Numbers in parentheses refer to benign tumors.

and Hussain, 1979). For the tests by van Duuren et al.
(1963) in the mouse and by Walpole (1957), β errors of 30%
and 40%, respectively, were estimated (Table 5). The
former value, where the compound was applied to the skin
in acetone solution and was probably partly evaporated, is
certainly an underestimate. The latter value is less certain
because of lack of knowledge of the details of the experiment.

J.A. Miller and E.C. Miller in Madison, Wisconsin (see
Ehrenberg and Hussain, 1979) have tested the tumor-induc-
ing activity of 2-hydroxyethyl methanesulfonate and ethyl
methanesulfonate in strictly comparative experiments.
Hydroxyethyl methanesulfonate introduces the same groups
into DNA as does ethylene oxide, but it is easier to handle
than the gaseous compound. The number of tumors per
group of 20 animals are presented in Table 6. Assuming
that the two compounds have similar retention times in the
animals, the number of tumors produced after treatment
with hydroxyethyl methanesulfonate could be estimated from
the corresponding data for ethyl methanesulfonate. Table 6
shows that the frequency found is close to expectation.
The number of tumors is low; but as there are no tumors in
the control group, only one at the low dose, and three at
the high dose, the calculated probability that there is no
response is about 5%. The experiment thus demonstrates a
significant effect of one hydroxyethylating agent, which
indicates that we have to consider this type of compound as
carcinogenic.

Preliminary epidemiological data further indicate that
ethylene oxide is carcinogenic in man. In the Hallsberg
case (see Discussion, Part 1), the number of leukemias
expected according to Equation 8--given an estimated risk
per unit exposure dose of 10 mrad-equivalents/ppm·h and a
likely value of the risk coefficient for radiation-induced
leukemia of 3×10^{-5}/man-rad--was, in fact, recovered
(Calleman et al., 1979). In this case, the population had
been exposed during the last 10 years, and therefore only
cancers with a short latency period, i.e., leukemias, would
be expected to appear. In the group of workers investigated by Ehrenberg and Hällström (1967) who were exposed
mainly in the period 1941-62, an increase in cancer of other
sites has now been observed (Hogstedt et al., 1978;
Hogstedt, Malmqvist, and Wadman, 1979). In this case, the
etiology is somewhat unclear because exposure to a few
other chemicals had occurred, too; but ethylene oxide is
suspected to have been the main alkylating agent at the
premises. The exposure situation is less well-known than
in the Hallsberg case, but a calculation backwards from the
increase in cancer incidence to the exposure concentration
(using the above ratio of 10 mrad-equivalents/ppm·h) gives

the reasonable average figure of about 10 ppm of ethylene oxide.

A couple of the leukemias in this group were of the chronic lymphatic type, which, because of its absence in the Hiroshima-Nagasaki material, is usually not considered to be induced by irradiation. A significant rise in the incidence of this disease has been observed, however, in patients who have received many trunk X-rays (Gibson et al., 1972). This could possibly be associated with lymphocyte stimulation, which was observed in radiation workers in the 1920s and 1930s and which is now found in ethylene oxide workers (Ehrenberg et al., 1974; Ehrenberg and Hällström, 1967).

CONCLUSION

Measurement of hemoglobin alkylation presents a monitoring method, from easily available blood samples, for the identification of populations at risk. The method is applicable to both primary and secondary mutagens/carcinogens. Applying some reaction-kinetics parameters, the same data may be used for a quantitation of the risk, e.g., using unit radiation risk as a standard. In fact, from the relationship given in Equation 6 the corollary follows that every compound that is or is converted in vivo to an alkylating agent is mutagenic and most probably carcinogenic. Hence, the demonstration of alkylation in vivo is a sufficient criterion of genetic risk (for a method to show alkylation in vitro, see Göthe et al., 1974). This is of importance because the resolving power of chemical analysis is many orders of magnitude greater than that of any biological test, and because risk estimates may be carried out directly in man without the uncertainties involved in making extrapolations from tests with laboratory organisms.

Reasonable agreement between estimated risk and found cancer incidence in human populations indicates (although the materials available for comparison are still sparse) that the error of risk estimates arrived at by means of Equation 8 is less than an order of magnitude.

Demonstration of hemoglobin alkylation is certainly a criterion of risk of heritable damage. The quantitation of this risk is much less certain, however, because the radiation risk coefficients have had to be based on animal experiments. Uncertainty about the gonad dose relative to the blood dose might be eliminated by measuring the alkylation of sperm DNA (Osterman-Golkar et al., 1976). In the case of relatively long-lived compounds of low molecular weight, such as ethylene oxide, the gonad dose is approximately equal to the blood dose.

Dosimetry of Alkylating Agents

WILLIAM R. LEE
Department of Zoology and Physiology
Louisiana State University

In estimating risk to humans, I would begin by assuming
that a substance that has been found to be mutagenic in a
variety of screening systems, if transported to human germ
cells in the active form, will also be mutagenic in humans.
But the substance could be valuable and difficult to
replace. If so, we face what B.A. Bridges (1974) has
called the third tier of estimating risk of this substance to
humans. I propose that risk estimation be done using
essentially the methods outlined for ionizing radiation work.
The first step would be to estimate the dose to the
human germ cells. The second step would be to determine
the consequence of this dose in test systems that can be
accurately analyzed in the laboratory. To compare estimates in systems that are physiologically similar to humans
with laboratory systems that can be accurately analyzed
genetically, we must use a common method of dosimetry.
To describe dosimetry, I will use the definition used in
radiation research, where dose is defined as the absorption
of energy at the area of interest. This distinguishes dose
from exposure. In mutagenesis, dose is the absorption in
the germ cells of energy in terms of rads. Using the Fifth
International Congress of Radiation Research as a receptive
audience, I defined dose as the amount of chemical that
reacts with the selected target molecule, thus replacing "the
area of interest" in the definition for the rad with "the
selected target molecule" (Lee, 1975).
This distinction between dose and exposure brings in
some interesting contrasts between chemical and radiation
research. Here, using the term of the Committee 17 (1975)
report on genetically significant concentrations, if you take
the exposure to a chemical mutagen over a period of
time--an injection or exposure by inhalation for an acute
period--the increase to the area of interest, to the geneti-

191

cally significant target, would probably continue even beyond the point in time at which you terminate exposure. We have shown in Drosophila, for instance, that alkylation continues in the sperm cell for at least 24 hours after we stop feeding the mutagen. For an interval after you stop exposure, you continue to accumulate the dose in the area of interest. Taking the integral under the time-versus-concentration curve as the dose, we would then estimate the dose as the cumulative assault on the germ cells that can be measured for alkylating agents by simply measuring the cumulative alkylation in the genetically significant target.

In my definition, where the dose is the amount of a chemical that reacts with a selected target molecule, I am using DNA as the selected target molecule for a number of reasons (Lee, 1976, 1977). It is a molecule that all of the test systems we are interested in have in common; it is at the area of interest in the germ cell; and it includes the genetically significant target. Total DNA alkylation is, of course, not always the genetically significant point, but it may be the alkylation on the O-6 in some systems or the alkylation on the N-7 in other systems. It depends on what you are measuring as your genetic end point. In any case, the relation between alkylation at one site on the DNA and alkylation at other sites on the DNA at low concentrations should be constant for a particular mutagen. As you change your mutagens to ones with different s-values (as used in the Swain-Scott scale [1975]), you change this distribution of alkylation sites. This can be resolved by using dose as total DNA alkylation and using, as we do in radiation research, a quality factor, such as linear energy transfer. For chemical mutagenesis, I would suggest, for example, that the s term be used to reflect the distribution of alkylation sites on the molecule.

Having selected DNA as the target molecule, we then must measure a selected reaction product; there must be some physical product to measure. Our system is that of Ehrenberg and others (Ehrenberg et al., 1974); simply to label the alkyl group, in the case of alkylating agents, and measure the total alkylation in terms of the cumulative level of label that one can measure associated with the DNA. A difficulty with this is that the selected reaction product is not always stable; as an example, alkylated bases are lost through hydrolysis and have a half-life in germ cells of about 2.8 days. So you do have to take into account the decay of the selected reaction product within the system.

Given a system of dosimetry like this, you can then choose the system for estimating a human dose on the basis of physiological considerations. Some reports, such as that of Committee 17, refer to human therapeutic doses in terms of Drosophila melanogaster. There is not really an equivalence between an exposure of <u>Drosophila</u> to a given concentration of gas in the environment and a human exposure to a similar concentration; you do not have the same system for transportation of the gaseous elements to the involved tissues. There is also not an equivalent in the circulatory system. The digestive systems are very different. So we really do not have a basis for comparing the exposure of insects with that of humans. When we go to mammals such as the mouse, the rodent is not the organism of choice for comparing or studying inhalation or digestion. (I understand that swine have digestive systems more like that of humans than rodents do). There are very valid physiological reasons for choosing systems that may not be suitable for genetic analysis in estimating the dose of a chemical mutagen to the germ line in humans.

If you measure the dose in some common unit, such as alkylations per nucleotide, you can choose the test organism for the physiological measurement without regard for its suitability for a genetic test. You can then choose the organism for the genetic test on the basis of your ability to classify the mutations appropriately by genetic analysis. With a measure of alkylations per nucleotide, you can compare dose with mutation frequency, as illustrated in two articles (Aaron and Lee, 1978; Lee, 1978). We find that exposure in <u>Drosophila</u> by the common procedure, feeding, does not have a linear relation to the dose in terms of ethylations per nucleotide on DNA in the sperm cell. The dose-exposure plot has an exponent of 0.8, and, for a variety of reasons, the curve tends to bend over. Principally, the flies do not like the material as we get to higher and higher concentrations and do not eat as much. This is the type of environmental problem that one has in measuring exposure. It illustrates the reason for basing estimates on the dose to the germ line rather than on how much the fly will eat in 24 hours or how much it will breathe a given exposure.

There are the same types of problems in the mouse, except in different directions. Work by Sega et al. (1974) shows an exponent of 1.5; in other words, using the standard intraperitoneal injection procedure for exposure, the curve goes up. In a sense, the relationship between exposure and dose was not linear in either case. This is the argument for measuring the dose to the germ line and using the dose-versus-mutation effect for comparative mutagenesis, rather than relying on exposure measurements such as milligrams per kilogram, concentrations in the atmosphere, concentrations in the media, and so forth.

Let us look at a specific comparison of dose and mutation frequency. Our recent work (Aaron and Lee, 1978; Lee, 1978) shows dose in alkylations per sperm cell compared with observed lethals. A linear relation was found between dose (measured as ethylations per nucleotide) and sex-linked recessive lethals. We are especially interested in the dose response at lower levels. It is linear with an exponent of 1 ± 0.1 over this range, and at the lower levels we find that the relationship extrapolates to the origin without any significant deviations from zero. In fact, it extrapolates slightly above the origin, giving no suggestion of a threshold or exponential type of relationship.

In the comparison among species, a common unit of dosimetry is needed. If you are measuring genetic effects of point mutations or small deletions, then alkylations per nucleotide is the appropriate measure of dose. However, if the genetic end point is chromatin loss or interchromosomal translocations, then alkylations per haploid genome would be a more relevant expression of dose. In the former case, correction must be made for the average size of the mutable loci in each species, whereas in the latter, the number of chromosome arms in the genetic test must be considered. The reason for using alkylations per haploid genome with translocation data is that two breaks within the same cell could potentially produce a translocation, regardless of the number of nucleotides per cell.

We used ethylations per nucleotide in Chapter 8 of Chemical Mutagens (Lee, 1978). We showed comparisons between mutation frequencies at different loci (in other words, mutations per locus per ethylations per nucleotide-- the same type of data that you can get in terms of mutations per locus per rad--for different loci in Drosophila). We do not have enough data to make those calculations for the mouse, and therefore, at this time, we cannot make a comparison between Drosophila and the mouse. Some specific-locus-mutation tests in the mouse have been done with EMS and MMS, but they are very limited in number, and the data were collected over a period of time, in a variety of experiments, with different germ-cell stages. We can go to chromosome breaks, but here, we too, have only limited comparison because in Drosophila most of the work with EMS has been based on point mutations.

In recent unpublished work, Dr. Ekkehart Vogel completed a series of experiments showing the comparison between sex-linked recessive lethals and translocations in Drosophila. Using the dose-response curve of Lee (Figure 4; 1978) and taking the sex-linked recessive lethal frequency as a secondary dosimeter, we can make computations for each of Vogel's experiments. We find that there is a nonlinear relationship between dose and translocations in Drosophila. The relation between translocations and dose in the mouse was shown by taking the data of Generoso and

Russell (1969) for translocations and the data of Sega et al. (1974) for determination of dose (as illustrated in Figure 6 of Lee 1978). A nonlinear relation with an exponent much higher than 2 was found between dose and translocations in the mouse or Drosophila. The consequence of this nonlinearity would be that were one to extrapolate to low levels of ethylations per nucleotide in the environment, those events that depend on chromosome breaks and rejoining for transmission would become very unimportant at low levels due to the shape of the curve. Those mutational events that depend on the point mutations, such as sex-linked recessive lethals, would, from the shape of the curve, be important proportionally at low levels. The type of risk estimate that one would predict would depend tremendously on the type of genetic end point we are interested in--whether we are measuring genetic end points that require chromosome breakage or those that do not require chromosome breakage, as in the case of the sex-linked recessive lethal test.

In our laboratory, we have recently determined a dose-response for MMS and EMS. In this experiment, we fed MMS at the same concentration as EMS in our previous experiments, except for MMS we fed for 8 hours, whereas for EMS we fed for 24 hours. MMS has a faster rate constant for alkylation than EMS (Osterman-Golkar et al., 1970) and is a more effective alkylating agent per concentration per unit of time. We observed a higher level of alkylations per sperm cell with an 8-hour feeding of MMS than with a 24-hour feeding of EMS but found a lower frequency of sex-linked recessive lethals. In other words, the MMS was less effective per alkylation, a fact which would have gone undetected had we not actually measured the dose as alkylations per nucleotide. EMS is more effective per alkylation with this particular genetic end point. If we had used translocations (a chromosome breakage event), MMS would have been more effective than EMS per alkylation, using Vogel's unpublished data on sex-linked recessive lethals as a secondary dosimeter.

BREWEN: What is the shape of that curve?

LEE: It is nonlinear, with an exponent much higher than 2.

BREWEN: The same as in the mouse?

LEE: Yes.

One other interesting difference between MMS and EMS is that in two experiments that we have done since to determine the shape of the curve for MMS, we have found that MMS gave a nonlinear relation between alkylations per nucleotide and sex-linked recessive lethals, whereas EMS gave a linear relation.

ABRAHAMSON: In what way is EMS linear and MMS not linear?

LEE: Figure 4 of Lee (1978) shows that the MMS curve is considerably below the EMS at low doses. With higher doses, we find MMS almost reaches the efficiency per nucleotide we get with EMS. It is a typical multi-hit curve, although the exponent is not as high as 2--but more like 1.5.

ABRAHAMSON: Does it have a linear component in the very low dose range?

LEE: You can always show mathematically that it does, but we do not have enough data at this time to say that it is a mixed curve.

BAUM: Does stage sensitivity enter into this picture?

LEE: All of this is done with mature sperm cells.

WALKER: As an aside at this point, in bacteria--E. coli-- EMS does not seem to be dependent on the functioning of the error-prone inducible repair system, whereas MMS is virtually completely dependent. That may have nothing to do with what is happening here, but there may be some fairly fundamental difference in the way the damage happens in the two types of process. I am sort of surprised to see that the difference shows up so clearly here.

LEE: Of course, MMS is a strong SN-2 type, and its pattern of alkylation gives very low levels on the ring oxygens. EMS is more intermediate, whereas diethylnitrosamine would be of the SN-1 type. We have not yet done any work with diethylnitrosamine. But we do find a difference in the shape of the curve as we go between EMS and MMS.

BREWEN: Doesn't Vogel argue that the higher the SN-2 value, the more efficient the compound is in breaking chromosomes? Perhaps you are looking here at recessive lethals with small deficiencies.

LEE: There is reason to think that is the case. Although EMS is intermediate in s-value and actually alkylates far more readily on N-7 than on O-6, the types of mutations that one recovers are perhaps best explained as being single nucleotide transitions.

BREWEN: What happens if you store these EMS-treated sperm? Can you change the pattern?

LEE: You change the pattern toward chromosome breaks;

the pattern with regard to the ADH locus has not yet been done. The pattern for complementation maps was done on nonstored sperm. A repeat of the experiment with stored sperm has not been done. There has been cytological work, not with EMS but with other mutagens, by Slizynska (1973) which shows that, upon storage, the cytological pattern approaches that of X-rays.

RAY: To lock this in, in the efficiency of EMS versus MMS for chromosomal level effects as related to the efficiency of alkylations per nucleotide, which produces the greater genetic effect?

LEE: Per alkylation, EMS is more effective than MMS. Because MMS is a nonlinear relation, the efficiency obviously changes with dose. At low doses, EMS is far more effective than MMS.

BREWEN: One more question. Do you get as great a storage effect with compounds with high s-values?

LEE: That is an important point. You get a greater storage effect with MMS (high s-value) than you do with EMS--that is Vogel's work, which should be published soon. That would fit in with the idea that as you go from EMS to MMS, essentially you are changing the basic mechanism of mutation production, where the alkylation of the ring oxygens is no longer sufficient to be an important component. Instead, you presumably pick up small breaks, which can also be detected in the sex-linked recessive lethal test.

ABRAHAMSON: Does that mean that the storage effect on MMS also increases sex-linked recessive lethal rates significantly?

LEE: With MMS, the storage effect is much greater than with EMS.

ABRAHAMSON: But does the sex-linked recessive lethal value go up significantly with storage of MMS?

LEE: No.

ABRAHAMSON: Only with translocation?

LEE: A series of problems involving mosaics should be considered. I do not think that we can really answer the question because the data collected so far are not clear. At the levels at which the work is done, you get a shift of some mosaics into completes. As you go up in level, more completes should begin to occur. This shift relationship requires an interpretation of the curve that we are simply not able to do with the present data.

WALKER: Does the number of chromosomal aberrations go up quadratically as a function of the storage time? It sounds as though you need two events.

LEE: That is right for translocations. It does go up--far more than an exponent of 2. It is very rapid. Of course, at the high level, there are only a couple of points on Vogel's data, but plotting those gives far more than a squared dose relation. The number of events that must be occurring to convert a single depurination, which is what we think is occurring there, into a chromosome break should be more than one. Then it takes chromosome breaks to produce a translocation. So there are many reasons for the curve to be so steep.

The second point is the differences in the germ-cell stage. The work we have been discussing here was all on spermatozoa, for the simple reason that that is where we have the methodology for identifying the specific germ-cell stage. This is done in the fly by treating the male and sampling sperm from the seminal receptacles of the female. In the case of the mouse, Sega et al. (1974) have developed a method for purifying spermatids from the epididymis and the vas, and those methods are therefore available. Unfortunately, we do not have a data base showing the alkylations in the different immature germ-cell stages. What is available is the alkylations that are retained from a particular cell stage until the mature sperm cell develops.

Sega and coworkers have reported a number of experiments in which the mouse was injected. After successive intervals of time, the alkylations that remained until completion of spermatogenesis were recorded. These were related to unscheduled synthesis (Sega, 1974, 1976; Sotomayor, Sega, and Cumming, 1978; Sega and Cumming, 1975).

This can be related to the unscheduled synthesis reported by Sega, Sotomayor, and Owens (1978). In a sense, as you go backward into successively more immature stages of spermatogenesis, you find a very strong shift in patterns. In stored mature sperm cells, back through late spermatids, the loss of alkyl groups in Drosophila (and apparently also in the case of the mouse) is no greater than what would be expected on the basis of hydrolysis. In fact, in a recent experiment over a 10-day period, Drosophila sperm stored in the female lost the labeled alkyl groups at a rate that would have been predicted by the average loss due to hydrolysis. This loss has a half-life on the order of about 3 days and therefore does not have an important role where fertilization occurs immediately after treatment. Hydrolysis becomes very important if you do a storage experiment in <u>Drosophila</u>, where you wait 7 to 9 days before the sample is taken for genetic analysis.

It was shown by Ehling et al. (1968) that in the first few days following treatment with EMS, a peak of dominant lethal production took place between days 7-9, followed by a drop in dominant lethal production after day 12. The peak of dominant lethal production would allow time for hydrolysis to occur, while in the still earlier germ-cell stages there is a period of unscheduled DNA synthesis (Sega and Owens, 1978; Sega, 1974, 1976; Sotomayor, Sega, and Cumming, 1978; Sega and Cumming, 1975).

Considering this great difference in germ-cell-stage response, I have suggested (Lee, 1975) that we should weigh the particular response in each germ-cell stage by the length of time of that germ-cell stage in the life cycle of humans. For example, EMS gives a two-orders-of-magnitude greater response in the postmeiotic germ-cell stages than in the gonial stage. If you take 20 days as the sensitive period for EMS in humans, a significant portion of the mutations that would be induced in the human population following exposure to this mutagen would be induced in the short 20-day period just following exposure. The majority of the mutations, though, would still be induced in the gonial stage if there were only two orders of magnitude difference in the response between the sensitive stage and the gonial stage. If there are three orders of magnitude of difference between the sensitive stage for 20 days and the gonial stage, then, for practical purposes, you need only consider the sensitive stage in considering risk.

The other deviation is that, whereas radiation produces all classes of mutations (the relative frequency and importance being a subject for debate), with chemical mutagens, some are known to be capable of affecting significantly only certain classes of genetic damage. Vogel has presented diethylnitrosamine as one case where he is only able to detect sex-linked recessive lethals, point mutations, and--in very large experiments--only one translocation, which is not significant.

In estimating risk to humans, one must compute the risk in terms of different classes of mutations. In some cases, we may find that a certain risk may be reasonably high--for example, in point mutations--and very low in immediate effects resulting from chromosomal aberrations, whereas some other chemical agent may produce an effect that is primarily immediate due to its efficiency in inducing chromosomal aberrations.

ABRAHAMSON: Do you know of such an agent?

LEE: Benzene has been reported (Lebowitz et al., 1978) to cause chromosome breaks. Certainly it is otherwise negative in the standard test systems. I think the regulatory agencies are going to face a very interesting ethical question: Which is more important?   One agent could produce an equal number of genetic deaths as another but could have its effect in immediately succeeding generations--say, a translocation effect that would reach equilibrium in three or four generations. The other chemical could produce only the types of events that reach an equilibrium in the population after quite a few generations.   Depending on your model of human populations in the future, you may have the same amount of genetic death, but a very different timing as to how that expense is incurred. It then becomes a question of ethics.

Are Benzene Effects Limited to the Chromosomal Level?

VERNE RAY

Medical Research Laboratory
Pfizer, Inc.

Benzene has received a lot of attention recently, after having been declared at least a suspect--and, in the minds of many, a bona fide--leukemogen. Apparently, benzene's chronic toxicity seems to focus on the hemopoietic system, and there is evidence of myelotoxicity and hypoplastic anemias, occasionally with acute or chronic leukemia developing. OSHA has estimated that about two million workers in the United States have a potential exposure to benzene-- this is a fairly substantial number of people who come in contact with it. As we try to deal with benzene exposure in the industrial workplace or at the gas pump in the local neighborhood, it would seem that vastly different approaches will have to be taken to control benzene exposure.

In terms of genetic data, as Lee said, the literature shows that in tests (for example, in Salmonella) with and without metabolic activation, benzene does not produce point mutations. From data in the literature and from data obtained from some people who have been doing research with benzene who have not yet published, it is my understanding that the mouse lymphoma model--a mammalian-cell point-mutation model--is negative for benzene. The literature reports one dominant lethal negative, and I know of another test that has been run that is also negative.

At the chromosomal level, you do find effects of benzene, both in vitro and in vivo. In human leukocytes, a considerable number of chromatid-type breaks have been found with benzene. Dicentric and ring forms have been reported, but they seem to be very sparse. Chromatid deletions have also been seen in metaphase chromosomes in rats, and studies have been done in rabbits which show both chromatid and chromosomal breaks.

Humans, the species of most concern, have also been studied. Two studies have been done by the Dow Chemical Company, and I think these have received quite a lot of publicity. One was on a group of 290 persons exposed to benzene over an extended period between 1965 and 1975 who were analyzed and found to be negative for cytogenetic effects. The paper is not all that explicit about exposures. It seems to me that the exposure in this group of 290 workers was less than in the second study which reported on 52 people (Table 1). There is another essential difference between the two studies: the manner in which metaphase analysis was conducted. In the first study, 50 metaphase figures per individual were used; in the second study, 200 were used. With time, it seems that the number of metaphase figures one analyzes has tended to creep upwards, and certainly the work of the Dow group suggests that at least 200 were recommended for their purposes. In the second study, people working in the presence of benzene over a period of time were compared with control groups, who, to the best of their knowledge, were not so exposed. (Considering that benzene is so widespread in the environment, one has to be a bit concerned about the lack of exposure assumed by the control groups.)

It is pretty clear that the declaration of a significant effect involves chromosome breaks and marker chromosomes.

ZIPSER: Is there any indication of how these effects are distributed over individuals?

RAY: You mean as to how many of the effects are seen in one individual? Yes, there were 59.1% of 44 control individuals without chromosome breaks and 40.9% with breaks. Among the 52 benzene workers, 26.9% had no chromosome breaks and 73.1% did. Although you may find that particular statistic interesting, I think that in the case of benzene, we do have an example of a

TABLE 1
Second Dow Chemical Company Study

	Group exposed	Group not exposed
No. of people	52	44
No. of cells examined	10,400	8,800
Chromatid breaks observed (%)	1	1.1
Chromosome breaks observed (%)	0.67	0.35
Marker chromosomes (%)[a]	0.19	0.06
Abnormal cells (%)	1.6	1.4

[a]Includes ring, dicentric, translocation, and exchange figures.

substance where, at least to date, the effects that we
see are somewhat limited to the chromosomal level, and
the data that have been obtained in dominant lethal
experiments have been negative. I do not have the
dose levels utilized in the dominant lethal experiments,
but I sincerely doubt that more than two have been
used.

I am not aware of any heritable translocation assays
that have been run to date. This presents an interesting
case for us. If you agree with the significance of that
level of an effect seen in individuals that have received (in
the study with 52 workers) "excursions" up to 100 ppm,
where the average exposures were considerably less than
that, certainly under 55 ppm, then we can approach this
particular substance in the way we discussed earlier. If
there is no evidence of point mutational activity, which is
remarkable in itself, the process of risk assessment here
could be applied along the lines we have discussed today.
This provides a reasonable way to model out, as we have
suggested.

I do not have much more information on benzene, but
the approaches that have been suggested are similar to
those outlined by Lee in that they focus on finding the
number of nucleotides affected by given levels of benzene.
In this case, we deal with a somatic-cell effect rather than
a germinal one. This should then offer an opportunity for
some interesting research models.

This is about the extent of the information that we do
have on benzene. A recent article by B.J. Dean (1978)
deals with benzene, toluene, xylenes, and phenols. I
recommend it for examination.

ABRAHAMSON: You described only two test systems--the
    Salmonella test and the TK test in mouse lymphoma
    cells--and both were mutagenicity-negative. These are
    point mutational systems. There was no across-the-
    board battery of tests run for point mutation?

RAY: Not to my knowledge. I do not know whether or not
    Drosophila has been run at this point. The Salmonella
    and mouse lymphoma have been run, although, to my
    knowledge, the mouse lymphoma data are not available
    in the open literature, and both are negative. There
    has been one study reported on the micronucleus test.

ABRAHAMSON: But again, that is a chromosomal test.

RAY: Right, and it was positive.

INFANTE: What do you think is the sensitivity of the
    dominant lethal test? Have any large comparisons been

made? What does the negative dominant lethal test tell you?

RAY: Looking at the negative dominant lethal and the exposure levels, I consider that a quirk. I think, in this case, that you are faced with a negative result just like with many dominant lethal tests of substances that produce both point and chromosomal level aberrations and may turn up negative in this assay. The dominant lethal, I think, has been demonstrated to be able to detect chromosomal level effects over any of the stages of spermatogenesis, including those preceding meiosis. There are substances that can produce dominant lethality which affects the spermatocyte phases.

ABRAHAMSON: When you have a dominant lethal, you are recording out of a spermatogonial cell. You are just recording the unbalanced translocation product, not a dominant lethal in the sense of a single chromosome break that has now persisted. So you are really recording translocation events.

RAY: There has been considerable discussion about that. I did not think that it was limited to a translocation event.

BREWEN: In the X-ray data of Ford and colleagues (1969), they can account for all of their dominant lethals by unbalanced segregates from translocations. One would presume that these large deletions will be lost in the 10- to 12-cell generations through cell lethality in the spermatogonial cells. This does not preclude the rare event that will survive and come through.

VALCOVIC: To come back to Infante's question. With the negative dominant lethal, in the absence of any metabolic information or any other heritable tests, you just have no determination whether the compound even got to the gonads.

INFANTE: The reason I asked about the sensitivity of the dominant lethal test is because I know the example of vinyl chloride. Sobels shows vinyl chloride positive for sex-linked recessive lethals and positive in Salmonella and Chinese hamster ovary tests. Chromosomal aberrations have been seen in workers in several studies. Yet vinyl chloride was reported to be negative in terms of dominant lethality.

BREWEN: You have a problem in a study like this. If the compound is not producing a long-lived lesion in the DNA, then, in order to be effective, the compound requires the act of DNA replication. Benzene may be an example of this, as a high positive result has been obtained in rat bone-marrow or spermatogonial cells that are going through a replicative process. Here we are looking at leukocytes; there are no replicative cells. The lesion that is responsible is not long-lived. By the time these cells reach DNA synthesis, the compound is no longer there, except perhaps for some residue that was in the serum and that might produce this very low--and I do not think significant--effect. The dominant lethal test would come up negative, because you are going to be looking at cells that are not replicating their DNA, and if the lesion does not persist in the chromatin, it will never be translated into something that will give a dominant lethal.

RAY: We are, in fact, looking at the tissue here, which has a very high mitotic index in the bone marrow.

BREWEN: Right. And a high effect is found.

EHRENBERG: If you ask what the negative dominant lethal test stands for, then the comparison with radiation could be useful. If you run a dominant lethal test on the normal scale, what you exclude is an effect comparable to that produced by some 50 rad of acute postmeiotic radiation. You could, of course, increase the number of animals and get it down to 20 or 10 rad-equivalents. This case with the workers is quite similar to what you would expect from another industrial chemical, which is also widespread in the environment: that is, ethylene oxide. All tests are negative, but, nevertheless, you can show a tissue dose in populations living in towns where, for instance, the annual dose might be on the order of the risk associated with the background radiation dose. You would never expect to detect that as an increased frequency of some kind of event.

When you come to vinyl chloride and the question of why a dominant lethal test was negative, although you find chromosome variations in various cells in the tissue, if you measure the dose just through alkylation after application of labeled vinyl chloride, you find that the dose in liver and blood is approximately the same. In the gonads, however, it is one order of magnitude less. The degree of alkylation of DNA or protein in the gonads is ten times less than what you would expect in the case of equal distribution over the body. You would expect this with a compound that is as short-lived as chloroethylene oxide, which seems to have a half-life of about 2 seconds in the mouse. We get more local damage close to the site of major conversion of the vinyl chloride.

NEEL: There are some tricky aspects to the statistical analysis of data like these.

General Aspects of Comparative Mutagenesis

LAWRENCE R. VALCOVIC

Public Health Service, Bureau of Foods
Food and Drug Administration

Test systems, especially the in vitro ones, are designed for sensitivity and are very helpful for determining whether or not a chemical has the potential to cause gene mutations or chromosomal aberrations. But, for mutagenicity risk assessment, the real questions concern how to derive quantitative data from "relevant systems." Brewen discussed this problem in relation to chromosome aberrations. I would like to refer back to the HEW document on mutagenicity (Flamm, 1977). In one section, we tried to give an overview of the approaches to risk estimation. We said: "The mutagenic potency of a chemical is a function of several factors--the overall absorption, metabolism, and excretion of the administered chemical, the transport of the chemical or its metabolites across the membrane of the target germ cell and its subsequent metabolism within the target germ cell, interaction of the chemical or an activated form of that chemical with the DNA to form a premutational lesion, and finally the fixation of the lesion, as a stable alteration in the DNA, to various replication or repair processes."

The latter two categories--binding to DNA and fixation of the damage with respect to replication and repair--are areas we have covered. Before we discuss comparative mutagenesis, we should briefly review the general factors concerning metabolism and what are referred to as pharmacology, pharmacokinetics, etc. I hope we can focus on mutagenesis, not carcinogenesis; that is, the risk to future generations and germ-cell effects.

Ideally, we would like to be able to combine sophisticated biochemical and pharmacological techniques regarding metabolism to identify metabolites and subsequently quantify dose at the target cell. In vitro mutagenicity data (so-called intrinsic mutagenicity data) are extremely helpful in risk estimation, but we must understand the differences between the metabolic patterns and processes of whatever laboratory organism is being used and those of humans. We do not have that type of understanding today. In mutagenesis, however, there is one advantage over other areas of toxicology: we are dealing with a process where we have a relatively firm understanding of the mechanism and target molecule. Lacking the detailed pharmacological information, we do have whole-mammal tests that measure genetic end points of sperm cells or egg cells or in F_1 offspring. Effects that are significantly above controls do provide us with a reasonable assurance that the chemical or an active metabolite of that chemical has reached the target germ cells. Often we do not have a clear understanding of where differences in metabolism may be.

I am not certain whether the needed pharmacological techniques are fully available to us or sophisticated enough to do the kinds of analysis that we would like to see done. Over the years, for sociological and political reasons, there has been stronger focus on carcinogenesis than mutagenesis. Therefore, much of the activity in the biochemical areas of metabolism and pharmacology has focused on many of the aromatic hydrocarbons, such as benzpyrene and aminoanthracene, the carcinogenic activity in their active forms, their activation, and so on.

As for mutagenicity, effort has focused on in vitro metabolic systems and their application for mutagenicity determination. Several years ago, there was hope that the host-mediated assay would provide a bridge toward estimating risks to humans, especially for mutations where mammalian data are effectively nonexistent. Basically, we have only the Russell specific-locus test data to rely upon. But the vast majority of people agree with Brewen that well over 50% of the mutants obtained in that system were probably due to short deletions. We have almost no measure of point mutations induced in a mammalian system.

Could the host-mediated assay incorporate whole-animal metabolism with the sensitivity of a number of the bacterial or microbial systems? There are several problems. One came to light several years ago when Malling attempted to employ Neurospora in the host-mediated assay. He wanted to maintain an organism within the mouse for longer than 3 or 4 hours--the limit at that time. Neurospora survived in the peritoneal cavity of mice, in the absence of a mutagen, for up to 36 hours. The mutation rate in these Neurospora was at approximately the same level as would be expected from a significant dose of X-rays. The interesting thing about this was that, with this equivalent mutation frequency, there was a very high percentage of deletions. Without a significant amount of supporting data, he attributed this to an immunological reaction of the mouse. There is quite a bit of emphasis now on modifications of so-called host-mediated assays to utilize mouse cells, say a mouse lymphoma line, as well as on other approaches to implanting the organisms into the mouse.

So far, these efforts have not developed much data, but for risk estimation we need to utilize the whole-mammal metabolism. The use of an S-9 liver microsomal fraction or other in vitro systems is satisfactory for asking the qualitative question in mutagenesis: Does the chemical have mutagenic potential? Then we want to know how the chemical might behave in a whole animal. There are so many soluble enzymes that can activate or inactivate, even in the microsomal system itself. Thus, in vitro data do not correlate completely with in vivo data. The mixed-function oxidase system in itself is very complicated. As we take membrane fractions as fragmented as an S-9 fraction or some even more fragmented, just how are these going to relate back to an in vivo situation?

In risk assessment, we must consider studies such as those of Felton and Nebert (1975), who have been looking at specific enzyme systems, such as aryl hydrocarbon hydroxylase (AHH), across a number of inbred mouse lines to examine genetic variation. The DBA/2 strain has very low AAH activity compared with strain C57BL/6. Therefore, the mutagenic response in Salmonella may differ by orders of magnitude, depending on the source of the S-9 fraction. Such genetic studies need to be used more in routine screening. When there are comments about optimization of the S-9, I cannot help wondering how one defines optimization. Are we going to select a rat, a mouse, a hamster; should it be induced or uninduced; and what inducer are we going to use? The utility of the Salmonella tests for risk estimation can be increased by incorporating different mouse strain S-9's or different inducers.

Being primarily a whole-animal geneticist, I am a bit critical of the utility of in vitro tests for risk assessment. There should be more emphasis on Drosophila. Drosophila has not been the subject of biochemical studies of the mixed-function oxidase systems as has the housefly and several other insects, but from the genetic data that have been obtained, primarily by Vogel in Leiden, it is quite clear that Drosophila does have a very potent MFO system (Vogel and Sobels, 1976). In the insect, this system is primarily located in the gut, the Malpighian tubules, and the fat body. The activity in the fat body, at least in some insects, is quite age-dependent, but as yet there has not been a really careful study as to its compartmentalization.

Clearly, there is a very significant amount of activity in the gut. When aflatoxin is fed, there is a significant induction of dominant lethals. In wasps, the mutagenic potency is just barely detectable (Valcovic, unpublished data). But Vogel's group and others have looked at a very large number of the so-called procarcinogens. With few exceptions, these have shown positive results in the recessive lethal tests. Perhaps Brewen could comment later about what recessive lethals in <u>Drosophila</u> really are, and I am sure Abrahamson has some numbers we can look at.

Brewen covered mammalian spermatogenesis and oogenesis. In other sessions we discussed what test systems exist within the categories of bacteria, fungi, insects, mammals, and humans that will be relevant in risk estimation. One approach that has been talked about by several people, and most recently by Sobels (1977), is a so-called parallelogram. One obtains in vivo data in somatic cells from mammals, germinal cells from laboratory animals, and the human somatic data and then extrapolates to the fourth point--human germinal cells. Of course, there are still a number of metabolic problems.

The human information certainly needs to be better. Heinrich Malling and others at the NIEHS are working on developing some systems for human somatic monitoring. Under an NIEHS contract at the University of Washington, researchers are working on producing monospecific antibodies to several human hemoglobin variants (Malling, personal communication). These monospecific antibodies are tagged fluorescently and could be put with a mixture of so-called normal cells and cells of exposed individuals. Any cells that have mutated to the specific mutation (the original ones utilized were hemoglobin S, and they are working now on hemoglobin Wayne, hemoglobin Cold Spring, etc.) would be detected as fluorescently marked cells. The analysis is done on single cells. This approach is far from being available for general use, but it has shown that, in artificial mixtures, the antibody is specific enough that it can also detect cells and is specific enough that the noise level is less than one in 10^{-8}. At dilutions as low as one in 10^{-8} of sickle cells with normal cells, the monospecific antibody does detect it.

WATSON: How does it do that without washing out?   How do you show that a red cell is a sickle cell?   Assuming you have an antibody against a sickle cell hemoglobin, how do you keep it in the cell so you can do the experiment?

VALCOVIC: I am not certain how they bind the fluorocene that remains to the cell and do the washing.

EHRENBERG: They produce a partial flowing out of the hemoglobin--some 20% of it, and they get the binding that way; a small break in the membrane.

NEEL: A hypotonic solution.   They partially rupture the membrane but still their problem is to get down to 10^{-8}.

WATSON: I should think with washing you would just wash it all away, so how do you just add the antibodies?   It seems to be quite a technical feat.

NEEL: It is.

VALCOVIC: It is.   They played for about 4 years with that aspect of it.   They have reached the point now of testing several people around the laboratory who are nonsmokers, etc.   The apparent mutation frequency is no more than one in 10^{-7}.   They are now identifying groups to see whether either chemotherapy patients or others who might have been accidentally exposed may show higher incidences.   This technique may fall down by not being sensitive enough.   Approaches such as this--monitoring humans for somatic mutations--are starting to come now.   These can add a bit to the data from the mammalian systems which were covered earlier.

DISCUSSION

PART 1, EVENING, MAY 15, 1978

HOST-MEDIATED ASSAYS

EISENSTADT: Going back to the host-mediated assay as an alternative to liver homogenate--trying to find creative ways in which one could monitor whole-body metabolism is doomed from the outset with the Salmonella system, as far as I understand it, because the strains that grow best in the peritoneal cavity are strains that do not have the lipopolysaccharide defect in them. They are not going to be very sensitive.

RAY: There are other ways to approach that, of course.

EISENSTADT: When you have used the deep rough mutants, they do not survive very well in the peritoneal cavity. Peter Goldman, for example, has done something rather creative. He did not do it as an alternative to testing--he had some questions he was trying to examine. He was able to populate the intestines of germ-free animals with the Salmonella strains and maintain them there for long periods. He monitored the mutation rates of the organisms being excreted in the feces. I do not know that anyone else has tried to exploit that for other purposes.

I would like to make a few comments about the suitability of liver homogenates. It is certainly true that the way the system is set up now, one is always making a compromise. You do what is most feasible, most easy to do. When it comes to any particular compound that you are interested in, there are a lot of different ways by which you can tune it up. For the purposes of screening hundreds of compounds, however, that becomes very unrealistic. Halothane, for example, is a compound that is totally missed by the Salmonella system except when it goes through the whole body; then you can pick up mutagens. One other example is an N-phenyl derivative of beta-naphthylamine. It is not mutagenic even in the presence of liver homogenate. Apparently, the whole organism can dephenylate that compound, giving rise to beta-naphthylamine. You then generate a mutagen. When you use the so-called bridge between the one test and humans and mammals, it looks promising. The complexities of liver homogenates (of microsomal metabolism) notwithstanding, there is a striking correlation between mutagenicity in this bacterial system and carcinogenic potency in mammals.

VALCOVIC: Unfortunately, mutagenicity in bacteria and mutagenicity in some of the other systems do not seem to correlate well. It has not been as carefully looked at as Ames has done with the carcinogenicity data.

EISENSTADT: But it is worth doing and worth doing well, given the striking correlation between bacterial mutagenicity and mammalian carcinogenicity.

WALKER: Just one more comment to finish that out. Maybe I did not stress strongly enough that Ames chose Salmonella because that was the organism he was working with. From what I have seen of Salmonella and E. coli, if he had started with E. coli, he already would have been in somewhat better shape than by using Salmonella. Part of the function of the plasmid was to catch Salmonella up to E. coli. That may extend the range of sensitivity somewhat. The situation may not be quite as contrived as it seems. I was questioned earlier about whether we have made things too artificially sensitive. The more I work with this, the more I get the feeling you cannot make a strain so sensitive that true nonmutagens become mutagens. It is difficult to extrapolate directly from the bacteria to an organism, anyway. If you are working with bacteria, you might as well take advantage of the genetic handles you have and ask whether this is a compound that can directly modify DNA to give a mutation, or whether it will give you a lesion that can be processed to give a mutation.

DETOXICATION

VALCOVIC: One of the real issues of risk assessment that we are forced to deal with for economic reasons is the detoxication mechanism. In the human systems, we are not going to be able to address this properly for many, many years. Scientifically, we can accept the straight-line correlation of data in a strain of Salmonella with carcinogenesis. For deriving risk assessments for regulation of chemicals, the strength of that correlation is not going to be suitable for the regulatory agencies for a great number of years.

NEEL: In that case, we should go out and get the kinds of data that really are relevant. You spoke about the somatic-cell systems that George Stamm is developing, for which I have great respect. It is unfortunate that he is working with the red cell, which is one of the few enucleate cells, so he cannot really test by the usual genetic procedures whether or not what he is observing is in fact a genetic phenomenon. No matter how much work is done there, you cannot use it for human problems until you have tied it in with germinal rates in humans. When you do that, you can begin to extrapolate from the somatic cell systems. I find geneticists the victims of a talk-big, think-little psychology--always looking for cheap, little ways to solve a very, very profound problem. You have talked yourselves and the public into a kind of psychosis. I keep hearing around this table, "Isn't there some cheap shortcut that will solve this great big problem that we've forced upon the public?" There is no other way but to get at the problem of human mutation rates and then, having related all of your test systems to human mutation rates, you can use them to extrapolate. But not until you have built the right bridges.

ABRAHAMSON: I feel as though we are back 10 years ago in some respects. I think we are confusing two things. One is a screening system that includes everything on our list plus anything else we want to put in there to tell us whether or not an agent is going to have a potential for mutagenicity. The second element is what systems do we use to make risk estimates? If we can use bacteria, then by all means we should use bacteria. At the present time, other than for the kind of potency you are describing, you can really divide that system in half; you can make extrapolations from mammals to humans, and presumably from humans to humans, although there are some who question that. Some of us would even argue that you could use insects and make extrapolations from the germ-cell systems of insects to humans. But that is where we are stuck right now in doing risk estimates. I assume we are talking about quantitative risk estimates.

FLAMM: One of the reasons why we cannot really interrelate the different systems is that, unlike with radiation, we are really at sea with respect to dosimetry. We have done little of the dosimetry that we are actually capable of, although Lee has made an effort, along with others. There really has not been enough of that kind of thing. I would add that we are never going to be able to do the precise risk estimating that we can with ionizing radiation, and I really do not think we have to. In doing risk estimation with ionizing radiation, people are normally correct within one or two orders of magnitude. If we could be correct within one or two orders of magnitude on human risk in chemical mutagenesis, we would have many, many of our problems solved.

As it turns out, we are pretty confident that the potency range on a per-molecule basis is at least 10^6 or 10^7, and we are trying to regulate chemicals over a 10^8 or a 10^9 range. Depending on what program we are discussing, these things can be independent, so we might be talking about ranges of 10^{-15} or 10^{-16}. A range from 1 to 10^{-15} would be from mutations in everyone to only one mutation at that particular site for 10 million years in a billion people--quite a range. When we go from things like artificial sweeteners to various common natural flavors in foods, we begin to encompass very broad ranges. It would be of tremendous utility to many of the regulatory agencies if they just had some idea of what ballpark they were in without the kind of precision that people had been trying to achieve with radiation.

HOLLAENDER: You forget that 25 years ago, when these estimates were made, we had much less information with regard to radiation genetics than we have today relating to chemical mutations--much, much less. Russell had no data at that time. We had some good information on <u>Drosophila</u> and microorganisms, but considerably less than we have now for chemicals. The problem is really much more complicated. We should end this conference with a definite statement of what we consider our estimates of risk. This can be a very guarded statement, very carefully worded. But it does not have to stand for eternity. It possibly will have to be changed in the years to come.

In the early stages of radiation research, we had these same problems. With very little data, we had to make a good guess. I think we should, right now, select the issues that require a definite statement. First, what are the limits of any risk estimates? All we can say is that we can recognize certain effects. If we do not recognize these effects, we can only state this fact. We have to give our limitations. With regard to background radiation, "doubling dose" was at that time very important. In terms of chemicals, we may have to take three, four, or five of them and try to establish some kind of a background to determine what the doubling dose is. This is just a suggestion. Otherwise, we will keep on talking in circles and we will not get anything out of this meeting. We want something very substantial to come out of this, even if it is very limited and shows weaknesses that we will have to adjust later.

ETHYLENE OXIDE

SUTTON (to Flamm): Is there any chemical that you would consider, on the basis of mutagenicity data, a risk to humans?

FLAMM: Yes, right now, based on the evidence at hand, I would say that current uses of ethylene oxide could pose a genetic risk to exposed human beings.

SUTTON: What are the data, what is the evidence?

NEEL: Could you give us the evidence?

FLAMM: One of the first things we have to address is what the human dose is. The human dose of ethylene oxide can be extremely high. It is a very commonly used substance; it is quite difficult to eat food that would be free of ethylene oxide (not chlorohydrin but ethylene oxide). It is very difficult to use a medical device that does not have it. IUDs are often sterilized with ethylene oxide and are placed in an area very proximate to germinal cells. Many drugs have been treated with ethylene oxide. And many workers, particularly hospital workers, come into contact with very, very significant quantities of ethylene oxide.

SUTTON: But exposure to ethyl alcohol is much higher. Now what is the evidence that ethylene oxide is a hazard to humans?

FLAMM: There is a lot of evidence.

VALCOVIC: On April 3, 1978, after discoveries at the Hallsberg Factory in Sweden, the Labor Union Association for Industrial Safety announced its decision to make a nationwide examination of all people working with ethylene oxide. This was caused by an alarm from an industrial hygiene medical clinic in Örebro which suggested that ethylene oxide might cause blood cancer.

SUTTON: That is cancer, not mutations.

VALCOVIC: In industrial exposure, chromosome aberrations.

EHRENBERG: Flamm mentioned the need for dosimetry on the chemical level. If we define the dose correctly as the time integral of concentration in cells--of ethylene oxide in this case (Ehrenberg et al., 1974) or of any other alkylating agent, whether it is primary or secondarily produced in the organism--it is possible in a rather simple fashion to relate genetic risk from that chemical to radiation risk. That is a procedure we have referred to as the determination of the rad-equivalence of the chemical.

   With regard to the Hallsberg story, the difficulty has always been to get appropriate exposure doses of persons; by exposure dose we mean the time integral of inhaled concentration, which should be given in ppm·hours per week or ppm·hours per year. A person working in an atmosphere containing 1 ppm of ethylene oxide will get 40 ppm·hours per week by inhalation. Taking measurements on some German workers where the concentration in the environment, and its variations, was fairly accurately monitored, it was possible to relate ppm·hours inhaled to dose in tissues. From that dose, we can express the risk in rad-equivalents. With ethylene oxide, which rapidly spreads systemically to all parts of the body, you would not expect to have cancer at some specific site. From the data we got, we calculated a collective annual dose to a group of about 100 persons during 10 years of work. We would expect within 10 years about half of the leukemias to appear (that type of cancer has the shortest latency period). Our risk estimate, based originally on bacterial mutation tests, was seven leukemias among the workers--somewhat less than half of which would have appeared. I must emphasize the uncertainty of this estimate, the uncertainty of the dose (a factor of two), and the uncertainty of the risk coefficient for leukemia incidence per man-rad (30 times 10^{-6}--that is, 30 leukemias per million man-rad). With our estimate of three cases, we called a plant working under those conditions we had calculated on, which corresponded very well to the German conditions. We asked, "Have you had any leukemias during the last few years among your 100-person personnel?" The answer was, "Yes, unfortunately, three." The expectation of these leukemias with regard to the age distribution is about 0.1 cases (Hogstedt et al., 1978). Statistically, it is highly significant. Of course, there could still be some other cause, but this is a plant working only with that chemical, sterilizing medical equipment. You do not have the bad situation for judgment that you have in the rubber industry.

We are discussing mutation risk now--the risk of heritable damage. I think this confirms, first of all, that mutation and cancer can be handled by one and the same rad-equivalent per unit tissue dose. At least this might be valid for certain relatively simple alkylating agents. Second, it confirms that risk estimation from laboratory test organisms is also possible with regard to heritable damage with the accuracy we have in the risk coefficients for ionizing radiation. Greater accuracy, of course, cannot be achieved by that method.

I think that is where we stand. There might be some difficulties with regard to the relatively large fraction of the number of mutations which become phenotypically manifested in the next generation. In the case of ionizing radiation, a fairly large fraction of them are due to chromosomal aberrations.

Ethylene oxide is to a very large extent radiomimetic, in that both point mutations and chromosomal aberrations are induced. The same is valid for all those unsaturated and aromatic chemicals detoxified via epoxides. This seems to be a general property of an introduced group that contains a hydroxyl group in the 2-position to the alkylating carbon. Of course, it does not work if you have rapid aromatizations, which you might have with benzene. I would not take this risk estimate to be valid for benzene without correction factors of some kind.

In a way, our approach, as described in my lecture, is unconventional. In the procedures followed by WHO or IARC, for instance, a compound is judged on the merit of that compound only. You need a complete evaluation of just the compound you are going to judge. This approach shows that if you express risk as a function of dose, you could use one and the same formula for all chemicals that are alkylating or transferred, i.e., converted by chemical reaction or metabolism to alkylating agents. Certain correction factors are required for difunctionality and such things, for steric factors when you have bulky molecules. But it is possible to do it, I think.

I think that is what I can say just now about that Hallsberg story. Ethylene oxide has generally been considered, at least in wishful thinking, as noncarcinogenic. Cancer tests, which are rather bad, have been negative. This is the first time that one could predict not only that it was carcinogenic but also to what extent it was expected to be carcinogenic. Epidemiological evaluation of other groups have started and they point in the same direction.

SUTTON: Is there evidence that it crosses the blood-testis barrier?

EHRENBERG: Yes, of course.

BREWEN: Has anyone done a dominant lethal test?

EHRENBERG: Yes.

HUNT: It is enough that the big chemical companies in the United States established a policy that women exposed to ethylene oxide would be removed from their positions. I do not know on what basis they made that judgment.

BREWEN: Is there evidence of fetal wastage in workers?

EHRENBERG: There is one study from Kazan (Yakubova et al., 1976).

NEEL: Was it a prospective or retrospective study?

EHRENBERG: The retrospective Russian study is extremely bad. In 50 control females, there is no spontaneous abortion.

NEEL: For humans, you must get a prospective study, not just a retrospective one.

HUNT: But that does not cause a chemical company much concern when they really want to replace these workers.

NEEL: We are talking about scientific evidence now and trying to provide a firm base for action.

RAY: I should comment briefly on some of the studies I just became aware of also out of Sweden. A regulatory group decided that they would administer $[^{14}C]$-ethylene oxide by two routes, one intravenously and the other by inhalation. They exposed animals, did sagittal sections, put them on a film as a function of time following dose, and showed the distribution of label among the various organs and the duration of those labels staying in those organs. Following doses that ran in the vicinity of 100, 50, and 25 milligrams per kilogram of body weight, which I must admit is a pretty severe dose, they showed that both testes and seminal vesicles became labeled in the period of time from about 20 minutes on up. Testes did clear radioactivity after 24 hours, but the seminal vesicles retained radioactivity. On that basis, they decided they had sufficient evidence to do a dominant lethal test. They proceeded to do the test at those levels and got negative results.

EHRENBERG: May I make just one comment on that?   They got a negative result--that was Appelgren's study (Appelgren, Eneroth, and Grant, 1977) in NMRI mice. If, however, you calculate the rad-equivalents of the chemical doses they applied, and from that the expected number of dead implants, it would be at the lowest dose one and at the highest dose four per female.   Over the studied dose range they had an average of three, if you pool them and look at the first 3 weeks.   Although there was no significance, they got approximately the expected increase. Calculated on the pooled doses, the effect they found in the first 3 weeks was significant.

RAY: Analyzed in that way?

EHRENBERG: Yes, analyzed in that way.   That requires knowledge of the independence of females; you consider the implants to be bi-nomially distributed over females.   If you consider that and make a chi-square test, then it is highly significant.

RAY: The only data available are from the study by Embree (1975) at the University of California.   He fed 1,000 parts per million for 4 hours.   That calculates to about 80 milligrams per kilogram, so the two sets of results are somewhat at variance.

FLAMM: He also got positive effects with 1 part per million.

VALCOVIC: No, 50 parts per million in the micronucleus test.

RAY: That was only one dose in the dominant lethal.

FLAMM: That was somebody else who did it chronically.

RAY: There was one dose in the Embree study and that was 1,000 parts per million.

EHRENBERG: May I say that Embree's studies were done at a dose four times higher than Appelgren's study

RAY: What did you calculate the 1,000 parts per million for 4 hours to be?   Isn't that in the vicinity of 100 milligrams per kilogram?

EHRENBERG: Yes, or a little more than that.   Embree's data agree very well with the same equation for the rad-equivalence that was applied to the human situation.   The interesting thing is that this equation (Equation 8) seems to apply to all forward mutation systems.   It does not apply at all to Salmonella or other back mutation systems, for reasons one can easily understand. This back mutation step does not catch the 30- or 50-fold increase in effectiveness of a difunctional agent--it responds to a difunctional agent by its monofunctional reaction with O-6 guanine, for instance.

ESTIMATING HUMAN DISEASE BURDENS
FROM TEST RESULTS

RAY: To diverge from ethylene oxide for a moment, let us assume that with chemical X we had heritable translocation test data on dose response showing a significant response by any set of criteria that we care to apply.   We presume that mice and humans metabolize this compound X in an equivalent manner.   What would be the steps we would have to follow to obtain some feeling for the impact of that chemical on the human genetic disease burden?   From that package of data and this last statement, what series of steps should we concentrate on to learn the lessons from radiation and from the other work that has been done?   Would that be a meaningful conceptual approach to risk assessment for cytogenetic or chromosomal level effects?   The point-mutational aspects of risk assessment are going to be even more difficult.   If you had those data, would it be reasonable to assume that it would produce chromosome level effects, that it is a heritable phenomenon, that you have some appreciation of the human exposure?

FLAMM: Are you including exposure to the germinal cells?

RAY: I am assuming that you have a heritable translocation, that mice and humans handle the substance in the same metabolic way, and that we know the germinal dose.   What steps beyond that point must we take to arrive at a risk estimate of the impact of that kind of dose on the frequency of human genetic disease?

SUTTON: You must add the impact of the specific mutations.   It has been pointed out that the missed implant is of absolutely no genetic significance to humans. The point mutation that causes somebody to require medical care throughout a lifetime is of much greater impact than a cell lethal.

RAY: I did not declare that the entire result would be fetal wastage.

SUTTON: You put the emphasis on chromosomal changes, and you brushed the point mutations under the rug because they are so much more difficult.   I think they are probably much more a burden to us than the chromosomal changes, which are so gross that they are eliminated.

ABRAHAMSON: Ray is asking what, given the inducement of reciprocal translocations in the mouse system at a given dose, and knowing the dose to which a human is exposed, would be the disease burden? It is that simple.

RAY: Right. What is the impact of that substance?

ABRAHAMSON: But that exercise has been done. The BEIR committee did it; we have done it with chemicals.

SIGNIFICANCE OF CHROMOSOME ABERRATIONS

BREWEN: A simple question to Neel. What is the frequency of newly arisen trisomy 21, which results from a spontaneous translocation in one of the parents and recovery of the unbalanced segregate?

NEEL: Unfortunately, Abrahamson and Brewen were not here when I developed a case for how very poor our information is on the impact of mutation on human populations. A whole new ballgame is opening up as it becomes possible for us to define more accurately what were previously called recessives--the null mutations with heterozygote effects. The BEIR and UNSCEAR committees concentrated on the dominants, but I think these are a very small portion of the total picture. If you are going to talk about extrapolating from anything to humans, first you have to know the total human genetic impact. We do not know that. I would think that this should be a very high priority--to get better information.

ABRAHAMSON: I am not denying that.

NEEL: We sit talking about how we are going to extrapolate to humans when we do not yet have any clear idea of the spectrum of genetic damage that requires extrapolation.

ABRAHAMSON: What is a human?

NEEL: That is just about it. What is a genetic human?

BREWEN: Are you saying that if you doubled the rate of missed segregates out of a B-G chromosome translocation and doubled that contribution to Down's syndrome, it is not a significant health hazard?

NEEL: Who is saying that?

BREWEN: You are suggesting that chromosome aberrations may not be very significant.

NEEL: What Sutton is saying is that if we knew the total picture, gross chromosomal aberrations would probably be making a relatively small contribution to the total genetic load, to use Muller's term, that humans carry. That is not to denigrate that contribution, but in the total picture it probably is small, especially if you take the social aspects into consideration. Even for Down's syndrome, for every fetus that survives there are at least two, I think, that are eliminated.

BREWEN: Eighty percent are eliminated.

NEEL: You contrast that with something like Huntington's chorea--the terrible example we always dredge up--and the impact of a single mutation that results in Huntington's chorea is way beyond ten chromosomal aberrations that result in death within the first couple of weeks, in terms of the cost in misery and suffering to all concerned.

BREWEN: But what is the rate in the population of spontaneously occurring Huntington's chorea?

NEEL: I wish we knew. This is not one of the more frequent mutation conditions, but when we talk about all of the degenerative neurological diseases, they begin to add up to quite a bit. We can now begin to put our finger on specific genetic entities with real accuracy; they are beginning to total to far more than we could visualize even 5 or 10 years ago.

ABRAHAMSON: I happen to agree with what he is saying but that makes no difference. I still will argue with him. If I have Ehrenberg's rad-equivalent, or my "rec," or somebody else's radiation-equivalent chemical value, and if you tell me that at this state of our knowledge this is the human genetic disease burden, and I apply a rad-equivalent value for a given chemical based on a translocation value, I am still prepared to take that rad-equivalent value and come up with perhaps a maximum estimate of the total genetic burden, recognizing that there will be a great deal of uncertainty in it. In other words, I can go from translocation to total genome damage based on what I do know in radiation of how many translocations I will include for a given dose of X-rays relative to how much gene mutation I will include. I will probably come up with an overestimate. I hope it is an overestimate; I would hate to underestimate, as a matter of fact. I can use the rad-equivalent approach to get today's value for genetic disease. If tomorrow you come up with a value that is twice as great, I will proportionately increase it by a factor of two.

NEEL: Why do you feel compelled to do that right now, tonight?

ABRAHAMSON: I will do it tomorrow morning if you wish. I have no objection.

NEED TO STATE COMPLEXITY OF PROBLEMS

NEEL: Now, just a minute. In your own lab you are pretty hard-nosed. We are talking about some major issues. My position is that there are no cheap, easy answers that are not wrong. We might do the science of genetics a greater service in the long run by stating the complexity of the problem and what it takes to get solid answers than by coming up with extrapolations that really do not meet your lab criteria when you make these extrapolations to humans.

WATSON: Do I get you? You would not ban anything now because you see the next 10 years as very interesting for finally determining the rates that you want to determine?

NEEL: Not quite.

BREWEN: But almost.

NEEL: I would certainly be guided by all kinds of screens against the more potent mutagens, but there are a large number of regulatory agencies waiting for quick answers so they can implement policies. Once we put those answers on paper, they get a certain sanctity. I maintain that anything that goes on paper ought to be so guarded, so cautious, in one big, compound, hyphenated sentence, that it cannot be misused. I have sat through 30 years of trying to make easy extrapolations and watching surprise after surprise come up. I had heard that the dominant lethal test was the greatest. Now I have heard all of these questions today about the dominant lethal test, the host-mediated assay, and its extrapolation to humans. I think that our technology has reached the point where, if we get with it, we can begin to get the kind of data we really need. As a professional human geneticist I do not see any reason to prostitute my profession any more than you would prostitute Drosophila genetics if you were faced with a problem dealing strictly with Drosophila genetics.

HOLLAENDER: With regard to radiation, you did it 25 years ago. We had to prepare some kind of a statement.

NEEL: As you may recall, I was a minority voice during much of that. In fact, we have now estimated the radiation risk downward very substantially as compared with 25 years ago.

ETHYLENE OXIDE EXPOSURE

EHRENBERG: What Neel said here about the difficulty of telling in figures what the suffering due to heritable damage really is from one rad-equivalent is very important. Very intensive research is required on, among other things, the possible role of what we called quanitative characters, which could be resolved into something on the molecular level--such as proteins that are changed. For that research, certain exposed groups, such as people working with ethylene oxide, should be used as study material. The annual dose that they get in these sterilization plants is on the order of 100 rad-equivalents.

WATSON: Per year?

EHRENBERG: Per year.

WATSON: Oof.

ABRAHAMSON: That is incredible.

EHRENBERG: That dose agrees well with the radiation dose--about 100 rads--that is causing a significant response in chromosome aberrations or dominant lethals in a stardardized test with mice or rats. On the other hand, in response to your question, one should use the existing risk estimates of UNSCEAR, especially and ICRP, as expected figures, with a note that a lot of things are overlooked and have to be studied further. In a way, it is much easier with tumors. You really have a radiation response in humans--you have reliable epidemiological data--so that figure is much safer.

NEEL: Let me agree with you on two points. First, it is much easier with tumors. Second, there is tremendous potential for studying the children of high-risk groups, such as the vinyl chloride workers in this country, and we have a number of other groups. The study can be made; with new techniques, such as two-dimensional electrophoresis, within a few years you will be able to look at a thousand different protein markers simultaneously. The data can be gotten. But it is going to take an effort.

EISENSTADT: But policy decisions need to be made soon.

NEEL: We should help influence these policy decisions in a sound way, in a scientific way, by recommending how we get the data we need.

EISENSTADT: That would be one way. The other way would be to make explicit what all the uncertainties are, but then to proceed.

WATSON: Let us put it this way. If you were a regulator, would you let people be exposed to ethylene oxide at this rate, would you say I need to watch what their children are going to do with that, or would you just be scared enough so that you would ban it? Is there anything that is so dangerous that you would finally cease being an academic?

NEEL: I might point out that I have been on that firing line perhaps as often as you and have, from time to time, ceased being an academic. As a professional, I am tired of geneticists talking about the big threat and then not having the guts to go in and get the kind of data we need. We talk big and we think little when it comes to action.

WATSON: Maybe you have to do both sorts of actions.

NEEL: Well, if I get that out of this group, I will agree.

ABRAHAMSON: I do not want to do epidemiology on this 10 years from now. We banned tris last year when we proved it was a mutagen in just about every organism it has been tested on.

EISENSTADT: But it took the carcinogenicity data...

ABRAHAMSON: That was also true of AF-2 in Japan. It took the carcinogenicity data to ban it finally. Fortunately, it was in mice and not in humans that they had the carcinogenicity data.

NEEL: You will not hear me argue against that, but you will hear me argue for getting a strong data base as soon as possible rather than pontificating.

ABRAHAMSON: I do not think we are in disagreement there.

NEED FOR MORE HUMAN DATA

NEEL: I have not heard too many plugs for the kind of data that we need.

HOLLAENDER: You are talking just the way Bill Russell did 25 years ago.

NEEL: You are absolutely wrong. I am talking the way H. J. Muller did 25 years ago.

HOLLAENDER: Russell said, "Let's wait 10 years until I have data. Why should we give a general statement about radiation now, because we just don't have the data?" But here, 25 years later, there are even questions as to whether his final data show real gene mutations. He did the best he could under the circumstances, with millions and millions of mice at a cost of about $25 million.

ABRAHAMSON: Per year?

HOLLAENDER: No, about $1 to 1.5 million per year.

NEEL: Look, my track record for putting my feet where my mouth is is pretty clear. I have spent 25 years in Hiroshima and Nagasaki trying to get decent data, and that is not being strictly an academic, Dr. Watson. I was working to get what we need.

WATSON: You cannot have it both ways. Your last speech before I made my statement to you was, "we've got to get more data and we shouldn't stick our necks out and ruin ourselves professionally by suggesting that we have enough data to ban anything." Maybe you did not mean to say that, but that is what I took your statement to mean.

NEEL: You are overinterpreting what I said. But I am reacting to making too many recommendations when the data base is as weak as it is. You should couple your recommendations with the proper respect for how weak the data base is, being very explicit about the uncertainties. The trouble is, if you give a figure to a regulatory agency, they will be off and running with it. It will take a major effort to get a revision in that figure.

HOLLAENDER: It was not so difficult to change the radiation figure.

BENEFITS FROM ETHYLENE OXIDE

EHRENBERG: In the ethylene oxide story, one should recognize two things. First, there is a great need for sterility. This has to be entered into the cost-benefit analysis: what harm ethylene oxide could do and in what way you could replace it. Sterilization of big equipment, such as a heart-lung machine, cannot be replaced by irradiation. Second, it should be possible to decrease the exposure to personnel, especially in the storage rooms. That is where they get most of it, handling the sterilized goods. Epoxide oven operators do not get a high dose.

RAY: This is very true. I think the benefits of this particular chemical are very high indeed. As you pointed out, the alternatives to ethylene oxide sterilization are not that readily evident for many types of work. Among the things that have been suggested is cobalt irradiation. Perhaps with tongue in cheek, people have talked about formaldehyde.

ABRAHAMSON: Cobalt irradiation is used in this country for sterilization of medical equipment.

RAY: We have not exhausted the uses of ethylene oxide. A lot of equipment is sterilized that way. Watson and others are pointing to greater protection of the individual working in those situations; that does not say you protect the individual by banning the substance. You go about it in a variety of ways consistent with your needs--with the utility of the substance and your responsibility toward public health. I very much agree with Brewen that this particular substance should be worked over as an example of how we go about risk analysis. It certainly is a public issue at the moment. All of us here are aware that it is going to require resolution. We should try to get at the concepts of how we can go about risk analysis and structure it so that we can apply the specific information we have. I suggest this because I view the process as more workable with chromosome-level effects. I am not trying to indicate that point-mutational effects are of lesser significance. If you would prefer, perhaps we could make basic assumptions on the evidence of a point mutagen as to the various systems in which it operated and the dose responses and some idea of the exposure of humans to one of those. Perhaps that would be a way to come up with the concepts for risk assessment in a realistic way. I was just trying to structure it. It is extremely difficult once you get to trying to relate these effects to humans, as Neel has pointed out. There is a tremendous gulf there. How do you go across it? That point alone could really consume the remaining time we have here.

INFANTE: But in the interim we need to determine what sets of data you are going to indicate would suggest that this chemical poses a genetic risk. That does not mean that we should not be getting other bits of information.   We do not know how to measure those end points.   We do not have to worry that the environment is going to get cleaned up in the interim.   We do not have to worry that we are not going to have anyone to study.   That simply is not going to happen.   I agree with Neel that we need to find something we can try to measure in humans as a genetic end point.   We need to indicate what data we can use to say that a certain chemical should be looked at as a potential mutagen.

HUNT: Could I have a small piece of historical information? When were the first papers published on the potential dangers of this substance?

VALCOVIC: Ethylene oxide was first reported as a mutagen in Drosophila in 1948 (Rapoport, 1948).

HUNT: I seem to remember--was it in Bar Harbor in the early 1960s?--that they had a severe problem with their mice that was eventually tracked to this agent. Did they publish that at the time? (See Allen, Meier, and Hoag, 1962; Meier and Hoag, 1966.)

VALCOVIC: I do not think so.   There has been an almost totally unpublicized situation in the past few years with sterilization of equipment in the animal facility of Research Triangle Park.   These not clearly defined reproductive problems in the animal facility were probably due to ethylene oxide residues.

HUNT: It is a pity that the mice scientists were not on the ball at that point.

SUTTON: I would be perfectly happy to use ethylene oxide as a model system.   I think it might be instructive to review exactly what evidence we have that leads us to this conclusion--expecially the mutagenic evidence.   We need the evidence that it reaches the sperm, the evidence on metabolism; the mere fact that something is a potent mutagen in the Ames test does not scare me at all.

PRIORITIES FOR IMMEDIATE ACTION

FLAMM: We are not saying that, actually.   In fact, this reminds me of the exchange when Watson said, "Does this mean that you wouldn't ban any mutagens?" and Neel said, "Only the very strong ones."   What we are really trying to do in this conference, as I understand it, is to get a fix on those that we ought to be banning right away.   Our methods to assess risk are going to be crude, and not terribly precise, initially. But we hope we can come up with methods that are good enough so we can eliminate some of the things that are clearly contributing to the human genetic disease burden. For the refinements, for better fine tuning later on, we will undoubtedly need more precise information on mutation rates in humans, involving correlations between humans and experimental systems, between somatic rates and germinal rates. Basically, the regulatory agencies today are trying to assemble the approaches and methodologies so we can do risk assessment. We are trying to come up with something so we can do what Neel said he would do.

WATSON: In relation to banning, we should say those things we should worry about, those things to which we may have to regulate exposure to.

LEE: In making statements about equivalents and hazard, we need to be careful and bring the variance and the uncertainties forward and make that a part of the statement. In practically any of these situations, there is going to be such a variance that it would be very difficult to argue against the value of one thing. Take something of value, like sterilization with ethylene oxide; if you lower that risk by two orders of magnitude, you are then into the range where certainly your alternatives are just as hazardous--if not more so when you talk about cobalt 60. The radiation people came up with a solution some time ago. They simply said that you can make your estimates but then you state that you should lower your exposure to the greatest practical extent; in other words, no unnecessary irradiation of women who did not need to be irradiated. You could say the same thing today with regard to those plants involved with ethylene oxide.

EHRENBERG: That is the statement the Swedish Board of Occupational Health will adopt. You know the permissible level of ethylene oxide in Sweden is 20 ppm; that is 40% of the American level. They are not going to change it with a formulation in those words you used. (The TLV for ethylene oxide was lowered in Sweden to 10 ppm as of July 1, 1978.)

ABRAHAMSON: As low as practicable.

RAY: You are talking about environmental exposure, obviously.

EHRENBERG: Yes.

LEE: Or industrial.

PART 2, AFTERNOON, MAY 16, 1978

CALCULATING RISK FROM EXPOSURE

HILL: Eldon Sutton has agreed to lead these discussions. We want to consider means of estimating heritable risk to humans from exposure to chemicals that have demonstrated mutagenic activity in some test systems.

SUTTON: No, you are already adding too much in. We are starting from zero with a chemical about which we know nothing. We may set as our purpose calculation of the inherited mutational risk from exposure to specific chemical agents. This calculation involves a number of steps, which I have grouped under three main questions:

1. What is the genetically significant exposure to the chemical? This must take into consideration routes of exposure, metabolism of the compound, the integrated dose, the cell stage, etc.
2. What is the spectrum of mutations produced in germ cells? They could be numerical or structural alterations of chromosomes or they could be point mutations. If the latter, is the effect dominant, recessive, or polygenic? What test systems should be used? Which in vitro and in vivo systems are most relevant? Are all members of the population alike in their sensitivity to a particular mutagen?
3. What is the impact on the population as a whole of the mutations produced? Early embryonic versus postnatal effects must be compared, as must mortality versus morbidity. In other words, there must be a cost/benefit analysis for the use of any mutagen.

HILL: We will start at square one. It seems that the

kinds of test systems that are available where we
might want to look at the results of testing would be
bacteria, yeast, insects, mice, and humans.

RAY: Did you mean to leave out human cells in culture?

SUTTON: That is included in the in vitro section. If we
intend to start at square one, I would like to back up
a little and imagine that I am working for a regulatory
agency.   What kind of information do we need in order
to draw conclusions about a particular substance?
Often we talk of calculating the risk and how we
should keep the risk low.   Ultimately, we should
remember that the drafter of the regulation is not
looking at one compound but at a series of choices of
action.   Not to use a given substance may mean to use
some other substance; we are always comparing.   It is
not our job here to make such comparisons, but the
data generated in answering this question must lend
themselves to that kind of comparison of choices, even
though the choices may be unpleasant.   Not to come
up with any kind of estimate, if in fact we have some
information that would give us a crude estimate, is to
make a choice based totally on ignorance rather than
on the best information available, no matter how bad it
is.   We should try to come up with a general approach.   If the results have a lot of error, we should
say so--and not in any sense generate a false confidence that is not justified.
     We have made conservative estimates, saying, for
instance, a straight line extrapolated to zero dose is a
conservative estimate.   That may make a lot of sense if
you are dealing with a single agent that you already
know you can do without.   But if you always make
conservative estimates, you have to keep in mind that
your other choice may appear unattractive, when in
fact it would be more attractive if you gave your best
estimate rather than just a conservative estimate.

EISENSTADT: What is the difference? Isn't the conservative estimate really the only estimate you can use?

SUTTON: The best estimate might involve a threshold, and
a conservative estimate might be an extrapolation
without a threshold.   On the basis of the nonthreshold
extrapolation, you might say compound A has a higher
risk than compound B, when in fact this is not true.

EISENSTADT: But when you have only one point, what
can you do?

SUTTON: I am assuming that you are extrapolating from
more than one point; otherwise, you can extrapolate in

any direction you want. But if your best estimate is low and your conservative estimate is higher, that gives you a very different risk in comparison with some other risk. So we should have all the information and not simply always make a conservative estimate--give our best estimate as well as the confidence in it.

BAUM: If you are starting from square zero, why do you leave out the plant systems? We have heard about very interesting work on barley, and at Brookhaven we tried Tradescantia, which is perhaps one of the most sensitive systems we know, and it seems a little early to rule these out.

PERTEL: We are planning to discuss the test systems per se.

SUTTON: Again, putting myself in the position of someone who has to make regulations, I can imagine that I would want to know several kinds of information First, what is the genetically significant exposure or "dose" (dose in quotation marks because it has been redefined)? We are interested in what is transmitted and in what causes mutation. We would like to know what actually gets into the gonadal tissue so it can do whatever it is going to do. Then, we would like to know what is the spectrum of mutational effects. Of course, the crux of a lot of our discussion has been how to determine the spectrum of the mutational effects. Having somehow gotten answers to that, we would want to know what is the impact on humans. This is where we are probably least prepared at this point to move forward with a lot of confidence. But we may be able to set some boundaries that are useful.

ABRAHAMSON: Do you want two components of genetically significant dose, such as occupational exposure and minimal population exposure?

INFANTE: What is the difference where exposure occurs? What are you getting at?

ABRAHAMSON: Simply that you may not have any real problem in terms of population. You may have only 200 workers in the entire United States being exposed to that agent. In terms of the genetically significant effects at the other level you are talking about, it would be miniscule. But you still might want to regulate the exposure--just like with radiation--so that it would be a maximum occupational dose.

WALKER: Societal dose versus personal dose.

METABOLISM INFORMATION

RAY: I would like to ask about one other component.
Wouldn't it be desirable, if not in many instances
necessary, to have metabolic information? The special
mutational effects can be related to the metabolism and
certainly to the impact on humans as you try to
extrapolate from test systems to humans.

SUTTON: The genetically significant dose means you have
to know what the germ cells are exposed to--that
includes the metabolism. Where are you going to get
that information?

RAY: It seems to me that you would want to know, if
possible, how the animal in which you have the most
confidence handles the compound. You might even
have some information on how humans have been
handling that compound, so that you can make that
comparison.

SUTTON: Perhaps we should list what kinds of information
on metabolism we want--what organisms we are
shooting for. Would that be useful?

LEE: First, I certainly agree with you that the questions
about metabolism should come under the question of
the dose, because that is where you ask what dose
gets to the place of interest. I would suggest, now
that you are an imaginary regulatory agent, that you
require that type of information from the companies
that produce this material. Why isn't it required that
they produce information on the metabolic fate of these
substances in mammaliam systems that are physiologically similar to humans?

RAY: If it is a new substance, that would not be much of
a hassle because the company that is developing it
would be required to produce certain kinds of information. If it is a substance that has been on the market
for a long time, however, and is produced by a
number of companies, the issue of who does the
testing is not all that clear.

LEE: I realize that there are problems there. But if we
could label the compound in various parts, we could
see where its different parts go and their fate in the
animal. You could begin to build up background data
that will help you all the way down the line.

HILL: Are you going to say just "metabolic fate," or are
you going to be more specific?

LEE: Of course, I would want to know the answers to

these questions: Does any part of the moiety complex with DNA or with protamines, what is its concentration in the gonads?

HILL: In the back of the guidelines for mutagenicity testing and the criteria for evaluating the data, there is a section on metabolism requirements that the EPA is putting out with regard to pesticides.

EISENSTADT: That is the requirement to use metabolizing systems that mimic mammalian metabolism?

HILL: This is a section dealing with gaining information on metabolism (that is, handling of the chemical) in mammalian organisms.

PERTEL: We do not mean to say that this is the be-all or end-all. It is more to develop what we really do need; that is, what sorts of organisms and what sorts of metabolism information are needed? All we said was whether it complexes with DNA, protamines, and, I guess, tubulin.

LEE: And the concentration in the gonads. These are the questions that one would start with.

SUTTON: We should list the minimal information we would like to have before we even bother with the next step.

EISENSTADT: It may be worth adding that, by and large, chemicals that tend to be carcinogens for one species also tend to be carcinogenic for many different species. To be sure, that is carcinogenicity, not effects in germ cells. But even though there might be metabolic differences across species, finding those differences does not necessarily help you very much with respect to determining mutagenicity.

HOLLAENDER: Doesn't the FDA ask what happens to the compound in the body as part of a company's application?

RAY: It depends on the compound. Certainly there are other things that you might not think about, such as chemicals for treating animals that end up as tissue residues--they want to know what those are. A lot of metabolic data must be generated.

HOLLAENDER: This is a basic requirement.

MEASURING GONADAL DOSE

SUTTON: But does this present basic requirement specify gonadal dose?

FLAMM: No. That is a critical thing, and I think Lee is on the right track in trying to circumvent getting into all the metabolic steps because it really is not all that relevant to mutagenesis. If you can look at where the action is, you simplify your job by orders of magnitude.

WALKER: I am not sure that your system isn't unique in that you have repair shut-off and you can assay the amount of alkylated damage present in the DNA and have a fairly effective dosimetry. If that were not the case and there were a repair system going in another organism or something, it would be the same as trying to estimate a UV dose in bacteria by following, say, how many thymine dimers are present in the DNA. At least with radiation, you can often put it in with a more or less instantaneous pulse. When you assay with chemicals, you are usually putting it in over a protracted period. If there were continuous repair going on and you based your dose estimates on the amount of damage present in the DNA, you would be drastically fooled--by orders of magnitude, depending on the particular repair system.

SUTTON: That is one reason I put dose in quotes.

LEE: With present techniques with mammals, you could determine the gonadal dose to the spermatozoa, say, in the epididymis. That is a system in which the repair systems are shut off and you have a decay over a period of days, so you could get a cumulative dose for an acute application. Considering dose to testicular DNA, which represents subcells that are undergoing repair, you will get a more rapid decrease, for example, in your alkylation when repair is going on. It is a more a dynamic system.
      Ideally, you would then consider individually the different cell stages in testicular DNA, spermatogonia, spermatocytes, and so forth. That type of work is being attempted, but it is not yet technically feasible-- at least not on a large scale.

RAY: I wonder, really, for the purposes that you intend to use the information, whether fractioning any further would be of that much value.

LEE: I think it would be very useful to fraction it down to the gonia and to get a gonial estimate.

ABRAHAMSON: You are ignoring the female.

LEE: We are ignoring the female because the female mouse is such a problem.

SUTTON: That raises another problem. You mention mice as if you automatically assume this is going to be done in mice.

LEE: I would prefer that it be done in systems physiologically similar to humans.

EISENSTADT: What are some mammalian systems that are like humans?

LEE: Physiologists would be better qualified to answer that. Primates are probably quite close.

EISENSTADT: Marmosets?

LEE: The digestive system in swine is more like that in humans than that in rodents. The Inhalation Toxicology Laboratory at Albuquerque uses beagle dogs for inhalation studies for plutonium (A.L. Brooks, Lovelace Foundation, Sandia Base, Albuquerque, NM 87108).

ABRAHAMSON: They have a long lifetime.

LEE: There are reasons for making these decisions that belong to the realm of the physiologist. If the dosimetry is done right, the geneticist does not have to get into the act at that point. Let the physiologist decide.

HOW MANY CHEMICALS?

EISENSTADT: Is it not unrealistic to hope that you could do that for all the chemicals about which decisions must be made?

LEE: I do not think it is unrealistic at all at this stage.

SUTTON: We have established that we are going to do it for some chemicals.

EISENSTADT: But that is thousands of chemicals.

SUTTON: The last I heard, it was 70,000.

LEE: For every agent that is being put on the market, for example, supposedly it should be required that its chemical structure be furnished along with the agent. The company that is going to produce the chemical would be in a position to label it. In fact, that company would be in the best position to actually do the labeling, if they would do it.

EISENSTADT: That is 5,000 chemicals a year--isn't that unreasonable?

BREWEN: It is unreasonable for the individual investigator, but not for the companies making the chemicals.

VALCOVIC: At this point, we are going along a single,
ideal track, and I think to go on the ideal track is one
thing, but if you are going to ask continuously how
are we going to handle 70,000 chemicals, you must at
that point deviate from the ideal track.   If we keep
mixing these, we will not get any place.   With several
kinds of chemicals for which these kinds of data and
information have not been available, we still have used
whole-animal test systems that measure germinal effects
and   concluded   something   about   the   mutagenicity.
Following the same pattern of analysis with every one
of 70,000 chemicals is not feasible.

EISENSTADT: But the regulatory decisions are going to be
made either on a one-by-one basis or on a class-by-
class basis.

VALCOVIC: There is a very significant difference between
the establishment of guidelines and the review of
individual chemicals that are currently in existence.

WHICH TYPES OF ANIMALS?

HUNT: We are on two tracks here at the moment, and I
think the basic physiologic track would be the best
way for us to keep going.   When we talk of the most
appropriate animal model for the particular system that
we have, is there anyone here who has information of
use to us on appropriate reproductive systems?   We
have used mice until now, obviously, and marmosets
have been suggested.   Is there any other animal that
will help us?

LEE: You could use the males of any mammalian species in
the same way.

WALKER: I think it would be better to take some loss in a
metabolic difference but at least still work with a
genetically tractable organism.   You could end up with
something that perhaps has a metabolism similar to
humans, but then the best you can ever show in that
system is some damage to the DNA.

HOLLAENDER: Stick to the mouse.

BREWEN: You cannot do genetic testing on pigs.

WALKER: But you weaken your case considerably, even
though you have improved it slightly.

ABRAHAMSON: I think I understand their problem.   Before we even get to the human, I think they would like to say, "What have we got in <u>Salmonella</u>? What have we got in some of the prokaryotes?" What do you have in your cheap eukaryote-prokaryote systems? Wouldn't you want to know whether there is some evidence of mutagenicity before you tested every damn thing in what would turn out to be a very expensive kind of approach?

WALKER: I would agree with that.   But that is a separate issue--the metabolic differences that affect how much reaches the gonads, that, I think, is most the important thing.

HOLLAENDER: Yes, stick to the gonads.

SUTTON: We have talked about measures.   What about species?   What is first choice?   Primates?

FLAMM: That is unrealistic, really.   It almost has to be the mouse.

EISENSTADT: As Walker says, something genetically tractable.

BREWEN: You have to be able to do the genetic test in the same organism.

EISENSTADT: You have to be able to do genetics on it.

BREWEN: What good does it do to try to relate a genetic effect to dose?

PERTEL: Just DNA binding.

FLAMM: But you have to have genetic end points that relate to binding.

WALKER: It is bacteria that are the model in that case because you at least have some genetic damage, which is a stronger case than for systems where the DNA is simply shown to be alkylated.

ORGAN SPECIFICITY OF DOSES

EHRENBERG: Lee and I agree completely on what you mean by dose, that is, the time-integrated concentration in the target organ or the target cells.   To determine this, you may classify chemicals, including reactive metabolites from chemicals that are by themselves nonmutagens, into two groups.   One group is chemicals such as MMS and ethylene oxide, which give the same dose in all organs of mammals.   There you need no special precaution with regard to the calculation of the dose to consider different stages, different detailed organs, and so on. The main thing to know about metabolism of chemicals of that group is the rate of elimination--the rate of turnover to nondangerous compounds. The constant is lambda--we could. also measure it in half-life, which is 30 minutes for MMS in the mouse, 9 minutes for ethylene oxide in the mouse, and also about 9 minutes for ethylene oxide in humans. It is essential to know the dose in the body in terms of absorbed concentration at a certain environmental concentration, given as ppm, for instance. It is also essential to know the rate of elimination, which is evidently very fast for epoxides as compared with alkanesulftonic esters. That gives one measure of something that is important to the risk estimate.

There is one thing more about these compounds which we have all mentioned: the possibility that they are converted to other compounds that are genetically active. So you should have the gonadal dose of the compound itself and of each possibly mutagenic species this compound gives rise to by metabolism. In the case of ethylene oxide, you have ethylene chloro-hydrin, chloroacetaldehyde, and ethylene glycol. You should know the gonadal doses of these species. Or else you have experiments showing that the risks from those metabolites are negligibly small, as compared with the risk from the main compound. This has to be considered in the evaluation. For compounds belong- ing to this class, it is possible, through measurements directly in humans who happen to be exposed acciden- tally, to determine the rate of elimination from tissues. You can assume from the animal model that in human gonads you also have the same dose as you measure, for example, in the blood. Another possibility is to measure alkylation of sperm samples--an idea we have played with.

When you come to the other class of compounds, such as vinyl chloride and benzpyrene, you have to determine the relative dose in different parts of the body--specifically, in the gonads--unless you can make measurements on human sperm. For such compounds, it is difficult to get access to the human gonadal dose unless you measure the rate of elimination--the lambda of the reactive species. But it is possible to measure the dose in different organs of an appropriate animal model and also in blood samples from humans. The blood dose and the liver dose appear to be the same for the reactive metabolite of vinyl chloride; they might be different with benzpyrene. The gonadal dose of the reactive species of vinyl chloride in mice is about one-tenth the liver or blood dose. We do not know to what extent this is due to conversion of vinyl chloride in the gonads or due to transport of a reactive species from other organs, especially the liver, to the gonads. One might suspect that if the latter is true--that it is a question of transport--the ratio of gonad dose to liver dose would be smaller in man than in the mouse because of the longer distance from the liver to the gonads. Perhaps one would make an overestimate by using the ratio from the mouse as a model.

There we could at least test the idea with a few important chemicals in pigs or monkeys to get these ratios. It could easily be done with labeled compounds.

WALKER: We are talking here about some basic research that should be done as opposed to what should be done in a more general sense.

EHRENBERG: I do not think this is basic research.

EISENSTADT: You would not want it to be done for every chemical?

EHRENBERG: No.

SUTTON: Other species in special cases.

EHRENBERG: In cases where you expect the dose to be different in different organs, it is important to have it.

HOW LONG CAN EXTRAPOLATIONS BE ACCEPTED?

SUTTON: One of the things we are supposed to do is identify major research areas as opposed to information needed to clear a compound.

NEEL: Ehrenberg has brought up the first of a number of uncertainties that are going to arise as we move across your schema. You are still a regulatory agent. Twenty years from now, Senator Proxmire is staring down your throat. He wants to know if you have really met your trust. With that schema, how are you going to be able to assure Senator Proxmire that you have done your job?

SUTTON: So far, we are only talking about the sequence of testing for mutagenicity.

NEEL: I am not sure whether we have already gone to the particulars or whether we are still talking about the general strategy. I am not quite ready to accept the general outline because I am not sure that you will be able to satisfy Senator Proxmire. Your impact on humans is your projected or estimated impact, correct?

SUTTON: In most cases, I think it would be.

NEEL: So how are you going to satisfy Senator Proxmire that your guesses were right?

FLAMM: The same way we do it now.

NEEL: The way we do it now is not very good.

FLAMM: We hope this will be a little better.

NEEL: Before we leave the general strategy, I think the Senator Proxmires of the world--and maybe some of the rest of us--will not be satisfied to accept these extrapolations indefinitely. Part of your general schema should be provision for evaluating what is actually happening to human populations.

WALKER: We have been this route several times before. Could you lay out the specific details into a projected big plan? If you have a point you really want to make, we could cover it specifically.

NEEL: I have a point I really want to make. It is in the literature and has been for about 5 years. Despite all of the projections you make--and I am all for them-- and all the screening, the question is, "Have you made the right moves?" I believe that at this point you can begin to monitor human populations for changing mutation rates.

WALKER: Could we take a few minutes to lay it out explicitly so it is on the record?

NEEL: I think the procedure is known to most of the people here. One samples blood for some 50 proteins on a sufficient scale to detect a mutational change at some specified level--there it is in one sentence. It can be done.

SUTTON: Would you accept adding an additional item as discharging our responsibility? Such as monitoring of populations.

NEEL: I am ready to subside.

SUTTON: In terms of making the additional step, that does not say that proteins are the only kind of monitoring.

NEEL: Right, other kinds of monitoring as well.

SUTTON: Are there major research areas that need to be developed, as opposed to just making measurements on specific compounds?

FACTORS AFFECTING VARIATION IN TISSUE DOSE

EHRENBERG: In what you refer to as basic science, for some model compounds one should see what the distribution of dose is in various tissues and see what factors are responsible for the variations you have. Could it be the size of the animal? Could it be some other factor such as metabolism in the gonads? We know too little about that.

WALKER: If you could say, for instance, that you have studied several model compounds, and the biggest difference you have ever seen between the liver damage and the gonadal damage is 20-fold, then you could say that in making an estimate on any tissue, the most we are likely to be off is 20-fold. The problem now is that only one or two compounds have been studied, so it is difficult to generalize.

EHRENBERG: We had no measures of the damage, but, comparing the number of relatively stable alkylating agents, which stay for minutes in the body--with half-lives of minutes or more--they give in the mouse the same dose in all organs, including the gonads. They are sufficiently small molecules--not very strongly lipophilic molecules that stick in the brain or where you have membrane-rich organs; they might cause something different. The dose of vinyl chloride in gonads is 10 times less. It has a half-life of 2 seconds in the mouse. If you take dimethylnitros- amine, the dose in the gonads is some 100 times less than in the liver and the blood. The life length of the transport principle, which is the diazotic acid-- methyldiazotic acid--which then gives rise to the alkylating agent, the carbonium ion or diazonium ion, is probably only milliseconds.

EISENSTADT: Not all metabolism goes on in the liver; there might be gonadal metabolism.

EHRENBERG: Perhaps. But then the gonadal dose is 100 times less--two orders of magnitude less.

LEE: What was the route of entry in administering the ma- terial?

EHRENBERG: Intraperitoneal injection.

LEE: It could be picked up and go through the liver be- fore it went elsewhere. If it came in through inhala- tion, it would perhaps be different.

EHRENBERG: It does not disagree very much as compared with inhalation.

COMPARATIVE PHYSIOLOGY OF TESTICULAR METABOLISM

HUNT: Do we face any problems?   I sense we do in terms of comparative physiology of reproduction.   We need to have some better information there.   It is certainly the case in toxicology of heavy metals, for example.   We see vastly different responses when we compare ovaries and testes with respect to lead or cadmium, for example.   It is quite likely that in cases of differential deposition we have not seriously considered the concentration effect in situ.   Whenever we look at these issues, we usually lack sufficient knowledge of the comparative physiology of the animal we are studying.   Where can we attack that in terms of the research needed here?

LEE: I was going to disagree with the majority here about the need for having a genetic system go along with the physiological studies.   I do not think it is necessary. I only want to point out that in radiation a great deal of work has been done with heavy particles by using plastic models to determine the penetration to certain levels.   Obviously, there was no genetic system to go along with that.   We could choose a physiological system for purposes of physiological research and determine the distribution to the germ line without the capability of doing the genetic test on that same species.

WALKER: Could you discriminate something where the damage had been removed in, say, an error-prone repair way, which introduced a lot of mutations but excised the damage, from something where no damage was introduced?

LEE: Yes.   That is why I suggested originally that you look immediately at two cells, one in which the repair system is metabolically inactive and one in which it is active.   If rapid repair is going on, you would, on the initial reading, perhaps get similarity between the testicular DNA and the spermatozoa DNA in the epididymis.   Then, very rapidly, a difference would develop between the two.   You could detect that in a beagle dog without ever doing any genetic tests.

WALKER: Only if the repair system undergoes something like unscheduled DNA synthesis or something you can get your hands on--this is not necessarily the way a repair system has to act.   Setlow talked about this If a repair system puts in one or two or four bases, you would not necessarily be able to detect its activity.

LEE: We are measuring here the loss of the labeled group, usually.   That is the way it is set up, and you can even pick up a zero patch in Setlow's system if you measure it that way.   That is the reason for measuring it by labeling the mutagen you start with, rather than by picking up the repair systems, as Setlow does.

WALKER: I do not want to overdo this.   When studying a low dose, you are putting your labeled compound in, mindful of the possible problems in getting it specifically and uniformly labeled.   It is going in slowly over 24 hours, or how ever long you are using for EMS. There is a certain amount of repair going on continuously that is putting in short patches: you do not detect it by unscheduled DNA synthesis.   It could be making a lot of mutations, but your sum of accumulated damage is very small at the end.   Unless you had a genetic system, how would you be able to detect it?

LEE: You have a system that is not metabolizing, which is the reason for using the spermatozoa of the epididymis.   That has not been included in these systems.   It should be.

BREWEN: I agree with you in principle, but in your elegant talk you showed that you can place no reliance on dose injected into a mouse or a fly.   If you really want to be able to do dose-response analysis, you have to do dosimetry at the chemical level on the target DNA.   If you do this in a species that is physiologically similar to humans, in which you cannot do the genetics, you are telling the drug house or testing house, "Now, when you do your genetic test, you have to do the same exact dosimetric measurements in the mouse or <u>Drosophila</u>."   So you are asking for two species and doubling the work load.   They are not going to like that.

LEE: I think we are saying that.   That is how we do it for radiation.   We measure the dose from radiation in a plastic model of the gonad and then measure the dose to the testis of the fly.

BREWEN: There is a difference between sticking a Victorine dosimeter in a plastic model and turning on an X-ray machine and reading it, in terms of labor and expense.

LEE: There is a difference, but it is worth it.   It is the only way I see that we can get the correct answer.

BREWEN: Ideally, I agree with you.   But in a practical sense I think that we are asking just too much.

EISENSTADT: There might be a chemical that, on the basis of its possible value, you really want to keep, no matter how bad it looked in <u>Salmonella</u> or yeast. Then you might bother to do that. I think many people would agree with this. But it is inconceivable to me that this is an operation you would want to perform on every chemical that comes down the line, unless you had some regulatory decision to make.

VALCOVIC: Doesn't that also come into play to a great extent when we are talking about impact on humans? You have gone to the point of identifying compound X, where in practice the first and second things may be reversed. You will not go through all the metabolism studies unless you have identified that this compound or something about it may have some genetically active component. You would do this in the relevant species in which you are measuring your genetic end points; then, depending on the other aspects of this chemical, you would require detailed metabolic information more analogous to a human situation.

LEE: On the practical question of economics as related to which to do first, I was under the impression that the regulatory agencies are going to require metabolic-fate studies anyway, for reasons that have nothing at all to do with genetics. If that is so, why not simply include metabolic fate? We are asking that when they do that study, they also include testicular DNA and the DNA in the sperm of epididymis. That is an additional two end points in a test already going on, already required.

SUTTON: Under research needs, do we need more general information on comparative physiology of testicular metabolism?

ALL: Yes.

ABRAHAMSON: We should get the oocyte in there, too.

WHAT DOES A CHEMICAL DO AND WHY?

EISENSTADT: Another general area, obviously, would be a detailed understanding of the repair mechanism.

SUTTON: That is the next step. Here we are just getting to the stuff where it does its work. Now let us get to the question of what does it do and why.

As a regulatory agent, I might want all this information, but that is not going to suggest to the companies what they should do first or second. Of course, they could certainly do a lot of this first.

EHRENBERG: You said "recommendations of what companies could do." Do you really...

SUTTON: What I said was that these are things that we would expect the company to provide us with, in effect, simultaneously. Isn't that about the way a regulatory agency works?

ANSWER: Sure.

SUTTON: Were I a private company, I would certainly do the simpler in vitro tests before I got heavily involved in more complex tests, simply because it is a lot cheaper.

HUNT: That is the difference between the way scientists and regulators think.

CLASSES OF MUTATIONS

SUTTON: With respect to mutational effects, several people have come up with classifications of types of mutation, along with various arguments as to how specific chemical mutagens are. One system we saw earlier had chromosome mutations, either numerical or structural, and genic, or point, mutations.

ABRAHAMSON: Nobody ever knows what that is.

SUTTON: There are various ways of classifying individual gene mutations: dominant, recessive, polygenic.

EISENSTADT: You do not want to distinguish between genotype and phenotype? The problem of polygenic and recessive is a question of impact, isn't it?

SUTTON: There is another way of classifying them that has to do with single-base substitutions, frame shifts.

NEEL (to Eisenstadt):   Delighted to hear you use the term phenotype.

SUTTON: I will ask at this point whether we should consider them as alternates in terms of assessing risk.

EHRENBERG: Dominant certainly counts, partly, at least, under structural or chromosomal effects.

EISENSTADT: You are talking about phenotypic expression when you classify things as dominant or recessive. That is not quite the same thing as characterizing the kind of mutational event that occurs following exposure of DNA to an agent, at least to my way of thinking.

ABRAHAMSON: Couldn't you divide those into intragenic versus extragenic, because that is about the best you are ever going to do in many of these systems?

ALL: Yes.

WALKER: I do not think so.

LEE: You cannot put anything past this group.

NEEL: The dominant/recessive bit might come under impact, so you could restrict the definition of mutation to what is happening at the DNA level.

ABRAHAMSON: If you can define it that clearly, but you may not be able to.

SUTTON: What are we going to need in order to go to the next step?

NEEL: Impact gets us to phenotype, which gets us to dominant/recessive, so maybe under spectrum of mutational effects you can talk about the DNA event. Then we will translate that into impact.

ABRAHAMSON: Right. I agree. Neel and I actually agree!

SUTTON: Are you suggesting that what we need to do is to split mutational effects into two steps, one having to do with kinds of chemical or genic changes and the next step being phenotypic consequences?

NEEL: I thought that when we reached the impact on humans, we would have to talk about dominant and recessive. So we can just delay that part.

ABRAHAMSON: That is right. We do not really care about that category now.

NEEL: Right. So your spectrum now is really what is happening at the DNA level--the things you call transitions and transversions and diversions and so on.

WALKER: It is independent of which gene undergoes alteration; the other classification scheme depends very much on how lucky or unlucky you are with respect to which gene gets mutated.

SUTTON: What is extragenic?

ABRAHAMSON: Intergenic refers to deletion mutational events that span more than one locus relative to the base substitution events or frame shifts that are restricted to a given locus.

WALKER: The term multigene is not very clear to me. That sounds like suppression.

ABRAHAMSON: In some systems, you obviously can make very refined classifications. At the higher levels, you cannot.

SUTTON: Let us say that we had reasonable estimates of the amount of mutation classed as intragenic versus intergenic.   Would that enable us to go on to the next step?

NEEL: You are interested in whether you are getting small deletions versus transitions, transversions; so that would come under the mutational effect spectrum that you want to know about.   I am not sure whether small deletions can be intragenic or intergenic.

ABRAHAMSON: The single-base deletion is obviously intragenic.   I recognize that the spectrum goes out beyond the boundaries of a given locus.   But many of the events Brewen was talking about yesterday were deletional in nature and extended beyond one locus.   That is sort of a different ballgame from what is happening within a locus.

WALKER: Deletions and superdeletions.

EISENSTADT: We would focus on something operational.   In bacteria, we can list the kinds of events that are detectable, scoreable.   We could list them for mammalian cells, too.

BREWEN: All you have to do is write them down.   Frame shifts, suppressors, base changes.

EISENSTADT: Deletions and insertions of base pair and frame shifts.

ABRAHAMSON: All of that is called gene mutation or point mutation in higher organisms because you do not have that much of a breakdown.

EISENSTADT: For mammalian cells, what are the categories?   Operationally, what are you detecting in higher eukaryotes?

VALCOVIC: Basically, intragenic and intergenic.

ABRAHAMSON: That is exactly right.

EISENSTADT: Chromosome aberrations.

ABRAHAMSON: That is another problem.

EISENSTADT: But are you detecting things at the gene level?

WALKER: Your criteria for discriminating between intra and inter--is it that intergenic mutations are visible in the microscope?

ABRAHAMSON: In some cases you can actually show that the mutational event covers more than one locus.

VALCOVIC: You observe something at a gene mutational level, as in the recessive lethals in Drosophila. You take the mutant individual and cross it with markers, identifying markers very close to that gene. Depending on the results, you can tell whether the mutational event that was induced was intragenic or intergenic. You cannot go much further than that.

EHRENBERG: In Neurospora, there are possibilities to decide what type of intragenic events have occurred.

LEE: Once we list the basic mechanisms in microbial systems, we then would point out that we wish to extend research to obtain that information in higher forms. In the meantime, you do your groupings as best you can.

MOLECULAR NATURE OF MUTATIONAL EVENTS

SUTTON: One of the next steps we have to consider is what test system we will require as providing adequate evidence on the spectrum. That is one reason why we need to think about whether we are covering all the possible things that can happen with any particular battery of test systems. Thus, we ought to specify the kinds of test systems that are available and what is the minimum that we would accept.

VALCOVIC: Maybe we could do that in reverse, by identifying research needs in this area of identifying the spectrum of mutational effects. By doing that, we will gain some idea of what sorts of test systems are available.

SUTTON: Name your research.

VALCOVIC: Gene mutations in mammals.

SUTTON: Can we be more specific than that?

VALCOVIC: Systems in which it is possible to determine the nature of the mutational event, primarily genic mutations. As Brewen has noted, well over 50% of the specific-locus-test mutants certainly behave as chromosome deletions.

SUTTON: You really mean, "What is happening within the existing test systems?"

EISENSTADT: We could call it the molecular biology of mutation in eukaryotes.

SUTTON: That is basically different from E. coli?

EISENSTADT: There are some interesting differences, very significant ones.

VALCOVIC: Neel has mentioned several times the situation with null mutants. We need better ways of identifying them in experimental laboratory animal systems.

ABRAHAMSON: The research should define the molecular nature of mutational events.

WALKER: Another critical point to decide about chromosomal rearrangements is whether it is a significantly different event that is causing all these effects you can resolve in the bacterial system, or is it just that you need two things that would cause point mutations, deletions, or whatever?

BREWEN: If you look at it in the ideal way, the events are the same in both systems, but all the deletions that we can recover in a mammalian cell, because of existing repetitive sequences, are absolutely lethal when they occur in bacteria. So you lose a very large proportion of your large-deletion mutants. In a mammalian system, you have an opportunity to recover them.

EISENSTADT: I guess that needs to be decided.

ABRAHAMSON: We do not know whether that is true. The target size looks different in our systems.

EISENSTADT: There are ways of detecting large deletions in bacteria.

BREWEN: With radiation it looks as though a very significant portion of them are deletions.

ABRAHAMSON: Not in their systems.

WALKER: But even with the Ames test there are ways to pick up large deletions.

VALCOVIC: Within the spectrum, we have large portions of repetitive DNA.

PART 3, EVENING, MAY 16, 1978

STRUCTURAL CHANGES

HILL: We are going structural.

SUTTON: It is hard to figure out how to assess the impact of structural changes. Having listed a lot of them, what do we do with them? It might be useful, since we have not solved the first two, to go ahead and look at some of the others and then discuss whether there are general ways of assessing damage. Is there a common currency, or do we have to put together each one piece by piece? In the first instance, we are talking about a rec unit, or a rad, or a man-rad or something. In the second case, we are saying that those are not very useful concepts. In the case of gene mutations, looking at intragenic changes, mainly single-base substitutions and frame shifts, where can we go with our test-system information in terms of estimating human load? I think most of us would agree that perhaps the primary effect is going to be on recessives and on the polygenic effects, rather than on dominants. In other words, you might find an occasional one that will cause a clear dominant effect. There is a big impact on the recessives and the polygenes in human populations.

ABRAHAMSON: You also want to include X-linked mutations for whatever they are worth. They make up a small component, but they will manifest themselves as if they are dominants.

VALCOVIC: Pseudodominant category.

SUTTON: That is the group of things we need to try and evaluate. In fact, can we assess with any sort of confidence the impact of those on the population? The presentations by Abrahamson and Neel paid less attention to these than they might have largely because measuring them is so difficult. It is quite unknown whether this polygene is really a large fraction or not. It was suggested that it may be a very large fraction.

ABRAHAMSON: Right now, it is the largest single burden component of the spectrum of mutational effects. Even if it has a small contribution in terms of incidence, that contribution is still going to be large because of the large bulk of that element. It is the iceberg below the water.

RECESSIVE OR POLYGENIC?

SUTTON: How much of that is new mutation?

ABRAHAMSON: Based on the way we handled it in the BEIR committee, we said it has an equilibrium level of ten generations. Therefore, one-tenth of them must be newly arising; that is, the first generation will show up one-tenth of the effect. We say the mutational component will be 5% to 50% of the induction incidence. If you plug in those two numbers, it will still have a very weighty value.

VALCOVIC: The mutational background of humans was discussed by Neel; it is uncertain.

ABRAHAMSON: There are 94,000 such cases per million liveborn, and if you have an incidence of that kind of mutational effect, it is going to influence those 94,000 cases.

SUTTON: Whether it is recessive or polygenic is immaterial. Can we go from those test systems that we have said are going to be our measure to some estimate of the impact on human populations?

BREWEN: You mean can you experimentally test the effect on a multifactorial inherited disease? No. You cannot do it.

ABRAHAMSON: But that is beside the point. If you have something like the rad-equivalent or rec or whatever equivalent you want, you will plug that in and then say, "This should be the contribution of polygenic mutations to the population." That is the way I would like to use your system.

RADIATION RISK EQUIVALENT

SUTTON: Why don't we hear about the radiation equivalent?

EHRENBERG: One may ask, with regard to the heritable
damage we are discussing here, to what extent the
rad-equivalent is needed.   I repeat the information
that we have.   The only factor in the environment for
which we have tried to quantitate human risk is
ionizing radiation.   In the risk equation I showed
(Equation 7), risk of stochastic effects with a genetic
mechanism is equal to dose times rate constant at n
equal to two times this factor, which is for frequency
of chemical changes at a certain nucleophilicity
corresponding to 1 rad times the product of correction
factors.

Equation 8 has been shown to be valid in several
forward mutation systems--in $\underline{E}$. $\underline{coli}$, in $\underline{Mycobacterium}$
$\underline{phlei}$, an organism with a completely different metab-
olism, and in barley.   In barley, it is a question of
mutations induced in the germ line long before meiosis
and which are recovered in the next generation.   In
the mouse, the data agree well for dominant lethals
during the first mating during the first three weeks.
These are postmeiotic data.   There are no good data
for MMS except for dominant lethals.

This product of correction factors in Equation 8
is equal to 1 for a number of monofunctional agents,
such as ethylene oxide, methyl methanesulfonate, and
a range of other compounds.   I specifically do not
mention ethyl methanesulfonate here.   In certain cases
you need a correction factor for that compound--it is a
little difficult to go into detail on that.

What do these data stand for?   The frequencies of
the very few specific-locus mutations so far induced in
the mouse do not disagree with this approach.   What is
of a mutational character in these animals is the tumors
instead of these events, which are all of the structural
kind.   This is what you score as intralocus mutations,
point mutations.

One required point.   Quite irrespective of the
unit you are using, when you go from animals to
humans the target dose per unit exposure dose might
vary greatly from animal to animal, especially with
compounds that are converted metabolically to active
principles.   There you cannot rely on animal experience for a quantitation.   You must have some kind of
direct value from human exposure, which one can get
from work environments, etc.

I thought of another thing when somebody asked
whether there are any other compounds that, like
benzene, only cause structural changes that are
negative as point mutagens.   Benzene is negative in
the mutation tests, but do we know that it is negative
as a point mutagen?   I tend to believe very strongly

that we would find that it has been just below the detection level of the test system.

A related substance, no doubt, is styrene. Many laboratories have tried to test it, and the tests have turned out negative. Yet some laboratories have demonstrated point mutation in the <u>Salmonella</u> test with styrene. So it is no doubt mutagenic, and it probably has the other properties.

In considering population monitoring, I would take the word <u>monitoring</u> differently from risk estimation. Monitoring would measure to what degree there is a dose contribution from compounds in the environment, and identify it. Risk assessment would then follow from Equation 8. On the basis of this equation, we would use the target dose per amount inhaled. The latter, of course, is less to a human than to a mouse, because the mouse inhales more air per kilogram of body weight per minute. We use this equation to calculate the number of rad-equivalents obtained from ethylene oxide in a particular work environment, multiplying it by a risk coefficient and by the number of persons, the time period they had worked, and a risk coefficient for leukemia. From this we conclude that the number of expected cases is around seven, about half of which would appear within 10 years. The found number was three. For ethylene oxide, therefore, this risk expression is approximately valid for humans with regard to cancer.

In the case of cancer, you cannot use the animal tests because of the enormous difference in dose-response curves, in sites. There are so few sites (tumor types) in laboratory animals that correspond to those in humans that one cannot use the laboratory tests for risk estimates. There are certain specific tissues in the lung where you can make predictions from data on the effects of plutonium, but that is an exception.

With regard to heritable damage, I would agree very strongly with Lee that if we use the rad-equivalence at all, we should remember that we are considering end points that are completely different. Only some of these could be called radiomimetic. The base-pair transitions, especially, and other such changes do not seem to be induced very effectively by radiation, but they are by EMS. You suggested that we employ a quality factor. One could include this in the product of correction factors in Equation 8.

I would like to add a quality factor that is a function of the substrate constant, as you suggested. This requires special consideration of compounds with a low s-value. Such compounds preferentially produce base-pair transitions. By contrast, epoxides induce multilocus deletions or intralocus deletions.

A prerequisite for the validity of this is the validity of the so-called A-B-C-W relationship (Abrahamson et al., 1973), which implies that at a given dose to the DNA multiplied by this constant (1×10^{-7}), the number of alkylations in the DNA will be proportional to the amount of DNA per genome. Effectiveness of dose per locus grows linearly with the amount of DNA per genome. That relationship is valid to some degree. Then this relationship has to be valid, too.

Heddle (1978) has plotted the number of mutants per unit dose of radiation against the number of mutants per unit dose of EMS. He gets some points that follow a linear curve. There are some exceptions. One of these is <u>Micrococcus</u> <u>radiodurans</u>, which is extremely resistant to radiation because it has a fantastic capacity for repair of radiation damage, but it lacks the extra repair capacity for mutations induced by EMS. Using <u>Micrococcus</u> for these experiments, you would get a completely wrong value by many orders of magnitude. A similar problem would be faced with the organism <u>Schizosaccharomyces</u> <u>pombe</u>, which has repair capacities intermediate between <u>Micrococcus</u> and mammalian cells.

You must choose standard organisms whose ranges of repair capacities resemble those of humans. This is the case with certain organisms. It is not the case with <u>Micrococcus</u> or <u>Schizosaccharomyces</u>. One should stick to rad-equivalence in dealing with all kinds of tumors. For expressing the risk of heritable damage, you might have to use some other unit.

An advantage of this system is that in a normal health investigation in a factory, you could monitor the dose of a compound and give a risk estimate directly in the environment from monofunctional alkylating agents, or compounds converted into them, at the level of 10 millirad-equivalents per week. This can be improved by one or two orders of magnitude.

SUTTON: The idea of converting to a common currency is terribly appealing, but I am bothered by the problems.

EHRENBERG: First, you need a common unit, because in most cases you have more than one factor in a given environment. You must be able to add them. Second, you need some scale you can easily interpret. If you are saying you would rather discuss the events than discuss millirads, I agree with you. But, third, practically all mutagens have to be considered carcinogens. You have to consider both effects.

Although here we are discussing only the heritable effects, you must also consider the somatic genetic effects in risk assessment and in the means you take to protect the health of the employees or the general public. For these three reasons, you need a common unit. If you could substitute another unit, I would be happy.

I will qualify it still more. You must consider factors in the environment from various sources, both radiation and chemicals. One of the worst problems concerns energy generation, where you have a large number of pollutants from fossil energy and burning biomass whose risk you must assess in comparison with the risks from nuclear energy. This is one reason the rad-equivalent has been selected as a unit.

SUTTON: You do not have to call it a rad-equivalent. You can call it a Muller or an Auerbach. But the damage from one mutagen would not equal the damage from another, depending on what systems you used.

EHRENBERG: We can just group together some of the cancer sites with some risk coefficients per million man-rad. This is from one evaluation I have done considering very low doses and from one evaluation of UNSCEAR. One could group these into digestive organs, pelvic organs, and so on. If you consider each of these an end point for describing the effects, it is easier to use a general unit of some kind.

BAUM: When those of us who work in radiation think of a rad it is more than just a rad; it is a unit of risk. The unit is 10^{-4} probability of mortality.

LEE: Let us consider three systems: changes in chromosome number, structural changes in the chromosome, and the combination of recessive, polygenic, and X-linked mutations. All the latter may share the same mechanisms. When you compare mutagens, the ratios between these change fairly radically. One must either feed other factors into the equation, as Ehrenberg has done, or simply, as I would prefer because of all the extra factors we now have in the equation, compute the risk for each of these three systems directly rather than go through the rad-equivalent. The ratio among the three areas is characteristic of radiation. The ratios characteristic of other mutagens are quite different, of course. The three areas represent different mechanisms.

BAUM: Either that, or build into this risk function a weighting function that has the radiation probabilities in it as well as similar probabilities.

LEE: The equation has become so long that it is no longer a convenience. One may as well go back to the original assumption. Another objection I have to the rad-equivalent is that it tends to mask or even deify the assumptions that went into the risk estimates of the rad to start with. I agree that we may take the radiation values of the risk assessment and carry those forward, but I would prefer to carry them forward within each of these three classes rather than as one uniform statement.

HILL: In the area of chemically induced carcinogenesis, the EPA has dropped rad-equivalents totally and has just looked at the individual expectation at a particular dose--that is, the risk at a dose to which people would be exposed. So there is no precedent, at least in that particular end point, for chemicals.

LEE: Don't you have to look at the risk of different types of cancers? Some agents are almost specific for a particular type. Others are not.

HILL: Yes, definitely. Site-specific.

LEE: This is one reason for speaking in terms of risks for a particular agent rather than going through a common unit.

EHRENBERG: May I say a word about site specificity? For carcinogens like ethylene oxide, which spread through-out the body, you have no prior expectation of any site specificity. (Recent epidemiological data indicate that ethylene oxide causes cancers other than leukemia in other sites [Hogstedt et al., 1978].) There probably will not be any unless you go to very high doses. At those very high doses, which change the physiology, the repair mechanism, and everything in the animal, you then start to get site specificity. That is how this idea of site specificity has appeared in several cases.

ABRAHAMSON: I am willing to accept what Lee suggests and try to make a risk estimate on the basis of polygenic inheritance only. I want him to tell me how to do it. On the basis of our test systems, we have established that we have produced single base-pair or frame-shift mutations in whatever test system we have. How do you want to extrapolate that to polygenic mutation? What is the procedure?

LEE: I will throw it back to you who have written the BEIR report and others. I said before that I want to use the assumptions of the risk that you have used without having to be tied to the distribution. So you come back to the doubling dose that was used a few years ago.

ABRAHAMSON: That is a rec.

LEE: You can apply the doubling dose. I am using the same assumptions, but within a class and not over the whole range.

ABRAHAMSON: We have now established that a given dose, by your definition, produces a certain frequency of base-substitution events, and we know the human dose exposure. We are going to say that that human dose exposure now has a probability of increasing the spontanous mutation rate of that type by a factor of some unit. The doubling dose is 20 times X. So 1 times X, which is human exposure, is going to give me 1/20 of the spontaneous mutation rate. Is that what you want? Am I on key so far?

LEE: Limiting it now to, say, polygenic inheritance.

ABRAHAMSON: That is all I am limiting it to.

LEE: Okay. This is fine.

ABRAHAMSON: We now have established that a given concentration will contribute 1/20 of the spontaneous mutation rate, to which polygenic inheritance is a major contributor. I now know that the current incidence of that disease is 94,000 cases. Right? Given that I have an exposure of 1/20 of the spontaneous mutation rate, I will now take 1/20 of 94,000, roughly 4,000 cases, which now will appear at equilibrium if there is an exposure to that. I will say that in the first generation we will see 1/10 of that, or 400 cases.

LEE: You did it as a class rather than across the board, which is exactly what I have been urging.

BREWEN: That is what we did with the rec, simply did it by class.

SENSITIVE SUBPOPULATIONS

SUTTON: What are we going to do about population heterogeneity? Suppose we have a population in which 1% is heterozygous for ataxia telangiectasia--that is, with a vastly increased sensitivity--what does that do to our calculations?

ABRAHAMSON: I do not think that at this stage of the game you can worry about that level of sophistication. That is my personal opinion.

SUTTON: Half the mutations induced would occur in that 1%.

ABRAHAMSON: I would then say that the other 99% of the population may have 1/100 of that chance, but they still outnumber the others, and therefore I am getting an average estimate of the doubling dose using your basis. It is an average doubling dose estimate.

BREWEN: Does the error of Sutton's measurement on the original mutation rate in the experimental system compensate for the 1% or 5% of elevated, sensitive individuals? Thus, when you talk about a mutation rate and put the confidence limits on it, you are including in that the possibility that it may be the upper level of the confidence limit.

SUTTON: No, I do not think it does, as I have found a group that is very much more sensitive.

ABRAHAMSON: Shelby just reminded me that one other element that was introduced into the polygenic component was a 5% to 50% contribution that is mutationally maintained; this is an order-of-magnitude range. We know it is not 100% contribution, and that would cover the extreme class, which would be the very sensitive one. The 5% contribution would be to the general public. That is about the best you are going to get out of it.

SUTTON: What about the fact that you have a very sensitive subclass? You would have to consider that mutations are clustered in those individuals. They will have a much heavier impact.

ABRAHAMSON: That is like saying that the equivalent dose is not the same to every individual. It is like saying that 10% of a population has gotten a tenfold greater dose, and if you want to factor it in on the basis of a greater dose to 1% of the population, I think you can do it that way.

LEE: Considering the heterogeneity of the population with respect to chemicals, it may be that only a 20-day period in the life cycle contributes a significant fraction of the mutants. If you are dealing with an environmental mutagen, so that the whole population is subjected to it equally, then this does not enter as a problem because it will be in equilibrium. It becomes a problem only if you deal with certain classes of people in the workplace and their reproductive stage in the life cycle. That is a higher order of sophistication, certainly.

HILL: Within EPA, they have said that the variability among individuals within a species is, say, tenfold, and the variation between species is tenfold, and therefore we will take a 100-fold safety factor to protect the population at risk. With a 5% to 50% range, that is essentially a tenfold factor. Until you have identified a subpopulation that is exquisitely at risk, maybe that does take care of it. We know from studies on a subpopulation of people taking drugs that they are at risk from hemolytic anemia because they have glycose-6-phosphate dehydrogenase (G-6-PD) deficiency. When you go into the workplace, where they are exposed to relatively high levels of all kinds of chemicals, the reports of problems in individuals with G-6-PD deficiency have been very limited. TNT factories are among the places where they have had some problems. Other than that, and maybe a couple of other citations, there has been nothing. This has been the one genetic condition in which we have been able to label a susceptible population with regard to intake of drugs, but, backing off from very high exposures at pharmacological levels, we have not been able to identify that these people are really at risk, even in the industrial situation. If we figure in a factor of 10, that may be adequate at this time, until we identify some supersensitive population.

ABRAHAMSON: I anguish with you on the question you have raised. I really think it can be an important problem, but I really do not think we have a resolution for it.

SUTTON: We will ignore heterogeneity.

BREWEN: We are not ignoring it; we are just saying we cannot deal with it.

HILL: Because we have some appreciation of genetic variability, we realize that there may be subclasses, and we should always be aware of them when they have been identified.

SUTTON: It seems this is one of the areas of research needed: the importance of sensitive subgroups due to both genetic and other reasons, such as age, concurrent exposure to agents, etc.

LEE: Particularly with respect to work allocations, because there you can really do something about it. Age or stages of the reproductive cycle; these things are factors that should be identified and taken into account in terms of work allocations.

SUTTON: The conclusion, I gather, insofar as assessing the impact on human populations is concerned, is that while within classes of compounds it may be possible to group risk estimates in terms of the unit concept (rad-equivalent or what you will), some persons are concerned about the spectrum effect and feel that the correction is perhaps more cumbersome than the summing together of the risks of different kinds of mutations.

LEE: That is a good summary.

SUTTON: It is easier to sum together the risks from the various groups than it is to try to combine them into an overall unit.   What additional issues do we need to consider in trying to estimate the impact on populations?   We have not talked about impact per se.   We have talked about how to measure the amount of these effects.   We have not talked about what is the effect on the populations in terms of health, survival, economic burden.   How deeply do we want to get into that?

RELEVANCE OF TESTS FOR GAUGING IMPACT ON HUMANS

HILL: The applicability of any one test system has really not been dealt with.

BREWEN: We have not dealt with the deficiencies in all the test systems.   Unfortunately, Walker and Eisenstadt are not here--they work with microbial systems.

INFANTE: Which test systems are going to be the most valid to make a risk estimate?

SUTTON: You do not expect us to go down the list and say, "Here is number one, here is first choice, second choice, etc."?

PERTEL: I think some of this, at least initially when we are working on a compound-by-compound basis, should be on a case-by-case basis depending on the compound.   Some tests obviously have a greater utility than others for certain effects.

SUTTON: When I tried to inject this earlier, I was assured that the committee had already prepared a beautiful report, and I agreed.   Now, are you suggesting that we go back and evaluate those test systems in terms of how much information they yield?

BREWEN: No.   For numerical, structural, and so-called

gene mutations, Neel has made a very appealing argument. My feeling is that we are lacking a lot of baseline data on gene mutations in the human population. But that applies not only to the type of mutation that Neel has been arguing for, the enzymatic variants, but also to the structural chromosome damage. The last 10 years have seen a tremendous advance in our understanding, in particular in cataloging--a term I hate to use because it implies boredom in the laboratory. But still we find out every month when we go to the literature that there is another human syndrome that is now positively identified with a structural chromosome aberration; up to now, it had not been identified, but now, with the new techniques, it can be. We still lack a large amount of baseline data from which we can begin to make risk estimates. You can go right down that whole list of genetic defects, and anyone in this room could suggest half a dozen criticisms of the techniques we have at hand for making quantitative risk estimations. That includes ionizing radiation. That issue is still not settled and we are 25 years into it.

VALCOVIC: I would think that we have an even greater gap in eukaryotic systems on gene mutational damage than we do in humans. At least in humans we have over 2,000 recessive diseases, whereas in laboratory animals, because of their highly selected and protected nature, we have a very small number of such recessive mutations. Effectively, we do not now have a method available for wide use for detecting such genic mutations.

LEE: You can take the recessive chromosome of Drosophila, mutagenize it, make it homozygous in different types of populations, and see what the effect on viability is--the total effect of all recessive mutants on that chromosome. Or in Habobracon you can do the whole genome, and study the effect in the homozygous male versus the heterozygous female. You can do your heterokaryote work with Neurospora.

BREWEN: The point is that you can do this sort of experimentation in many of the organisms that we use day in and day out. But we do not yet have the concrete baseline data in humans so that we can begin to apply our information.

LEE: There certainly has been work to get that. One can go back to the work of Morton, Crow, and Muller (1956) to see the effects of homozygosity there. Basically, if you are asking what the effects of the recessives are, you are asking what effect homozygosity would have.

ABRAHAMSON: We are even more concerned with the heterozygous effect of recessive mutants.

LEE: Well, yes. The ratio between the homozygosity effect and the heterozygosity effect would tell you a lot about whether it is going to be an immediate effect in the next few generations or one that extends over a very long period of time--the equilibrium time, to put it in your terms.

VALCOVIC: What don't we have in humans? We have well over 4,000 documented cases of single-gene mutation recessive diseases. Are you saying we do not have any induced cases in humans?

BREWEN: That is right, and we do not know the spontaneous frequency of these recessive diseases in humans with a great deal of accuracy.

VALCOVIC: What do you anticipate is the probability that we will ever be able to obtain such data?

BREWEN: Do you want a number? I can give you one.

VALCOVIC: Given the total number, given the generally accepted spontaneous mutation frequency, the total number of genetic loci, and the total number of gametes that one may sample in the human population, what is the probability that one would ever ascertain with any degree of frequency the new mutational level?

SUTTON: When you say "spontaneous occurrence," are you talking about mutation or just simply the frequency of these rare diseases?

VALCOVIC: Are you talking about incidence or mutation rate?

BREWEN: I am talking about mutation rate.

SUTTON: We do not have incidence, either. We do not have the incidence of homozygotes.

VALCOVIC: Without going through the calculations, one probably needs a number of new births per year in the neighborhood of 200 to 300 million--I do not think one is going to find that--in order to get reliable data.

SPONTANEOUS MUTATION RATES FOR HUMANS

HILL: Are we at a stage where we can say from testing that a chemical is potent or is not very potent? Is there evidence with regard to mutagenicity saying that it takes a small or a large dose to produce mutations in test systems? Can we get a statement with regard to relative potency of various chemicals? If yes, can somebody run around in a factory, run around out in the environment, and say that the exposure is some level, that the individuals or workers are exposed to this chemical at a certain level? Can one then combine the information on potency and exposure and come out with a risk estimate? You know what it is in your control animals, don't you?

ABRAHAMSON: Usually you have some estimate of current incidence of disease. That is one thing you do have.

HILL: Incidence means the number of new cases in a given period of time.

PERSON: And it does not reflect mutation frequency.

ABRAHAMSON: You do have a range of spontaneous mutation rates for humans. That was the figure I gave in my presentation: 0.5×10^{-5} to 0.5×10^{-6}. Current research will improve on those numbers, but that is the range you are stuck with. There is no way you can develop a new one right now. That is the range that you have.

HILL: How about in 15 years?

PERTEL: How much is it going to change?

ABRAHAMSON: I do not care whether it changes or not; that is the number you have. That is the number Brewen is saying we do not have, and I am saying that is the number we are stuck with. If you ask me what is the relative potency of the drug or chemical or thing, we do have that incidence in experimental animals and we can extrapolate it. We are going to have a spontaneous incidence or spontaneous mutation rate in human per locus, and we are going to have an induced rate per unit dose for the experimental system. That is how we got the doubling dose in the first place.

BREWEN: Within an order of magnitude.

ABRAHAMSON: Within an order or two of magnitude.

HILL: The way EPA is dealing with carcinogenicity information is to say that there is some risk associated with exposure to the chemical over and above whatever that control rate is. In other words, that delta is added to the control rate. I do not give a doggone what that control rate is; it can be 10^{-6}, 10^{-8}, 10^{-5}--does it really matter? What you are doing is adding on an amount to whatever that background is. That is the risk; that is the change. That is the amount of risk you are contributing to the next generation because of exposure to the chemical. Is that the number you want? I do not know.

ABRAHAMSON: That is the number we use.

LEE: No. You used the doubling, didn't you?

ABRAHAMSON: When you ask me to give you the doubling dose, I put spontaneous incidence on the top of the equation and induced rate on the bottom.

LEE: You are saying spontaneous is not important.

HILL: I am asking whether it is.

ABRAHAMSON: As long as you have a number, that is all that he wants. I have just given you the number, because that is the number you have.

DOUBLING DOSE AND RISK ESTIMATES

LEE: There is a philosophical difference here as to whether you start out when you can know the delta above or whether you start out with the idea of the term being the relative increase over what you are already getting. This is a very different philosophy from the history of radiation genetics. Genetics starts out with the idea that any increase in the mutation frequency is harmful, and therefore we measure the relative increase in the frequency in estimating risk. This is going back many years, I realize.

ABRAHAMSON: What do you think the doubling dose is? That is what you are defining. It is the inverse of the doubling dose that is the risk per unit dose exposure of the population. That is what you are dealing with. Doubling is one way of getting to it. Invert the equation and you have the other element that you want. It just happens to go through a doubling-dose concept.

HILL: But do you have to?

ABRAHAMSON: No. Put 1 over the doubling dose in the equation to obtain the effect per unit of mutagenic dose. I am saying that if you want induced rate per locus per concentration (dose) over spontaneous rate, which is 10^{-5} to 10^{-6}, rounded off that is the value you are interested in. That is the inverse of doubling dose. You need the denominator I showed, because this is the human genome. You are interested in estimating human risk. If you want a mouse genome rate, you can put it in and decide to extrapolate a mouse-induced rate to a mouse spontaneous rate to humans. I am not in favor of that. Obviously, we would like a value in humans. We cannot get this value in humans yet, so we use the organism or system that we do have that is nearest to humans; that is the animal rate. We apply the human spontaneous rate and assume we are at least halfway to the answer. It is not going to be too different, if it is a mammalian system in which we are· establishing this, whether it is somatic or germinal.

BREWEN: Naive as it may sound, a great deal of concern has been expressed over the years about doubling the frequency of our mutational load. Abrahamson's equation says that we have room to increase it by one log and not even detect it. If we are so concerned about doubling it or tripling it, why are we not concerned about a one-log difference that we would never know existed?

ABRAHAMSON: The equation says you have a one-log difference. That is the range that we have in terms of the spontaneous mutation rate. You improve one range and you improve the value.

BREWEN: That is all I said; I would like to see that improved.

SUTTON: It is not obvious why this rate is important. It is historically important because you could establish the doubling dose in mice, you could establish the ratio in mice, and then apply the ratio to a different species.

ABRAHAMSON: That is not what we did; we never did that. We always took the spontaneous rate in humans and divided it by the induced mouse rate. That was the way in which we established doubling dose. When you turned that equation over, it gave you the effect per unit rad. This is X-rays; I hate to throw X-rays in, but that is how it was done. You are going to do the same thing with your chemicals. This inverted system gives you the effect per unit dose of the chemical. Because I want it in humans, that is the end point I am looking for.

SUTTON: That comes out expressed as a fraction of the spontaneous rate. Why not express it as so many people per million?

ABRAHAMSON: As you well know, mutants per million

provides no estimate of human harm. I do not know what a human mutant is in terms of its incidence of harm or in terms of human disease burden. I can go from there to disease burden by saying that if the value I now calculate--one unit of concentration--is going to increase the rate by 1/20, or 1/100, or what have you, I now have that current incidence of disease. I am going to plug it into the appropriate place that Lee is asking me for. That is all I want to do; that is all you want me to do.

VALCOVIC: Mutational mechanism is not easily translatable to...

ABRAHAMSON: Harm.

VALCOVIC: Phenotype.

ABRAHAMSON: That is precisely right. You can tell me you induced 10,000 new mutants in the human population and I do not know what to do with them as mutants. I do know what to do with them in that current incidence of disease.

LEE: This is the reason why mutagenesis developed along different lines from the carcinogenesis matter, where you deal only with the numerator. In carcinogenesis, you have an end point in terms of human deaths.

BAUM: The absolute risk is the one you concentrate on.

ABRAHAMSON: The relative risk gives you a two- or threefold greater value. When you look at relative risk figures, which is what the BEIR committee report primarily is about, the risk estimates for carcinogenesis are much greater than when you look at absolute risk values.

HILL: We can look at something like structural chromosome aberrations that brought an estimate of 2×10^{-4} as the spontaneous incidence. At this time, that can be somewhat easily converted into some sort of load, some sort of disease burden, can't it?

ABRAHAMSON: That is right. In that one category.

HILL: In that particular instance, we do not have to diddle with spontaneous background, do we?

FREQUENCY OF BALANCED TRANSLOCATIONS

BREWEN: We do not know. That is the whole point. It is one of the points I made when I talked about it. We are given a figure of 2×10^{-4} spontaneous balanced translocations with liveborns, and I maintain it could be as high as 10^{-3} because of our detection techniques. If I do an experiment in an organism like the mouse, where I have 95% confidence that I can detect a translocation, how do I translate that into the effect on a population in terms of recovered translocations when the true spontaneous rate is unknown? What you have to do is accept a 400% error.

ABRAHAMSON: Your level of spontaneous incidence today for balanced translocations in 1 or 2×10^{-4}. You have a suspicion that it might be as high as 10^{-3}. Until that suspicion is verified, I am going to use 10^{-4} because it is the only number I have.

BREWEN: No. I can tell you that 2×10^{-4} is incorrect just based on the fact that that number was determined by karyotype analysis of cord blood of newborns. In a fertility clinic they do a somatic chromosome karyotype analysis and pick up approximately 40% of the balanced translocation carriers in the male population when compared with a meiotic chromosome analysis.

ABRAHAMSON: But you are looking at a very specialized ascertainment problem. You now are going into a group that is medically deranged in some way, or disturbed. It is like going into the criminal population.

BREWEN: Wait a minute. Everyone who carries a balanced translocation has a fertility problem; it is simply a problem of the efficiency of detecting it by cytogenetic means.

ABRAHAMSON: I do not know where you are coming from again. If you want to change the current incidence, I am happy. Give us a value.

BREWEN: If you carry a balanced translocation you are in all probability a semisterile. That goes for mouse and human alike. If you go to a fertility clinic and you look at the male population that comes in, and you analyze them karyotypically, somatic chromosomes, you pick up an incidence of translocation carriers. If you then take a testicular biopsy, you triple the incidence of translocation carriers based on translocation configurations at meiosis. The incidence in liveborns, which is determined by somatic chromosome analysis, is off by at least a factor of three or four.

ABRAHAMSON: Then apply that. That does not bother me. Brewen is trying to say that the testicular biopsy has a better ascertainment level than does analysis of the cord blood, and I accept that. If he is telling me that the current incidence of balanced translocations is off by a factor of three, then apply the factor of three. That is no great problem. Pat Jacobs said that her risk estimates were probably underestimated by 75%. We applied that correction factor.

RISK ESTIMATES SUBJECT TO CHANGE

LEE: I know you know you are doing this: you are taking the best value available and, as you say, applying it. If one carries the variance of each of those values along through the whole calculation, it becomes very disturbing. The philosophy developed many years ago was that alteration in the mutation rate as it has evolved, whatever it is, is a disturbing thing. This is perhaps a very good philosophical basis to come back to. Consequently, if you are wrong--and you may well be--in your absolute calculations, your calculation that a certain substance is a high risk, or medium risk, or a low risk on the basis of this would not be too greatly off. In other words, the relative risk of certain compounds, as long as they are within the same class (that is, causing the same types of events), may be accurate, even though the error on the absolute value may be quite large.

ABRAHAMSON: I do not think we have any disagreement there. Nobody ever asked that a risk estimate be engraved in stone. All we are doing is making the best possible estimate with the information available today, not in Neel's terms of 10 years from now. Ten years from now I will be happy to modify that risk estimate if you give me better information. That is all I am trying to do.

VALCOVIC: Some have argued that mutagenicity testing is not validated because we do not have a human mutagen. Edinburgh attendees will remember that carcinogenicity testing in laboratory animals is okay because we have human carcinogens.

ABRAHAMSON: I disagree. We do have human mutagens-- X-rays are one of them. You can show chromosome aberrations induced...

VALCOVIC: Point-mutation mutagens.

BREWEN: You have not found one in the mouse yet, either, so do not worry about it.

VALCOVIC: Procarbazine is pretty good.

HILL: HGPRT.

BREWEN: That is somatic.

ABRAHAMSON: When you point to a child that has a genetic defect, you can always say there are many other
possibilities that may have caused it. That is begging
the issue. I do not accept that argument.

VALCOVIC: The argument is that mutagenicity cannot be
incorporated as a portion of the regulated aspect of
toxicological phenomena until such time as there is a
clearly demonstrated induced point-mutation mutagen.
This is a real question. As Abrahamson said, because
of what all of us understand about DNA and mutagenesis, because of the number of genes, the spontaneous level, and the number of occurrences that one
might see of a particular type, it is always very easy
to reconcile that it could have been a spontaneous
occurrence. That sounds like a very trite kind of
thing to a geneticist, but it is an argument that has
been put forth.

ABRAHAMSON: You could have raised that argument before we started here. We could have disbanded if that
is the argument that is going to rule the day. It is
obviously one that we are not going to accept. That
is a platitude as far as I can see.

BREWEN: Then rely on structural chromosome aberrations
because we do have a lot of mutagens for humans in
that respect. Sutton and Neel, who is not here,
would get upset with that decision.

LEE: I would, too.

DATA TO IMPROVE RISK ESTIMATES

SHELBY: I wonder if Abrahamson could take a few minutes
to make some specific suggestions as to what kind of
data could improve the risk estimation that comes from
the equations we have seen.

ABRAHAMSON: I do not think, unless Neel is really going
to turn the world upside down, that you are going to
get a better estimate of the...

SHELBY: Denominator.

ABRAHAMSON: ...of the denominator.

SHELBY: Of the numerator then; that is where we can
fund and support research.

ABRAHAMSON: That is precisely right. The best estimates are going to come from the higher organism systems.

SHELBY: I am asking for specific data that you want in order to improve that risk estimation.

ABRAHAMSON: Do not put me in the position of God; obviously, I would like germinal mutations in mammalian systems. I do not think I am going to get them. I would be delighted to settle for good estimates and good dose/frequency relationships for mammalian somatic cells at this time.

SHELBY: In vivo.

ABRAHAMSON: I do not know whether I can get them in vivo, but, if I can, that would be fine.

QUESTION: How do you relate that to the germinal...

ABRAHAMSON: I am prepared to make extrapolations.

BREWEN: You cannot do it with chemicals.

LEE: You can do that with radiation because there is only this order of magnitude difference between the germ-cell stages. But when you get to chemicals, some or all...

ABRAHAMSON: Remember that I am dealing with two metabolically active cells. I am dealing with a gonial cell and I am dealing with a metabolically active...

SUTTON: That is the key to this entire meeting.

FEW EVENTS RECOVERED IN GONIAL CELLS

BREWEN: That is the key. One of the big points about chemical mutagenesis is that they have yet to recover a significant number of mutational events from spermatogonial cells. Where they are recovering them is in the metabolically inactive cells.

LEE: Yes, where the things have been turned off.

QUESTION: Are you trying to say that one mutation in a somatic cell equals one mutation in a germ cell?

ABRAHAMSON: I did not say that I would go that route. I said I would extrapolate. But I would have to build in certain extrapolation bridges.

QUESTION: What are the bridges?

BREWEN: One of them at this point is infinity. Because the mutation rate in spermatogonial cells is infinitely lower than it is in late spermatids and spermatozoa with practically any chemical that has been looked at, it is infinity.

LEE: That is true even in germ-cell stages, where you have a great deal more sensitivity than in the mouse.

ABRAHAMSON: Then tell me the test system you want.

LEE: Fly. Vogel has a whole series of things. This is very serious. The differences are so great that one has to make estimates in different germ-cell stages. This is an essential part of the numerator in Abrahamson's equation.

ABRAHAMSON: But if you do not have that value and you do not have it out of the mouse, then I want to get some way of getting to it in the mouse.

BREWEN: We should start looking.

VALCOVIC: This is what Malling and I are developing in the mouse (Valcovic and Malling, 1973). The kinds of systems that do not have quite the uncertainty and at least have the capability of molecular follow-up that is not available in the classical specific-locus systems. Granted, that system has developed more slowly than I had hoped.

ABRAHAMSON: But that is exactly where we are with Neel, also. I have to make the risk estimate, today, on the basis of some system. I will use Drosophila in the risk estimate.

VALCOVIC: The question is where do we go, not what do we do today.

ABRAHAMSON: I will use Drosophila and try to see how I can extrapolate via the mammalian non-germ-line if I have to. And I will have some fudge factor in there; most of you will jump all over me about it, but it will still give me some element of risk.

TEST A FEW COMPOUNDS ON MANY MICE

LEE: I want to make one comment about the germ-line data in the mouse. We could get that kind of data for, say, four or five model compounds and get those same data in the germ cells of the fly and perhaps other systems. I would not be at all surprised if we were able to make for many classes of compounds a good enough comparison to calibrate our fly and other sub-mammalian systems with a mammalian system so that we could make very good risk estimates on the basis of, say, the knowledge (for an alkylating agent) of the distribution of the alkylating sites, the s-value, the response in the different germ-cell stages in the fly, and calibrations between similar systems and the result in the mouse. But we do not have these data to calibrate with in the mouse. One of the great disappointments to me is that when the mouse people went into chemical mutagenesis, instead of doing the type of experiments they did with radiation, they decided to test all these many compounds with very small numbers. It does not work that way. You have to do the kind of experiments that you did with radiation on a relatively few compounds.

EHRENBERG: These compounds should be selected very carefully to be good models.

ABRAHAMSON: If you ask me what I want to see funded, I would fund a tris experiment, because that is one of the best environmental mutagens that we know has been in the marketplace.

QUESTION: In the Russell test?

ABRAHAMSON: No. I would do it on an enzyme system analysis.

LEE: I think the Russell test should be used, too.

ABRAHAMSON: And do an embryo spot test. Why not do them both together in the same system? Do everything you can get.

BREWEN: Look at every type of mutation--numerical, structural, so-called point mutations, if you want to put quotation marks around specific locus. Do them all.

PERTEL: All in one animal.

ABRAHAMSON: I can tell you that tris produces sex-linked recessive lethals. It produces translocations in the germ line of Drosophila.

VALCOVIC: Procarbazine is another interesting compound.

SHELBY: In the biochemical specific-locus test, we have data on one compound, triethylenemelamine. In the Russell morphological specific-locus test, which has been around for 25 years, we have marginal data on ten compounds. We have good data on one or two compounds. Why is this? These are the data that people keep turning back to again and again. You ask why, and they say because it is an expensive endeavor. It costs less; it costs a fifth of what it costs to run a carcinogenesis bioassay--even to screen 50,000 offspring.

BREWEN: The problem is that after they screened 5,000 and found no mutations, they put a 95% confidence interval on it and said, "It is not higher than the spontaneous rate; shut the doors on that animal room, and let us go to compound Q."

ABRAHAMSON: We are talking about Russell's program.

BREWEN: Russell's specific-locus test.

SHELBY: This is what Abrahamson mentioned that he would like to have data on to improve his risk estimates.

MORE WORK NEEDED ON GONIAL CELLS

ABRAHAMSON: We have said that if we had the right
   systems, we might have some index of harm or human
   detriment associated with these elements.   We argued
   about how we go to a risk estimate for humans.   We
   finally agreed that one approach would be to use the
   doubling-dose concept and get per unit concentration
   of effect; then we would apply this to the current
   incidence of genetic disease for this category of
   polygenes and recessives as best we could.   One area
   that concerned both Lee and Brewen very much was
   the fact (and I think this becomes part of where we
   need to go for more useful research) that we have not
   yet gotten mutation rates out of gonial cells, either
   Drosophila or mouse; these are critical.   One major
   effort on these two systems should be either to find
   the mechanism for this or to get a very expansive set
   of data (which I think was Lee's point) with a few
   critical chemical mutagens.   We are not dealing with a
   case of just too small a number base to work from.   In
   outlining research needs, this would be one area of
   great concern--getting good test systems.   This would
   include the electrophoretic approach, the biochemical
   mutants in spermatogonia, and perhaps the specific-
   locus test system, but expanded to 200,000 cells to be
   looked at under these circumstances so that one could
   establish whether or not there is a frequency to be
   used there.
      I think we agree that this is critical.   If you try
   to make risk estimates for humans, that is one of the
   two germ-cell stages of great concern.   You can make
   risk estimates on the other stages, as Lee pointed out
   yesterday, but they are not going to accumulate much

harm (except for the exposure). They are not stem-cell populations as the gonial cell population is. They are not long-term cell stages, I should say, as in the oocyte. The total amount of harm would be rather small relative to the two stages that most concern us. Am I expressing that in about the way you would like to see it?

BREWEN: No, I would disagree with that last point. With some systems it may well be that the major contribution to human hazard will come from one of these short stages. Consequently, I would like to see included in the test a measurement of these postmeiotic stages that no longer have repair, weighted according to their shorter time.

ABRAHAMSON: I assumed that was implied in what I was saying. We can already get that kind of mutation-rate data.

LEE: We do not have it in the mouse with a series of chemicals comparable at the specific-locus point. The electrophoretic variants and so forth are still for the future. I have heard that one set of data is coming out of the National Center for Toxicological Research soon, but it is very new material. So we need all stages, I would say.

ABRAHAMSON: We need the weighting factor.

BREWEN: We may apply a weighting factor, which means you do not need 200,000 in the postmeiotic stage if you have 200,000 in the gonial stage. But you do need all stages weighted according to their respective lengths of time in humans. We also need a better estimate of the length of time of each of these stages in humans because that will be the weighting factor. We have data on that, but the data should be presented in this way by those expert in that area.

STAGE SENSITIVITY

ABRAHAMSON: Let us assume for a moment that that kind of data base will exist and that, in fact, we still will not observe significantly increased mutation rates from gonial cells. If one of Brewen's models is correct, the sensitive component of that stage will not be there long enough to get much of a dose to it, or the system repairs itself almost effectively by dealkylating the nucleotides that have been alkylated in the first place.

PERSON: Either that, or you have a situation of 99.9% cell lethality.

ABRAHAMSON: Any one of these situations could apply.
    Therefore, when you do measure a mutation rate, you
    do not find anything above control.   You are left with
    essentially negative data for a critical stage.   You will
    have positive data that you will weight, but these will
    not contribute much in the way of mutation to the
    human genome.   What, then, do you do?   Do you have
    an expression of risk?

LEE: You said that that much is not important, but it
    could be very important.

ABRAHAMSON: That is one possibility.   There is no prob-
    lem if you have a very important mutagenic component
    to it and then have a reasonable risk estimate.   You
    have essentially a series of test systems that have
    been run through the guidelines, and these things
    have come up positive across the board until you get
    to mammals.   There you have no mutations in the
    spermatogonial population (or oocyte population if you
    have done it there as well), and in the postmeiotic and
    meiotic germ-cell stages you have an insignificant
    component.   You will now be faced with a very critical
    decision, as I see it.   How do you weight the two sets
    of data?   That is the main point that should be
    discussed. At this point you can make a risk estimate,
    saying that there is essentially a very small probability
    of harm to the human population on the basis of the
    mammalian results, although, based on the other
    evidence, we have a reasonable probability of damage
    in everything else that we see.   You cannot make a
    risk estimate on that basis--you have two different
    levels.   Do you agree with what I am saying?

BREWEN: Correct me if I am wrong.   My impression is
    that with radiation they do recover mutations from
    postmeiotic stages.   In the attempt to establish an
    upper limit, they took into consideration that the ratio
    of mutational events recovered between the postmeiotic
    stages and the stem cell in the male was not sufficient-
    ly high to warrant disregarding the gonial stages.   In
    other words, the time of contribution over the repro-
    ductive lifetime was so many orders of magnitude
    greater by the stem cell than by the postmeiotic stages
    that this is the one you worry about.   We are saying
    now that we have the reverse situation.   Even if you
    get a small effect in the postmeiotic stages, that may
    be a very significant contribution to a health hazard.

ABRAHAMSON: That may be one possibility.   In the case
    of the mouse gonial versus mature germ cells, the
    mature cells are twice as sensitive as immature cells.

Here you may have ratios of 100:1, where the post-meiotic cells may be 100 or 1,000 times more sensitive than the gonial cells. You weight that relative to the duration of those stages, which cannot be much more than 50 to 60 days. The whole gonia to mature sperm cycle is in the range of 100 days.

LEE: The spermatogenic cycle, measured by equilibrium time in the thymidine experiments, was 75 days. That point does need to be determined. It would be somewhere between 17 or 18 to 25 days for the period of the midspermatid on. This is the period of great sensitivity when you no longer have the repair systems going. I have discussed this with Gladhill. I do think that type of thing needs to get worked out by those who are expert in the field and put into the record because it is an important thing.

ABRAHAMSON: But those data are readily available.

LEE: They are available, but they need to be presented from the existing data base.

PERTEL: Would it be possible for somebody to work this up?

LEE: I would suggest Gladhill.

ABRAHAMSON: I have attempted to summarize where we are and what problems we face with respect to the kind of thing we will see in terms of data. Now where do we go?

LEE: There is a way out of your dilemma that would, in a sense, put the burden of proof on those who wish to establish a license for a compound. Suppose you find that a substance is mutagenic, say, in late spermatid and spermatozoa in the fly. If an experiment of reasonable size shows that that stage in the mouse is also sensitive to mutations, then you can estimate the component to human hazard that that would contribute by weighting with that short cell stage. The type of experiments that are usually done would have detected a positive effect in the gonial stage if there were only an order of magnitude difference.

In most of the results that come out of Oak Ridge, the gonia are much larger than the late spermatid stage because they breed them for a longer period of time. They get more data there. It would detect a tenfold difference as positive in the spermato-gonia. If that is negative, the safest thing to do is assume a 100-fold difference. This would work because if you do assume a 100-fold difference and some length of time for these germ-cell stages, the gonial stage is still the more important contributor with reference to human health. Assuming that there is a 100-fold difference, you end up with a contribution to compute. It may not be correct, but if it is not, it will most likely be in the direction of where there might be a 1,000-fold difference or more, and therefore the gonial cells would not contribute at all. If you wish to prove that point, you simply have to do enough gonial stages in mice to show statistically that there is less than two orders of magnitude in difference--three orders of magnitude, in which case you would be safe in ignoring the gonial stage and basing your estimate entirely on the postmeiotic stages.

EHRENBERG: There is a very important issue here. I wholly agree with carrying out such studies. Without going into details, there are several indications that you have to work at low dose levels that are valid for exposure situations when you evaluate this difference. This difference between gonad stages and sperm (postmeiotic) stages might be exaggerated at higher doses (unrealistically high from the exposure point of view) because of aberrations that appear in the gonial stages and that cannot pass through meiosis when you use the higher doses. This has to be done in principle by evaluating the shape of the dose-response curve with each of the stages. This can make it possible to estimate what the ratio of the sensitivities of the stages would be at realistic exposure situations. Then this experiment would really give guidance to further estimation of risk in humans.

LEE: There are other reasons besides chromosome breaks for this difference between the stages. The repair system has a great deal to do with it. In the gonial stage, where there is a matter of days between alkylation and replication, there is adequate time for repair, whereas in the case of the spermatozoa stage, repair could not occur until fertilization. Minutes after fertilization, you also have DNA replication, which means an overrunning of repair with replication. I think there is a difference in mechanism there that needs accounting for. But chromosome breaks can also be a larger component of what you are measuring if you limit yourself to certain stages. Ehling has pointed out (personal communication) that you have very few chromosome breaks in the first few days after treatment. Looking back at the data for a review article (Lee, 1978), I found that taking the data of Cattanach, Russell, and Generoso (i.e., Cattanach et al., 1968; Generoso and Russell, 1969) for dominant lethals and also for translocations, there was no evidence at all--even at their high doses of EMS--that they were able to get chromosome breaks, translocations, or dominant lethals within the first two or three days following treatment. By days seven to nine, they reach a peak. If we break the data up into the mutations that were observed with EMS in the first three days, compared with the mutations that occur in the next four and then the next four--in other words, if we do the breeding and accumulate the data in this way--the difference suggested by Ehrenberg would become apparent because the increase due to chromosome breakage should occur during about days eight through twelve, rather than in the sample one through four.

ABRAHAMSON: I have no argument with what you are saying, but I do have a problem with what Ehrenberg is saying. You are basically asking for a dose-response curve to be done in the mouse for each of the chemicals under consideration, at low doses. In an ideal world, that would be magnificent, but when you are dealing with a potentially large number of chemicals, you cannot conceivably expect to get a good dose-response curve.

EHRENBERG: I suggested this because if you only do this with one dose, but pretty high, for six chemicals, you will still know very little of what you want to know. I did not say that you should establish a dose-response curve at realistically low doses; that would get into the trouble of mega-mouse experiments and such things. Instead, you need a pretty good dose-response curve where one or two of the chemicals you have been discussing are carefully selected. This will permit you to draw some conclusions as to mechanisms. If you have a theory or hypothesis that you will have a different mechanism at low doses, you should apply it. But if you do not, you can extrapolate down. This should be worked out at doses where you can realistically carry out experiments within the limits of funds and so forth.

ABRAHAMSON: I stand corrected. I am glad we have had that clearly stated; now we can see where we are.

SUTTON: It should be emphasized that in making these tests in mice, we must not rely on the existing specific-locus test. We must have some measures that are likely to pick up transitions, transversions, and frame shifts.

ABRAHAMSON: I said that we should use the specific-locus test last; the other tests would supersede it.

SUTTON: Of course, some people might say, "But we have the specific-locus tests and we do not have the others yet."

ABRAHAMSON: Yes.

LONG-TERM BUILDUP OF DETRIMENT

NEEL: One of the long-standing dilemmas that has come out of the work in radiation genetics is that in long-range chronic exposure to radiation, generation after generation, there was still no net dominant deleterious effect. Populations of either Drosophila or mice simply did not collapse the way we thought they would under that much radiation. There is still no satisfactory explanation of what happens to those mutations. In setting up this research, even at the risk of creating some future embarrassment, perhaps we could think of that type of experiment with some of the chemical mutagens. For instance, Spalding and Green's experiments (Green, 1968 a, 1968 b; Spalding and Brooks, 1972) have not been mentioned at all. This may only be inviting trouble, but our job is to find out what happens.

ABRAHAMSON: That is right; a good point. If you are going to recommend that kind of experiment, with 40 to 50 generations of mice, each being exposed to radiation (without looking at the breeding scheme), being looked at to see if there is any accumulation of detriment over the generations, it will have to be in a laboratory where support is guaranteed for the 40 generations. This is critical; you cannot have fluc-tuations by the whim of the agency that originally put up the money.

NEEL: At least an unusually long contract or grant.

ABRAHAMSON: There are very few places in the country where you can get support for such a long time. Oak Ridge, NIEHS, or Los Alamos, as in the case of the Spalding experiments. Have we now summarized what we are recommending as valid research programs to get to the point where we can make the risk estimates?

OOCYTE REPAIR OF SPERM DAMAGE

BREWEN: Have we ignored the female? One of the inter-esting things about the female is the tremendous stage sensitivity that Generoso and colleagues (Generoso and Russell, 1969; Generoso, Huff, and Stout, 1971) have demonstrated in dominant lethal testing with chemical mutagens. We have not discussed this at all. It appears to be the reverse of the case with radiation where the most mature stages are the most sensitive. This has been verified both cytogenetically and by the dominant-lethal test with the agents MMS and TEM.

One finding by Generoso et al. (personal communication) is very cogent to the whole problem. He reported at a recent subcommittee meeting that there is apparently a very large difference in the ability of various strains to "repair" the damage introduced into the sperm after sperm penetration and fertilization. If this is repeated and shown to be a highly variable phenomenon in various mouse strains, we will have a very serious problem in most of these tests, particularly if it appears that we are going to be concerned principally with the situation Lee has described, where the postmeiotic stages are the most sensitive. You can conceive of a situation in which you would get a zero effect with one combination of male/female and turn around and do the same experiment with another combination in which you would get an effect two orders of magnitude higher. This would be just because of the situation in the female oocyte and its ability or inability to repair premutational damage in the sperm.

NEEL: A recent meeting in Ottawa (see Pegg, 1978b) on repair mechanisms was absolutely fascinating in terms of the ferment in that field right now. Depending on the nature of the damage, maybe 90% is getting repaired. There was discussion that some of the enzymes involved might be inducible, but no one is quite sure how. Wouldn't that be an appropriate topic? A small shift in the efficiency of those repair enzymes could have to do with the apparent doubling of the mutation rates.

ABRAHAMSON: You and Brewen are both correct. Some important information can be gotten not only from the mouse female, but also from the human female. Ovary studies can be made from hysterectomy patients, so we can get some information on repair enzymes, for example, in various stages of oocytes--in what is the most important stage, the equivalent of the immature stage from the standpoint of mutation hazard. You may not agree with that, but the female should be emphasized as an area of research needs because it is half the human genome, without a doubt, and we have

the least information on it. Where we do have information, it is either the most sensitive stage from which
we have mutation rates or the least sensitive.

EHRENBERG: The possibility that repair enzymes are inducible should be a field of research. If you want to
extrapolate down to low doses, especially in chronic
exposure, you might have theoretical reason to believe
that the dose-response curve behaves otherwise at the
low doses. I refer to those curves I showed with a
"hump" in the low-dose region--around 0.5 rad--in the
plant experiments where they were irradiated before
and during meiosis. This involved the male side. One
hypothesis to explain this has been that sensitive
stages are eliminated at high doses. That cannot hold
when we find the same things in chronic exposure.
You cannot have elimination of sensitive stages when
you find the same hump in consequence of chronic
exposure. There are a number of reasons to believe
that enzyme induction is responsible for this. At the
same time, the hump could go in the other direction.
If you have another pathway for mutation induction,
you could have a negative hump. Such results have
been obtained with EMS in bacteria by Mohn (1977).

LEE: I had hoped for future research emphasizing the
tracing of labeled mutagens into the oocyte and
following their fate. We do not have that kind of data
at all--how stable are alkylation groups, which stages
will remove alkylation groups and which ones will not?
This basic material needs to be obtained for the female
side to match what we are now attempting to do with
the male side.

BREWEN: Can you get the material hot enough to study
autoradiographically?

LEE: Yes, and I was thinking in terms of an autoradiographic approach.

MUTAGENS ACTING AWAY FROM DNA AND GONADS

ZIPSER: Although most mutagenic substances obviously
interact with DNA, it is perfectly clear that a chemical
could be mutagenic not only without interacting with
the DNA but also never getting anywhere near the
gonads. One can imagine a situation where repair
enzymes are turned on or off by signals coming from
other organs, such as hormones. Therefore, chemicals
that interact with that system could easily affect the
level of repair. If it is true, for instance, that 90% of

all mutations are repaired, then it could increase the spontaneous level up to 90% without ever getting any place near the gonads. Obviously, that will not be a common situation. Most chemicals will, in fact, mutate by interacting with DNA, and of course there are chemicals that might enter the cell but not go near the DNA and simply inhibit the repair system. Chemical mutagenesis does not have to occur in any other system besides mammals or even humans. Any kind of screening technique must have some cognizance of that. You cannot define dose, for instance, on the basis of binding to DNA, although in most cases that is a very reasonable approach.

ABRAHAMSON: How would you go about demonstrating these kinds of unusual but possible mechanisms?

ZIPSER: I do not know anything about demonstrating them, but it is clear that it is a logical possibility; it is not completely without foundation. The promoters of tumorigenesis almost certainly do not bind with DNA, as opposed to the initiators, but one of their permanent functions might be stimulating mitotic recombination, or recombination in general, which would lead in somatic tissues to a much higher frequency of homozygotization, as we say in bacterial genetics. The effect of such compounds on reproductive cells is unknown to me, but such things exist, and there is now good reason to believe that that is how they operate; they could quite clearly be mutagenic without attacking DNA. Presumably, any experiment that tested chemicals on mice would tend to alert you to this. I was just worried about the definition of dose.

LEE: What would you substitute for it?

ZIPSER: There is no obvious substitute.

PERSON: So your objection is to compounds that might not depend on that as a mechanism?

ZIPSER: Right. For those compounds that do depend on it for a mechanism, for the accurate study of those compounds, that is a perfectly reasonable thing. For a general screening (for instance, if you screen by binding to DNA and ignore all compounds that do not bind to DNA), that might be an error.

LEE: I should emphasize that this would be applicable for alkylating agents. That needs to be underlined.

ABRAHAMSON: If you had a chemical that in a variety of test systems proved to be mutagenic and was still mutagenic in a <u>Drosophila</u> test such as Lee might run, and yet was never found in the cell itself, that might give you an indication.

ZIPSER: Obviously, substances like this are not going to be mutagenic in bacteria.

ABRAHAMSON: I realize that.   But the original screen system is not exclusive to bacteria.

ZIPSER: Of course.   I am trying to say that something can be mutagenic to an organism, in principle anyway, without ever entering the gonads.   This means chemicals, of course; obviously, radiation is probably different.

LEE: I want to emphasize that.   I was referring to EMS and the data I had reviewed for EMS when I made the comment about the lack of dominant-lethal effects in days one through four.   That was what we found for EMS.   For MMS, there is a positive effect at the highest dose level.

HUMAN POPULATION MONITORING

ABRAHAMSON: The next topic is human population monitoring.

NEEL: I get the impression that some of you feel I am here to subvert this meeting, but I would rather think of it as an effort to extend the horizon of the meeting.   I have always supported all the basic investigation one can dream up that is relevant to our problem.   But there is an additional dimension to which we must give adequate attention.   I guess I am the only one of us here who was involved in the early work on radiation in the 1950s.   At that time, there was a great deal of pressure from AEC and so forth for quick answers.   A group of strong-minded scientists (Herman Muller and Sewall Wright, for example) met under the auspices of the BEIR committee and quickly got off into research policy.   They spoke to the issue of the complexity and what we needed, and out of that came the kind of research support that did a great deal for Oak Ridge and the other national laboratories.   At the same time, they recognized that we should take maximum advantage of the opportunity to study human populations exposed to mutagens, because of their rarity, and because this was the kind of data that some people would demand.   Out of that came the support for a fairly extensive follow-up study at Hiroshima and Nagasaki that continues to the present time.

It has been suggested that perhaps the studies in Japan did a disservice to the cause because we had not shown anything, and this absence of clear effects is constantly quoted in Washington. When we first went into Japan, some people feared that humans might be unusually sensitive to the genetic effects of radiation and were willing to consider doubling doses as low as 10 R. We have now demonstrated that the doubling dose cannot be that low, or we would have picked it up, and I take that to be a significant contribution. More than that, in everything that I have ever written I have been extremely careful to use compound sentences that say "There is nothing here at the level of significance; on the other hand, there is still a great area of uncertainty that we are seeking to dispel." One of the occupational hazards of making a contribution is being misquoted; one has to live with that and attempt to correct the record.

The uncertainties of radiation were great, but here there is an additional level of uncertainty. With radiation you knew that the dose got to the gonad; but here there is an extra layer of uncertainty in any effort to extrapolate, particularly because the human gonad is going to be exposed to any potential mutagen for a much longer period than any experimental organism with which you are apt to work. You just do not know how chemical doses might accumulate. There is a new public mood abroad these days, and in the absence of the best data you can get from humans, imperfect though they may be, you are open to attack. EPA is vulnerable to attack from two sides. A group of environmentalists will say, "All right, you cannot prove that you really have protected human populations by these measures. Here are the uncertainties." The people who say this are very intelligent and have done their homework well. Another group will say, "You have not proved anything has happened to humans, and these regulations are really excessive." These pressures will only increase in the next 10 to 15 years. The country will be in such an energy crunch that the pressure to relax standards will be absolutely enormous. The burden of proof is going to shift to those who say this is going to hurt people.

The present screening programs will help to flag really potent mutagens and will help guide industry in making choices early in their developmental programs. But it must be accompanied by some kind of effort to get at people so that there will not be a whole string of lawsuits when abnormal children appear--as they will--in the families of exposed workers. There is no pat, precise answer. We and other groups are trying to see what is the most efficient way to monitor populations for relatively small increases in mutation rate. The technology is changing very rapidly; protocols that would have seemed inconceivable 10 years ago are now within the realm of possibility. For instance, we have been using the old-fashioned method of trying to look at enzymes one at a time for variants. I just saw the new two-dimensional polyacrylamide gel and its resolving power--and what it may do for us. The gels are beautiful, with enormous resolution. Out of the nerve cell and muscle cell, the investigator can pull several hundred proteins that can be scanned for evidence of differences from some standard type. Significant progress has been made toward computerizing the readouts. We are really looking at an order-of-magnitude change here. We want to extend the horizon to give EPA and other agencies the chance to protect themselves.

ABRAHAMSON: Are we talking about newborns? Who are we monitoring?

NEEL: There are two basic strategies here, and it is going to be very difficult to decide on balance which is the better way to go. One way is to obtain a placental cord blood sample from a series of newborns in, say, Newark, New Jersey (which has a high record in terms of cancer), Detroit, Michigan, and some rural areas and make observations, continuously monitoring for changes in frequency. The other way is the obvious strategy of contrasting high-risk and low-risk groups. For instance, we are in the middle of a second look at the problem in Japan, now using these new technologies. So far, it is a matter of screening a battery of some 30 enzymes for electrophoretic variants, but we have known all along from mouse work that perhaps we should be looking for the null mutants. We now have the fast centrifugal analyzer that lets us look for half-activities in the screening mode, and I hope that we get the two-dimensional approach in there as soon as possible. That is a contrast between a high-risk and a control group.

In this country, it will be very difficult administratively to do a high-risk/low-risk contrast because you have to set up this enormous field mechanism to go out and get the children and persuade them that they really want to have their blood drawn, and so on. We do not have that problem with the placenta studies, where, incidentally, we have informed consent and it is all done very legally. If we are to go that way, looking at high-risk groups, it probably cannot be done unless we have something like the two-dimensional technique, because we have to extract the maximum information from each child. Even our worst experiences in this country are not yielding very many children. There has been considerable discussion of this on an international level, such as at a recent meeting in Oslo on Genetic Damage in Man Caused by Environmental Agents, and one can visualize an even longer meeting, with international collaboration among the industrialized nations. There is already a great deal of discussion in West Germany, Norway, and England. You can pool the high-risk groups. For instance, Lars Beckman reported at the Oslo conference on his work with arsenic smelters, which is a very interesting population to study. They could be brought into this picture.

EHRENBERG: May I make a comment about the arsenic smelters? There is possibly combined action of lack of selenium in that area; that seems to contribute, as it does in Finland (Schrauzer, 1976; references in Frost, 1975).

ABRAHAMSON: Obviously, there is no shortage of high-risk groups in industries or "cancer-alley" areas of the country.

NEEL: You must put <u>high</u> in quotes; it is a relative term. If you were going to go that route, you would want to define the populations with great care. For instance, the children of vinyl chloride workers would be a high-risk group, but it would not be a large sample of children for some time. In Michigan, we have this weird PBB situation, which is still poorly understood, but I will give you any odds you want that in the next 10 years there will be suits when one of these people has a defective child. Unless there has been some kind of monitoring program to show that as a group there has been no increase in defects, the state (or the nation) has no defense. You could be in trouble in any individual case, but if you have general data on what is happening in the population, you will be much stronger than if you have no data whatsoever.

ABRAHAMSON: What is your assumed population size to be run in things of this sort?

NEEL: We assumed that we really should not miss an increase in mutation rate by as much as 50%, and we assumed a spontaneous rate for our indicators of 0.5×10^{-5}. We also assumed an alpha or type-I error of 0.05 and a beta or type-II error of 0.20. Under these assumptions, one can detect a 50% increase with two samples of 313,000, if each child is examined for 20 different proteins. You could do the same thing with 150,000 births, each child examined for 40 proteins; the total number of observations is the important factor. Obviously, one will not attempt year-to-year monitoring with a requirement for numbers like that, so we thought in terms of five-year cycles, treating the data with either running averages or contrasting successive five-year periods. Under those circumstances, of course, the need was for a sample of 60,000 births per year studied for the 20 indicators. This would be based on the frequency of electrophoretic variants. If one could search for half-normal enzyme levels or kinetic variants with the fast analyzer, one would get a lot more information per system. This technology is all in a state of great flux.

I would urge in the strongest terms that there be somatic-cell studies to parallel any germinal study. Once you build a bridge between somatic- and germ-cell rates, you can rely on somatic rates. You know what the conversion factor is, and you can get away from the terribly expensive and laborious germ-line studies. Somehow the bridge has to be built that will let you extrapolate from monitoring for somatic cell rates to monitoring for germ-cell rates. The best system for somatic-cell rates now looks to be the one George Stamm is working on at Seattle. Ray Popp (Popp et al., 1975) also has a system. Since both these systems involve the enucleate RBC, we may never prove the precise genetic basis for the changes they study, but if we can make an empiric relationship between the increase they study and some measure of germinal rate, we have an indicator.

WEAK MUTAGENS

EHRENBERG: You mentioned that by new test methods you easily handled and maybe also clarified the strong mutagens. As I have stated--perhaps I was not understood--it is the concern with weak mutagens that has led to the development of the method I tried to describe. I am thinking of mutagens for which you could never measure a doubling dose for various reasons but which might nevertheless occur and be

important components in our environment. You might
not even get positive tests in any of the systems, but
from a study of the resolving power of these test
systems and some knowledge of the metabolism of the
compound, you would guess that it is mutagenic. I
can mention two examples. One is ethylene, which is
representative of a whole series of 1-alkenes that are
converted to epoxides in the body. These do not
belong to compounds where you could not enrich the
metabolite and study it. Ethylene and propylene, for
example, are very important compounds in the petro-
chemical industry, where you have high exposure
levels, and in the urban environment, where you have
exposure levels some 50 times higher than in rural
areas. Ethylene is no doubt converted to ethylene
oxide in vivo. I mention this compound because we
know that it is metabolized to something known to be
mutagenic.

From another example is nitric oxide, which, through
five or six different pathways, leads to alkylation of
DNA. We do not know which will operate in humans.
It is very difficult to study this in any model system
because the pathways would be completely different.
It is important to see these compounds in their
relationship to nitrate used as a fertilizer and nitrite
used as a food additive. The problem has to be seen
as a whole. When we handle such compounds, we may
use the equation I showed earlier (Equation 8), not for
a risk estimate, but for a very rough estimate of what
kind of risk our negative test is excluding. This
should obtain a scale on the order of magnitude. The
problems may ultimately be solved with the kind of
investigation suggested by Lee, the importance of
which is agreed upon by everyone.

From what Neel has said, it is only through
measurements in humans themselves that we can get
information on the levels of alkylating compounds
generated in the human population. Through methods
of chemical analysis that are available, but in some
cases need further development to improve sensitivity,
we can measure the compounds. Such measurements
on blood samples, which could be done in connection
with any medical examination (therefore, not doing any
experimental biopsy), could identify populations at risk
as one of the parameters involved in the kind of
genetic studies mentioned by Neel (proteins). You
could introduce these as one of the variables. One of
the possible developments of this technique is that you
need not necessarily deal with known compounds. If
you measure alkylation products in blood samples,

chosen because they are so easily drawn, it is possible to transfer the alkyl groups to carriers suitable for analysis. These carriers could be radioactively labeled; they could be suitable for gas chromatography or mass spectometry or some other technique. We already have the methods for a few compounds. We have shown that it is possible in principle to do this transfer to a carrier suitable for analysis where you determine not only the amount of the foreign compound, but also which one it is. From that you can draw a conclusion as to what villains in the environment we should look for and try to eliminate at the same time that we introduce a chemical background of the genetic monitoring of populations. We should do cancer monitoring at the same time, I think.

ABRAHAMSON: Am I understanding this? In Neel's system, we are looking at the offspring of possible high-risk populations. In your system, we would be looking at the high-risk population itself in the factory, the workplace, studying the possibility that their somatic cells would be alkylated and removed onto some other carrier molecule and determining what the chemical is. Am I correct?

EHRENBERG: This is correct in a way. There are not many steps left until we can, for instance, enter into the rubber industry and try to identify the compounds there that give rise to a dose of something in the body. Then, of course, in critical cases, we can go back to animal experiments and see whether they can pass through the barrier to the gonads, what stages are sensitive, and so on. But for a first provisional estimate of risk, we could use the rad-equivalence to see of what order of magnitude it is. But I did not mean only that. If you go to populations in general, the method might be made sensitive enough for a monitoring of mutagenic factors in the outer environment, for instance urban pollution.

NEEL: May I extend one aspect of this? Earlier we heard a presentation on chromosomal damage in a group of 52 people exposed to benzene and 44 controls. There was a very marginal difference between the two groups. There is an analysis that just screams to be done: to look at the distribution of damage by the Poisson approach. Are there just two or three people responsible for that increase who would be susceptibles? One way to go is to identify the susceptibles. Setlow gave some of the cited data about the inheritance of defects in DNA repair mechanisms that we now recognize; there are at least five. He did some calculations about the heterozygote frequency and extended them by pointing out that the complementation groups suggest that these are not homogeneous but heterogeneous entities. This means that the carriers are two to three times more common than what you anticipate on the basis of homogeneity of each entity. It is perfectly possible that these carriers are going to be unusually susceptible (predisposed) to damage to DNA.

ABRAHAMSON: Sutton raised this point earlier in your absence.

NEEL: Another point is that if one went to monitoring newborn infants, it would be natural to plug in cytogenetics. You would have the problem of optimizing the research design so as to get the most bang for the buck. A good cytogeneticist will want to band and look for smaller and smaller defects, but if you can show that actually 80% of what you have picked up are aneuploids, which are very easy to screen for, you might do a subset for the really detailed studies.

EHRENBERG: There is another aspect of this direct monitoring of people. When you come to compounds that are metabolized into alkylating agents in the atmosphere, the environment, food, and so forth, and especially to compounds that are converted to mutagens, you may commit very grave errors if you rely on animal doses in the estimate of human risk. This concerns not only the weak mutagens, of course, but any mutagen. Therefore, if you can establish an exposure-concentration/target-dose relationship for some important chemicals directly in humans, it would make the risk estimate on the basis of the animal data, and so on, much safer.

In a recent French report on micronuclei produced by benzene and benzpyrene, benzpyrene gave a dose-response curve with the points close around it; by contrast, there was an enormous scattering of the benzene points around the curve. (I do not remember whether the mice were hybrid or not.) This really calls for some kind of detection of the sensitivity of people just by tissue monitoring of the benzene to see what the distribution of ability to convert it to an alkylating or arylating agent is.

ABRAHAMSON: A question for Neel. When you gave us the N sample sizes, you were talking about 60,000 per year on a five-year run, on your previous testing of 20 proteins per sample. Now you are talking about gels that will run several hundred proteins. What do you estimate your sample size will be, if you get the technique going?

NEEL: With the improvements in the old-fashioned technology, we are now up to about 40 enzymes in proteins run in the lab in one-dimensional gel, which would halve the sample size. So you could do 30,000 people for 40. If we go up to 100 tests per individual (being conservative), then the sample size is more like 12,000 per year on a five-year cycle.

ABRAHAMSON: And that need not be done exclusively in the United States; in fact, you would prefer to see that distributed over several countries.

NEEL: This is one of the beautiful opportunities for international cooperation. I will suggest this in Moscow this summer.

TESTING FOR NULL MUTATIONS

LEE: Are you including in this a test for nulls?

NEEL: All of this new technology has to be worked out. Harvey Mohrenweiser has screened a whole series of enzymes to get those with the smallest coefficient of variation, so you can be pretty sure you can detect with accuracy a decrease to 50% activity. (When I say "coefficient of variation," this is always standardized against red-cell hemoglobin; you must not take an unstandardized value.) Mohrenweiser now has adapted 15 enzymes for activity studies in the centrifugal fast analyzer (Mohrenweiser, unpublished data).

LEE: But with the fast analyzer, you would be able to pick up an inactive protein--or the absence.

NEEL: Over the past 15 years, we have built up probably the best collection of genetic variants at this level in the country. We want to use them to determine the sensitivity of the methodology in the detection of new protein variants. We do have some nulls and will be able to determine exactly where we stand in their detection and how far we can trust the new methodology.

ABRAHAMSON: In other words, you will put up a positive kind of control?

NEEL: You are absolutely right.

ABRAHAMSON: How many do you have now, of a positive control type?

NEEL: We must have in the freezer variants of 30 different

systems that would be useful in either the standardiza-
tion of studies using the fast analyzer or the two-
dimensional methodology. We are just now beginning
to work with white cells, harvesting them from the
cord blood samples. A lot of the enzymes in red cells
are in white cells, so we can use the same enzyme to
control both sets of cells.

LEE: I have been anxious to ask one question. What is
the conceptual difference between a null enzyme, as
you define it now, and the old Mullerian terminology of
an amorph for a morphological mutant?

SUTTON: The difference is that we now know what we are
talking about.

LEE: I grant that. You are identifying a protein. Scientifically, it is far preferred, from the standpoint of
assaying a mutagenic hazard; is it possible that
Russell's system of picking up the white mouse may in
a sense be picking up the same type of mutagenic
event as a null?

NEEL: We know now that most of what Russell picked up
were homozygous lethal, pretty clearly deletions, and
those operationally would be nulls.

ABRAHAMSON: Would you repeat those last two sentences
for the record?

NEEL: We agree (and the Russells would probably agree)
that most of what they found was homozygous lethal.

BREWEN: That was 50% in the oocyte, 50% in postmeiotic
stages, 20% in gonia.

NEEL: It is now clear that some of their "point mutations"
result in loss of activity of several different enzymes,
which is good evidence for deletion.

ABRAHAMSON: Seven percent of the chromosome.

NEEL: This is additional evidence that these really are
deletions. You will agree with that?

PERSON: Absolutely.

NEEL: In coming back to nulls in general, we should be
careful. These are not always necessarily mutations in
structural genes. A mutation in a controller or
operator gene would also register as a null. If we get
null-mutation rates, we must be careful not to equate
them to specific-locus rates. On the other hand,
there were similar problems in Bill Russell's work--his
rates were "specific locus," but in a rather broad
sense.

LEE: It would probably detect mutations in the whole oper-on. As a means of assay, is just simply looking at the F_1 mouse and saying you have a white mouse still a valid and useful assay for mutation?

NEEL: I have never argued against that. You people keep trying to make this an antithesis; I see it as an extension.

LEE: I am highly pleased with that statement.

NEEL: These are not competing technologies; there are as many observations that we cannot make in humans--that we will not try to do with humans. For 30 years I have supported every piece of fundamental research to understand radiation mechanisms.

SUTTON: But that cannot substitute for point-mutation tests because they are not all point mutations.

LEE: But they may take up point mutations along with deletions and all the other things, too.

NEEL: If one does observe an increase in mutation rates, this calls for some real detective work. You have to go back to the bench and reexamine what is in the environment, what may have slipped through the screening systems. Ehrenberg talked about a com-pound, ethylene oxide, that might have some effects we cannot anticipate. You go back and worry about that one and develop test systems that will show, with due attention to the metabolism, what may be happen-ing to that compound in the animal metabolically most similar to humans.

LEE: The electrophoretic variants should be added to the existing data base on specific-locus tests. We are not proposing dropping the specific-locus tests, but adding this other bit of information to that standard test that has been used in the past.

NEEL: As you know, the NIEHS has put a fair investment into developing a test strain where you have hetero-zygosity at eight isozyme loci in test animals. In the fly you have the same thing.

VALCOVIC: In Chuck Langley's Drosophila work there will be about 30 loci (Langley, personal communication). The two inbred lines were nine loci, and with the efforts going on now, that will be close to 25 where one can perform the electrophoretic approach as Malling and I have presented it for the mouse system.

NEEL: This may be the new specific-locus test. I have been asking for years that we pick a series of structural proteins in the mouse, the human, and <u>Drosoph-ila</u>, and get spontaneous rates on these proteins. We have all these problems of extrapolating because we are comparing pink eyes and curly wings with kinky tail and retinoblastoma. Now we can work with the same structural proteins in diverse organisms. We desperately need the comparative mutation rate; this work is not spectacular and it is laborious, but it bears on one of the great enigmas of genetics. Didn't Abrahamson say that the average <u>Drosophila</u> rate is 0.3×10^{-6}, the mouse rate 0.5×10^{-6}, and the human rate 0.7×10^{-6}? Aren't you amazed that for humans who live a thousand or more times longer than <u>Drosophila</u>, at a 10° higher average temperature, the rates are so similar? This is a screaming mystery that we have been walking around ever since genetics began to study mutation rates.

ABRAHAMSON: It has bothered me for 30 years.

NEEL: We should get comparable protein studies.

LEE: To me, that has an obvious answer in that all of us have only one early cleavage.

NEEL: Wouldn't you like some evidence to back up your...

LEE: I think there is evidence in the fly that the mutations are fixed spontaneously at that stage. That is hidden in A. P. Schalet's unpublished dissertation at Indiana University.

SUTTON: In terms of monitoring, I would like to emphasize one point you made about the Japanese studies. Most of the participants in this conference are too young to remember these events, but over the years since the atomic bomb explosions in Japan there have been a whole series of reports from obscure people and laboratories of some very large effect in the radiation survivors and their offspring. The only reason these things have not gotten anywhere is because there existed this very large, very public, study that simply did not show it, and thus the other efforts never got off the ground. If we do not have some kind of comparable baseline here, we will see exactly the same thing among those people who do a very small, dirty study and find some outlandish result--if, indeed, that is the way it is. Another point on research interests is that we could make the best of both worlds if we could find a good way of testing sperm for mutations--chromosomal and especially biochemical. I would give that research a very high priority in the general area of monitoring.

ABRAHAMSON: Brewen is now looking at chromosome ab-
    normalities induced in human sperm after the sperm
    has fertilized the egg and through the first few
    cleavage divisions.

BREWEN: It has been published (Yanagimichi, Yanagimichi,
    and Rogers, 1976) that one can fertilize hamster ova
    with human sperm.

SUTTON: Perhaps you should use the term hybridize in
    public statements on that?

BREWEN: Pronuclei are formed, and rumor has it that
    these interspecific hybrids manage to go through at
    least one or two cleavage divisions, so that you get
    two- and four-blastomere-stage embryos.   Theoretic-
    ally, they should make it to the eight-cell or sixteen-
    cell stage, which is the point at which the paternal
    genome begins to be transcribed.   If this is the case,
    then it is possible to take a sperm sample, treat it
    with a mutagen (or take a sperm sample from an
    individual that has been exposed to a high level of a
    mutagen), and simply do the in vitro fertilization,
    grow them until the first cleavage division, and make
    direct observations on the chromosome abnormality--or
    sister chromatid exchange, which would be highly more
    sensitive in terms of the sample size that you would
    needbecause of background noise.

EHRENBERG: A short question for Neel.   What frequency
    of nulls, where you have half the level of enzyme,
    could you detect?   What is the coefficient of variation?

NEEL: For a series of enzymes, which Mohrenweiser is
    looking at, the coefficient of variation is about 12% of
    the mean, so two standard deviations would take you
    down to 75%--you are looking for 50% levels.   So we
    think we can pick up nulls.   Some enzymes are so
    variable that they cannot be used in this system.   I
    am talking about a special tissue: the erythrocyte,
    which is an end-stage cell where everything that will
    be induced has been induced, and there is not much
    change by the time they get into circulation.   There is
    a real problem with some tissues, particularly the
    fibroblast growing in culture.   It is now becoming
    apparent that subtle differences in the culture media
    may turn proteins on and off.   Many problems must be
    checked out very carefully, enzyme by enzyme.   We
    now think that for the erythrocyte we have a battery
    of about 15 where the coefficient of variation is small
    enough that one can detect nulls.   In fact, nulls are
    being detected--not very many yet, but when you find

half-normal levels in a child and go back to the parents, one of them will show a half-normal level. It does work.

LEE: I would like to ask your reaction to a test for nulls only as a useful mutation assay. If you are able to pick up only the nulls, is this too narrow a spectrum or is it useful, in your opinion?

NEEL: My own thinking is in a stage of rapid evolution right now, I confess. My introductory paper quoted Drosophila data indicating that null mutations, which may now result from mutation at several different loci in addition to the structural, are five times greater in frequency than mutations giving an electrophoretic change. This is surprising. If you extrapolate it to humans and pick some 5,000 proteins, as I did, then the nulls are a very important group. It could be that that is the way to go; we should forget about at least one-dimensional electrophoresis. On the other hand, if the two-dimensional method lets you look at 200 proteins at a time for electrophoretic variants, then you have a very powerful handle for looking for electrophoretic variants. We are interested in determining whether the reading of two-dimensional gels can be computerized. There is a terrible data-management problem here in dealing with these numbers.

LEE: I was thinking in terms of a screen where with Drosophila you pick up the nulls and all the others die--the positive-selection system for nulls.

INDEXES OF HARM

ABRAHAMSON: May I refocus one aspect that is part of monitoring but not quite as you are envisioning it? Ben Trimble's work just before his death--not his survey of the British Columbia population, but on the index of harm of various genetic diseases.

NEEL: I quoted that earlier, but it does not hurt to re-iterate. The impact of a genetic disease is not measured simply by its frequency, but by hospitalization, as shown in the work of Trimble and Smith. I think Martha Smith is going to try to extend that paper.

ABRAHAMSON: We had data where there were five times as many hospital days spent, five times as much death associated with the dominant diseases in the first five years of life, up to twelve times as much of this or that--I have forgotten all the indices that were investigated--and it seems to me that an area of great concern is the cost, not only in dollars, but also in terms of the anguish of ill health at the level of genetic disease versus nongenetic disease in the population. I would also call your attention to a study done by A.D. Little & Co. for EPA about four years ago looking at radiation. They did a balance of cancer cost versus genetic cost, surveying all the genetic diseases and giving them each a dollar cost, concluding that for every severe genetic disease we had listed in the current-incidence board, the cost to society was at least five times as much (in dollars) as the equivalent cost for a given cancer.

NEEL: Where did you see that study?

ABRAHAMSON: I was a consultant to them, telling them about the BEIR committee report, and their experts published this report in which they cost-accounted two kinds of diseases--somatic versus genetic--and came to a dollar figure of five to one. (For those who have not seen the report, I will circulate my copy.)

HILL: I know of two other studies, one by Childs, Miller, and Bearn (1972) and one by Day and Holmes (1973), where they were looking at the frequency of admissions to various kinds of wards--pediatric and adult medicine--looking for the impact of genetic disease. They felt that there was an overrepresentation of admissions for these various diseases in comparison to their frequency in the general population.

NEEL: The Childs-Miller-Bearn study yielded a numerator, but they never had a denominator to go with it--in other words, the size of the population they were sampling. So they could not know how disproportionately these diseases were represented. But those studies show, for instance, that nowadays in a pediatric hospital 25% of admissions are for clearly genetic conditions and another 25% are perhaps genetically related. For instance, if a child with cystic fibrosis comes in with a pneumonia, the pneumonia is the proximal cause of admission, but you still have the underlying genetic factor.

ABRAHAMSON: If we have exhausted the monitoring area, can we move on to the next sector?

BREWEN: Have we reached a consensus that we do need more background information?

ABRAHAMSON: I thought that was what this discussion was all about.

NEEL: We have not spelled out the research needs for this area--we have them for the other areas. There is not yet a scheme ready to be put in place. No one came here with something cut and dried. One needs to see how to optimize, to get the most bang for the buck in any monitoring program. My philosophy would be to let many flowers bloom now and experiment with several different approaches to see which is most cost effective.

HILL: I would like to go out on a tangent from that and refocus on things that have come to the fore. I see the real value of the population monitoring studies, but when it comes to the individual chemical that we have some information on and we may not have sample sizes anywhere near adequate to go in with that method and set up the appropriate kind of contrast that you want to run, we are left with just a spectrum of data from various systems.

ABRAHAMSON: It would seem to me that this group could not sit down and design the research needs that would be optimal--more bang for the buck--but a small group of individuals who were concerned with it could develop those kinds of research programs as a separate workshop with a restricted number of people in that area.

NEEL: I think we have funding from DOE for just that kind of a workshop, where all points of view are going to be represented. We should, for whatever comes out of here, recognize the area--it is big enough that probably you can share among various agencies--so that EPA recognizes this would be a legitimate area in which to buy a share if quality standards are met.

WHAT DECISIONS FOLLOW POSITIVE READINGS?

ABRAHAMSON: Let us move on to the kind of question Hill just raised. What do you do when you consider a given chemical, possessing a series of test data--albeit imperfect at the present level of knowledge--and a decision has to be made by EPA? Pretend that you are all part of the regulatory agency, that you are sitting around a table and have been told that you must make a decision, restricting decisions to mutagenic effects and using certain data bases to make decisions. For instance, you have a compound positive for DNA damage in vitro and in vivo. It shows gene mutation damage in vitro in both eukaryotic and prokaryotic systems; it is positive in the <u>Drosophila</u> sex-linked lethal tests, positive for chromosomal damage, positive for in vivo translocation, and even positive in the disputed dominant-lethal test--positive across the board. That is for one test compound. Looking at some of these, what decisions would you come to on the basis of the information present?

BREWEN: Earlier we heard a presentation about benzene being a clastogen. It would have been noted as a positive on cytogenetic effects, and it was not. What does the plus mean? Does the plus mean what I saw yesterday for benzene?

PERTEL: No. You are to assume that there is sufficient power in these tests for them to be scientifically valid.

ABRAHAMSON: You are dealing with statistically signifi-cant results based on a large data base sample. Is that a fair statement? How would you respond as a regulator to a chemical, or are you prepared to make a response? Obviously, there is an index here saying that we are dealing with a presumptive mutagen with respect to humans.

HILL: There are different levels of investigation. One is qualitative--is the compound negative or positive in a given test?--and the other is the consideration of at what dosage was the effect observed. This is getting into the relative potency of the chemical.

ABRAHAMSON: We are playing a game right now. Assume that we have a reasonable data base with reasonable potency, expressed when we put down a positive without specifying the dose levels.

DOSIMETRY

SUTTON: Such a compound is clearly a mutagen, but what you do not have is the information on exposure.

ABRAHAMSON: You mean in the human population. You do not have human dosimetry, for example.

LEE: Such a compound, which is positive in mutagenicity tests, is a perfect case for simply requiring dosimetry, and because it is DNA-binding, the methods are available; from that one should be able to go straight to the system and come out with an estimate using essentially the logic that has been used for radiation. That would apply for those substances that are DNA-binding. It would not apply to the others, but it would apply to this one very nicely.

SUTTON: One of the things we have ignored in this discussion is routes of exposure. We should keep in
mind that in a real situation, these are not wholly
equivalent, and the data on exposure must be done in
a proper way.

LEE: This route of exposure would be the area where I
would prefer that physiologists be given a free hand
to use the organisms of their choice for estimating
dose to the germ line since the model for inhalation
studies is different from the model for digestive
studies.

ABRAHAMSON: If you take the hypothetical cases that
give the largest number of positives, in each case you
would conclude that you have a considerable amount of
evidence that indicates it as a presumptive mutagen,
but you do not have dosimetry studies and you do not
know how to make an effective risk estimate based on
the kinds of analyses we have discussed. Up to that
point, you really want to get the next base level.
You might have to try to make a risk estimate on this
basis and extrapolate it, but it would not be the kind
of risk estimate this group would consider appropriate
at this stage without further information.   Is that a
fair statement?

SUTTON: I think we could say, "It is a potential hazard."

ABRAHAMSON: Yes. I was using the word presumptive.

RISKS VS BENEFITS

EHRENBERG: You need the quantitation of risk. That is
the only thing that can enter into the cost/benefit
evaluation, with the risk as one component in the cost.

ABRAHAMSON: In some situations you might clearly have a
no-benefit situation under any circumstances. For instance, if we are dealing with a food coloring where it
is only a cosmetic phenomenon, it has no benefit one
way or another and no health benefit; we do not have
to worry about it.   If we are dealing with an industrial chemical that is of great consequence--tris, for
example--where we do have a very clear-cut benefit
and nothing to replace it with (a clear-cut benefit of a
certain number of deaths from fire in children's
clothing that could be avoided in any given year, or
severe burns or associated illnesses), we would have
to look at the cost in terms of the risk associated with
the next generation or future generations.

OSTERBERG: Of course, in the case of tris, we have replacements that might be safer.

ABRAHAMSON: Of course. I was trying to put it in a situation where you might not have any replacement for the time being, and you would have to make a decision of how long you want to leave it on the market, how quickly you want to move into some replacement compound if that were at all possible. I do not know how far we can push this kind of data base at this point because we obviously have not read the complete workups on each of these things, and we have not sat down and tried to develop them.

PERTEL: You do get into a borderline situation. You begin to call in expert groups at that point.

ABRAHAMSON: Clearly, this is the way screening has been going for the past several years--when it has been going at all--and this is the kind of data base that has been developed up to now.

LEE: What we have done, if this is the consensus of this group, is take a step beyond what has been the case so far, saying that given this type of qualitative screening, you now have a basis from which you may ask for additional work. On the basis of that, you can proceed with dosimetry. We know the type of information one needs for those compounds where you do show DNA-binding. In other words, we are dividing chemicals into their various classes and saying that for one class the methodology has developed to a point where we can ask for the kind of data that will lead to a risk estimate and for other classes we still have not reached that point.

A TIER SYSTEM OF TESTS?

ABRAHAMSON: Let me turn the question around a little. Is there a more efficient attack that could be undertaken both from the standpoint of both industry and from that of government? Would you always want to get the screening base before you go for the next step? Would it not be more efficient to operate a tier system: get the DNA damage, the in vitro damage-- some of the inexpensive, good cytogenetic data in vivo or in vitro--without going into heritable translocations, ignoring the dominant lethal test for the time being (which most of us seem to want to do), and get that data base as a first step? Second, having that kind of information where you would have a series of positives, would you then move into, say, <u>Drosophila</u> and mouse simultaneously, with the view of doing risk-estimate work simultaneously with getting mutagenic data?

LEE: The question of the order in which things are done is very important from the standpoint of economy. This is an industrial decision or an administrative one for the head of a granting agency, but you will often find that in the process of development, the appropriate labeling and tracing work of the label where you are essentially building up part of the data base and the dosimetry, can fit into the actual research and development very economically early in the process. That was not always there in the past, but I think it will be economical in the future simply because you are building up the molecule, labeling it, and finding out what it does as a means of developing the process and also perhaps developing analogs that may be more effective.

ABRAHAMSON: I think regulatory agencies can help shape the program or protocol procedures that would be involved here.

LEE: It would be particularly useful if government could rebut the cost question that would undoubtedly come up by saying that a large part of this cost should be a part of the development and not attributed to only this particular purpose--that it is a useful data base other than just for mutagenesis.

EHRENBERG: Lee mentioned yesterday, in suggesting this research program on a few well-selected compounds, the importance of intercalibration of the systems. As long as you consider minuses (i.e., negative tests), which you have for some of these compounds, it would be extremely important as a basis for judgment to have some idea about the intercalibration of the systems. You should provide the negative results with a confidence interval. If a minus tells us anything, it is the acceptable level of effectiveness of the compound should it be outside a certain confidence interval of the negative test. There, this study you have suggested might lead to certain rules of intercalibration. There are some indications that for whole groups of compounds you might have the same intercalibration factors, at least approximately enough to consider this side of the problem.

LEE: Earlier we went over what would essentially be required for the next series of steps. Should we move on?

SHELBY: What have we decided?

LEE: I thought we simply said that you would insist on quantitative dosimetry and from that type of information, since they are all DNA-binding, or at least do damage to DNA, one can essentially quantitate this type of damage and from that plug in the type of procedures that have already been developed for radiation and end up with a risk estimate.

VALCOVIC: I think I see a difference. Maybe we are not interpreting in the same way what DNA-binding means here. I thought that we could assume that there had been complete studies. If it were just a qualitative finding--if we are talking about DNA binding...

PERTEL: Assume that these are good studies with dose responses.

VALCOVIC: What does DNA-binding mean? Is that in vitro?

PERTEL: No, in vivo. With DNA binding you can obtain sensitivities of 10^{-15} g/kg more, giving you a level in the gonads. The fourth one is also in vivo by the appropriate exposure route. These are givens--that this is the optimal source.

LEE: May we assume that if there is damage to DNA that can be measured quantitatively, it could presumably be measured in systems that were given exposure similar to what humans are given, and thus dosimetry could be determined; one could also determine the level in the test systems for which you are measuring the mutation consequence. This gives you the background information to make a risk estimate.

VALCOVIC: I get the impression from this that all the appropriate experiments have been done, that all I need to do is sit down with a paper and pencil.

LEE: There is nothing as to the levels that would be encountered by the human germ line, and therefore until you get some estimate of that level, you have no basis for making a risk estimate.

PERTEL: Some of the component in here is human exposure.

LEE: The exposure of humans and the resulting level of dose to the germ cells that would grow.

ABRAHAMSON: I think that if I know what the mouse mutation rate is per unit dose, I can then establish, with the human spontaneous rate, what one unit dose contributes in the way of genetic disease. You are asking for an additional step that asks, "What human exposure?" Under human exposure I can put down what the actual risk to humans is, not from one unit but from exposure to one-thousandth of a unit. We could take it through, "One unit is equivalent to this much genetic damage, and what is the human exposure?" It is either one unit, two units, or one-thousandth of a unit of that. The final figure of human genetic disorder is determined by the number you want: the human exposure rate or real dose rate.

VALCOVIC: I think that in a practical sense you are going to do it on a basis of per potential exposure. You are therefore not going to wait until all of the comparative human metabolic studies have been done on each and every chemical. Granted, those things will reduce your level of uncertainty.

SHELBY: That kind of information is not necessary to produce a risk estimate.

BREWEN: May we go back to the information Lee gave us the other day where he plotted the dose of a compound fed to flies, measured the mutation rate at each of those doses, and got a dose-response curve, which we might say was linear. Then, when he looked at the amount of alkylation in the sperm, he found that there was not a linear relationship between concentration applied and amount of damage to DNA. When he then plotted his dose-response curve against alkylation, the curve was no longer linear; it was quadratic. These tests are done, I assume, at reasonably high doses-- much higher than the human population will be exposed to. Without the dose-response data you will extrapolate back on a linear curve and come out with a risk estimate that may be two logs too high. You can be in error in the other direction and come out with an estimate two logs too low without the dosimetry data.

ABRAHAMSON: I do not think we are arguing about that point. I think we are accepting the fact that we want the dosimetry data. We should recognize two elements here. A risk estimate for a given human exposure is the risk estimate we really want, but we can develop a risk estimate per rem or per 5 rem of radiation as an example, whereas human exposure might be, on a yearly basis, 0.2 or 20 millirem. You get that once you know the per unit concentration and once you know the dose-response curve--and the dose. You are asking for the absolute risk estimate per unit dose. That is of less value until you know the human exposure for the reproductive life span. Then the risk estimate tells what the actual burden will be.

LEE: You could have a situation where you have determined that the chemical or its metabolite binds covalently with DNA and yet the Drosophila tests, the in vivo cytogenetics tests, the heritable translocation tests, and the dominant lethal tests are all negative, this is quite possible, because if you look at the numbers we have on ethylations per nucleotide versus sex-linked recessive lethals (Aaron and Lee, 1978; Lee, 1978), we estimate that we would require 4×10^{-5} ethylations per nucleotide to double the spontaneous frequency. Most tests for screening mutagens do not have the sensitivity to permit detection of doubling the spontaneous frequency. There is a lot of room beneath the end of our observed data for agents that could ethylate in the same way as EMS, producing exactly the same consequence on DNA, and would presumably have a linear relation, at least from extrapolation above, and not be detected as positive in any of the test systems (except for bacterial) simply because they were not sensitive enough, as Ehrenberg pointed out.

In those cases, we need to have a series of model systems where we know essentially what level of hydroxyethyl groups must be added and what level of methyl groups must be added with a certain distribution in order to give positive levels of mutation in Drosophila sex-linked recessive lethal tests, in dominant lethal tests, and in other tests of this type. Compounds can be listed as weakly mutagenic when they are doing exactly the same thing chemically that EMS does but for some reason their toxicity is such that we cannot give a level of alkylation required for a positive test or that they simply require metabolite to be metabolized and are not metabolized in sufficient quantity to give an aklylation level in our test systems that puts us into the plus category.

The public would surely not accept this now, but I think that in the future, if we do our basic research well now, we will be able to establish curves where the distribution of alkylation and groups added to DNA can be computed and a certain level could be considered a risk that is not acceptable. In other words, a hazard could be put onto a level of ethylation if you knew the distribution of the ethylation on DNA and the amount.

We cannot do that now, we should emphasize, and before we can do it, we would need a series of model compounds that were adding covalently binding to

DNA. But it is possible to do the research that will give that kind of information.

Then one would use what I choose to call a "secondary dosimeter." Ehrenberg has made a very useful suggestion of using substances in the body that are alkylated and can be measured at levels more sensitive than you could measure DNA. I prefer not to use the term dose for alkylation of hemoglobin because this is not the area of interest. However, it may be extremely useful as a secondary dosimeter. By this I do not mean a secondary dosimeter is of lesser importance; I am simply noting that one must know the correlation between alkylation of hemoglobin and alkylation of DNA. This is distribution between certain sites that might be found in blood cells and distribution among certain sites in DNA.

Such things need to be determined with in vivo experiments. With that, as Ehrenberg has pointed out, one could, in the future, actually obtain a risk estimate for these compounds that are negative across the board with all of our systems except possibly the Ames system. It would take a lot of basic research on model compounds. Even then, the results would apply only to those compounds that did fit within the range of the models that had been tested.

ABRAHAMSON: That covered the opposite extreme. Anything in between you would have some other level of action on. Perhaps that is the best way to end it.

SUTTON: Isn't sterility more of a problem? Of course, sterility kind of takes care of the genetic burden.

BREWEN: Is that permanent sterility of the exposed animals or sterility in their offspring?

ABRAHAMSON: In fact, sterility is a situation that was reasonably common. I do not know whether this came out of the data base. It was the case when a whole group of laboratories tested some 20 different pesticides. Two were positive in the Ames test. The same two were positive with Drosophila, positive with unscheduled DNA synthesis, and, I believe, positive in the yeast test. But two others were positive with Drosophila, positive in yeast, and positive in unscheduled DNA synthesis. Finally, one more was positive in unscheduled DNA synthesis. So you had five positives going across, only two of which were positive essentially across the board. The Ames test picked them up. The Ames test missed at least 50% of the mutagens that were being picked up by higher eukaryotic systems in this batch of 20 chemicals.

LEE: What was the <u>Drosophila</u> test?

ABRAHAMSON: The <u>Drosophila</u> test in every case was sex-linked recessive lethals.

BREWEN: Was it positive in all broods?

ABRAHAMSON: It was positive in sperm/spermatid tests. The data base on spermatogonia would not be enough to allow you to go on to it. I think only 1,000 chromosomes were tested in spermatogonia. At the level that these things were being funded, you could never have done a spermatogonia test that would be valid. You should understand that. Twenty compounds were being run through in 18 months in <u>Drosophila</u>, and you were detecting a doubling in the spontaneous mutation rate. On the level of the mature sperm/spermatid tests, we were able to detect a doubling. That is the information that did exist.

LEE: Here again, since there is a plus for DNA damage, there is the opportunity to ask a question as to the dose level to the germ line in <u>Drosophila</u> as compared with in the mouse and to have some handle on this question as to whether the sterility really would take care of it. In other words, below the levels that cause sterility in the mouse, would you predict a significant mutation frequency using sex-linked recessive lethal tests? If that is so, it is not proof, but it is a strong indication that at substerility levels you have a real mutagenic hazard. You need to have some idea of the dose and dose-response curve in order to get a handle on that question.

EHRENBERG: I think it is a common situation. You might expect--and you have found--that you would get in vivo effects on chromosomes, but you do not get anything in the Ames test or in in vitro tests where you have this artificial situation where the enzymes are producing and destroying the active principle. If you could only make dosimetry in that environment by some good technique to see whether you catch a metabolite according to the principle we described for vinyl chloride, you could see whether you would have detected the standard error--the confidence interval of a particular negative result. Then you could go on for the dominant lethals and see whether there is the usual correlation between in vivo cytological disturbances and dominant lethals--for instance, as obtained with methyl methanesulfonate, X-rays, and so forth. You put up the hypothesis of what frequency of dominant lethals you would expect. Do you exclude that by a negative result in the size of test you have run? If you do not exclude it, then this minus (negative result) does not mean anything.

ABRAHAMSON: A minus is not necessarily a minus; it only tells us that we do not have much confidence in the size of the test, if we can have another approach to it.

LEE: If you do the proper dosimetry, a minus could mean simply that it does not cause mutations in that system or it could mean that you simply have not done a test with the sensitivity to detect it. You can distinguish between those two with the dosimetry. There are two kinds of minuses.

ABRAHAMSON: One is a minus and one is a question mark.

LEE: That is right. Actually, you might even say that one is a zero and one is a minus, because you just have not done the test that would give you the answer in one case.

PERSON: Are you saying that with the dosimetry you can get an absolute minus, that you are 100% sure it is not?

LEE: You could get confidence limits on saying that the mutation response in this system is significantly lower by a certain quantity than the mutational response in another system, because you had a given amount of genetic damage to the DNA that in one system was recorded and in another system was not recorded. That type of minus could be stated quantitatively.

VALCOVIC: It is not saying an absolute minus. It is having a greater biological and statistical confidence or explanation of the disparity of the data.

SUMMARY

HUMAN GENETIC LOAD

In the course of the last 10 years, advances in medical genetics have resulted in a doubling of our estimate of the human genetic "load" representing serious genetic disorders suffered by the population. Our present estimate of these genetic disorders indicates that about 10% of all liveborn will manifest (either at birth or during subsequent life) a wide variety of serious genetic diseases. Neel, in reviewing the United Nations and National Academy of Sciences estimates, suggested that for at least one category of diseases, e.g., recessively inherited conditions, these are grossly underestimated. The bulk of this currently recognized disease burden, some 9%, comes from the category of congenital malformation and multigenic conditions that have not been amenable to simple Mendelian analysis. Opinion is still divided as to how large the mutation component is for this category. Recent national and international reports assessing the impact of mutation in increasing these diseases are at variance. Some suggest that the mutational component may range from 5% to 50%. Assumptions here can greatly affect the projected number of disorders resulting from environmental mutagens.

Two clearly determined disease categories that are mutationally maintained are monogenic disorders (including dominants) and X-linked recessive diseases; together, they contribute 1% of the liveborn disorders. Also well recognized are two kinds of abnormal chromosomal conditions, which collectively contribute 0.5% to the disease burden. These diseases result from individuals inheriting either one too many or one too few chromosomes from their parents and from inheriting chromosomes that have lost important blocks of vital genic material. These conditions usually lead to severe mental and physiological disorders, including sterility, infertility, and much-shortened life span. If past experience is a guide to the future, we can expect to identify even more of these conditions as a variety of medical genetic techniques detect more subtle chromosome derangements and their associated effects.

Finally, many leading geneticists are disturbed by the great uncertainty about the impact or detriment resulting from the heterozygous effect of recessive gene disorders. The BEIR committee of the National Academy of Sciences suggests that perhaps an additional 2.5% of all ill health may result from this heterozygous effect, and Neel (this report) conservatively estimates that future biochemical research will demonstrate that the impact of recessive diseases outweighs all the other contributions.

Within the last decade we have also learned that genetic, primarily chromosomal, disorders are responsible for about 50% of all spontaneous abortions. A small shift in intrauterine mortality, as Neel points out, can have enormous consequences on the postnatal genetic load.

Clearly, such a statistical treatment of the genetic disease burden cannot adequately describe the personal tragedies and suffering associated with this burden--nor an impact on future generations such that the number of affected persons collectively overwhelms that resulting from any natural catastrophic event. Moreover, it is in the nature of genetic disease and selection that the less severe the disorder, the greater the number of individuals who will be afflicted with time, whereas the more damaging the disorder, the shorter will be its persistence in time and therefore the fewer the number of individuals who will be affected.

If only 20% of our total health costs, roughly estimated at some 160 billion dollars per year, are attributable to genetically related diseases, we see that a substantial social burden is involved in the treatment and maintenance of afflicted persons. The recent studies of Trimble and Smith (1977) already have demonstrated that children with well-defined genetic disease entities are admitted to hospitals five to ten times more frequently than the average, and their days of hospitalization are ten times greater than stays resulting from nongenetic causes. Moreover, the limited studies of Day and Holmes (1973) show that 17% of all pediatric in-patients are hospitalized because of disease of genetic origin. Compositely, then, these studies suggest that one to two times as many health dollars are associated with genetic-disease-related pediatric conditions than with all other causes combined.

In all likelihood, environmental mutagens contribute to a large and costly genetic health burden. The manner of evaluating how much contribution will be made by any specific agent was the major area of discussion at this conference.

SPECTRUM OF MUTATIONAL EFFECTS

A mutagen may be defined as a substance (or a mixture of substances) that induces heritable changes in the genetic material (mutations). When the mutations are produced in the genetic material of somatic (body) cells, they may ultimately affect the exposed individual in diverse ways; for example, in terms of cancer, accelerated aging, congenital birth defects, and other diseases such as atherosclerosis (for which a mutational involvement has recently been suggested). Such somatic-cell mutations are not transmissible to future generations. When mutations are induced in the genetic material of germinal cells (egg or sperm), however, then they can be transmitted to subsequent generations and contribute to the genetically determined disease burden discussed above.

The mutations may be restricted to individual genes. They may also involve changes in the number or structure of the chromosomes containing these genes.

These inherited changes result from the interaction of the mutagen with DNA (deoxyribose nucleic acid), the macromolecule that encodes the genetic information. In addition, changes in chromosome number may also result from the interaction of a mutagen with specific proteins of the spindle apparatus. The spindle apparatus is responsible for the precise distribution of sets of chromosomes to dividing cells (somatic and germinal).

Testing systems have been developed to detect and characterize the range of genetic effects that may be induced by a mutagen, as well as the type of chemical interactions that may be involved (see Flamm, Setlow, Brewen, Eisenstadt, Walker, and Abrahamson).

Concordance of test results from different species is a strong indication that a given mutagen is potentially a mutagen in the human also. Of particular importance is the method of action of the mutagen in the variety of test systems. In some cases, the action is very direct, leading to substitutions, additions, or deletions of DNA bases. In other cases, the mutagen may modify these bases through ethylation, methylation, adduct formation, etc., and, in general, cause disruption in the normal functioning of the genes and their products. Some of these lesions, when acted upon by DNA repair systems, may then be converted into an altered DNA sequence. Setlow's discussion centers around DNA repair systems, which themselves are under genetic control, and the relationship between recognized genetic abnormalities in repair and their association with cancer.

Differential mutability and/or sensitivity of the varied germ-cell stages within an organism was the subject of extensive discussion. Such stages as spermatocytes or spermatids are found to be inordinately more sensitive than the spermatogonial stage for most mutagens. The spermatogonial stage, however, is of greater importance in accumulating and transmitting genetic damage, primarily because, as stem cells, they (or their descendants) persist for the reproductive period of the individual. As Brewen and others point out, there is also great concern that the mouse ovary may not provide an appropriate model system for evaluation of the human ovary response.

CARCINOGENESIS VS MUTAGENESIS

The relationship between mutagenesis and carcinogenesis has lately attracted a great deal of attention. There are now considerable data demonstrating the correlation between a chemical's ability to produce mutations in in vitro tests and in in vivo bioassays for cancer. The most appealing interpretation at present is that induced cancer involves somatic mutations. This meeting discussed risks to future generations, in contrast to the individual risk assessment involved in carcinogenesis studies.

While there are other, perhaps superficial, differences between the mutation and cancer end points, such as the long latent period required for the manifestation of cancer, it should be remembered that the cancer cells are competing with normal cells. Their ultimate fate is determined by a number of selective factors, in the same way as the persistence and spread of a new genotype in a population are mediated by selective factors operating at the organismal level, where there is also a long latent period, which is measured not in years but in generations.

ELEMENTS OF RISK ASSESSMENTS

In dealing with toxic chemicals, a distinction should be made between qualitative hazard evaluation and quantitative risk assessment.

Hazard evaluation is the review of pertinent toxicological literature on a given end point, such as cancer or reproductive effects, to ascertain whether the chemical does or does not produce the effect under study. In studying the mutagenic hazard of chemicals, all data bearing on their ability to induce mutations must be reviewed, including exposure not only to the parent chemical, but also to contaminants, degradation products, and metabolites. In hazard evaluations, multiple test systems are used to determine whether the chemical can interact with or damage the genetic material (DNA) so that mutations and chromosome aberrations will be induced or such genetical processes as crossing over, gene conversion, or sister chromatid exchange will be altered. In the application of the mutagenicity data to humans, one must determine the manner in which the compound will be metabolized by humans or related species--whether, in fact, the compound or an active metabolite will reach the gonads. Collectively, these items constitute a qualitative assessment of a potential hazard to humans.

After the hazard evaluation, a risk assessment may be made. The quantitative statement of risk estimates the probability that the hazard will occur in exposed popula-

tions. A crucial part of any risk assessment is an estimate
of human exposure to the offending agent. It is hoped that
these values will be translated into a more useful measure--
population dose. It should be noted that, from the
standpoint of genetic implications, and provided that the
response is linearly related to dose in the range considered, the same amount of mutation will be produced in
10,000 individuals receiving 100 dose units of a mutagen as
in one million individuals each receiving 1 dose unit of that
mutagen. The risk assessment includes appropriate data
and spells out all procedures. In such risk assessments,
one must use data from the appropriate test systems,
including the potencies of the chemical in those systems,
estimates of the size and composition of exposed human
groups, and estimates of the dose levels and frequency of
exposure. One must also consider specific storage systems,
such as the accumulation of chlorinated hydrocarbon
pesticides in human fatty tissue or the slow release of such
accumulations in mothers' milk to infants. These factors
contribute to the exposure levels and gonadal dose levels.
All this information is then combined with a reasonable
model for extrapolation to humans to generate the quantitative risk estimate--namely, the expected increase in the
genetically determined human disease burden resulting from
the population exposure.

   The final report on a chemical thus consists of two
parts: a qualitative estimate of the likelihood that the
chemical is a potential hazard to humans and a quantitative
estimate of the probability that the chemical will induce the
hazard.

   The practical (regulatory) application of risk assessment is the establishment of the "allowable dose," and it is
recognized that a different level may be set for occupational
groups relative to that set for the general population.

DETERMINATION OF MUTAGENIC DOSE--
EVALUATION OF HUMAN EXPOSURE LEVELS

Exposure to synthetic chemicals has increased greatly in the
last several decades, with up to 70,000 of them in commerce
and around 1,000 new ones introduced yearly. There is, of
course, enormous variability in individual exposures, which
results from a constellation of factors, including social,
physical, and biological ones. Where one lives, works, or
travels and one's age, sex, eating preferences, smoking
habits, or state of health, including inherited differential
sensitivities, are just a few of the myriad of interactions
influencing exposure and the subsequent effects determined
by that exposure. This human exposure dose estimation
generally requires a number of assumptions. It should be

noted that the degree of uncertainty in estimating human exposure dose is often greater than that of the biological test results for effects such as mutagenicity.

The determination of the germ-cell dose of a chemical mutagen relative to the human exposure dose, discussed above, is another essential component in establishing human genetic risk. Only mutations in the germ-cell lineage can be transmitted to subsequent generations. The dose of a mutagen to these cells is, of course, related to the exposure and the route of exposure (feeding, inhalation, surface contact, etc.), but it is also related to any metabolic and physiological alteration the mutagen may have undergone before reaching the germ cells and to the persistence of the mutagen in these tissues.

Thus, the mutagenic dose will be the amount of chemical that reacts with the target genetic molecules to produce a measurable selected reaction product that has a relationship to the mutational process. The dose, then, is the time of integral concentration, which is similar to the way in whch the dose of ionizing radiation is derived. Lee's discussions deal with specific methods of establishing this measure of germ-cell dose. A more indirect measure of dose can also be obtained by measuring the reactivity of a mutagen with other kinds of cellular molecules that have a constant relationship to the genetic material (see discussions by Ehrenberg).

EXTRAPOLATION FROM ANIMAL AND CELL-CULTURE RESULTS

The approach of estimating mutagenic risk from adequate human data, that is, from epidemiological data from large-scale population monitoring, will not be available to us, it is hoped, because it would mean that important regulatory and experimental testing procedures have failed in alerting us to the specific mutagenic hazard. Thus, in the near future, the major methods of deriving risk estimates will all entail extrapolation either from mammalian or other whole-animal experiments or from somatic cell cultures of human or other mammalian lines. Of course, it should be remembered that chromosome aberrations may alert us to hazards a long time before a mutagenic effect is recognized in the germ cells.

The shape of the mutagenic dose-response curve and its importance in extrapolation of risk assessments to humans at low dose exposures receive considerable discussion in the presentations by Hoel on chemically induced carcinogenesis and by Baum on radiation-induced carcinogenesis. Hoel deals primarily with the existing statistical procedures that have evolved to relate carcinogenic response to dose and the refinements that have been introduced into the mathematical models as basic underlying biological mechanisms have been elucidated. Hoel's discussion provides an important critique of some of the existing models and their likelihood of underestimating risk in the low-dose region of the curve. A clear message from Hoel is that response in the low-dose region is best depicted as being approximately linear, and that even for very complex models, the linear (no threshold) extrapolation does not overestimate the risk. It would appear at present that linear extrapolation is not excessively conservative.

Most workers in the field of mutagenesis and carcinogenesis recognize that the shape of the dose-response curve may take on complex forms at very high exposures to chemicals or radiation and will often appear to saturate or assume a hump configuration as a result of cell-killing and differential sensitivities of heterogeneous cell populations. An important caveat ensues: high single-dose exposure levels are inappropriate regions from which to extrapolate to determine the response at low doses. A number of points are needed on the mutation curve before conclusions can be reached.

In Baum's discussion on radiation-induced carcinogenesis, many dose-response curves are developed, but they frequently have a linear contribution in the low-dose region of the curve. Where initial studies do not always show this, Baum provides evidence that the studies may have been truncated too early, and that longer studies of the populations in question have tended to demonstrate a trend toward linear response.

Finally, at this point we have had extensive mutation studies on a wide variety of organisms, from viruses to mammals, showing that, with respect to a variety of ionizing radiations, a linear dose response is obtained in the low-dose region of the curves or when low dose rates are applied (see, for example, UNSCEAR, 1977, 1972, 1966, 1958; BEIR 1972; BEAR, 1956-1960). Thus, the conclusion is that a single energy quantum is capable of initiating the lesion that results in the mutational end point.

Chemical mutagens operate in similar fashion in the low-dose region of the curve, as has already been demonstrated in some experimental systems for a few well-studied mutagens, ethyl methanesulfonate (EMS), for example, and it would appear that the same applies for the less extensive data base of other laboratory mutagens.

One can expect to obtain estimates of mammalian germ-cell mutation rates for some select group of chemical mutagens, but because of the expense, time, and difficulty of obtaining reasonably large samples, it is unlikely that reliable estimates of induced gene mutational damage will exist for the thousands of chemicals of interest. Data for even a small set of defined chemicals will be of great value, however, because they can be almost directly extrapolated to the human situation after applying appropriate corrections for metabolic and other factors. For these same chemicals it will be easier to obtain mutation data on somatic cells of animal test systems as well as on human somatic cells treated in equivalent fashion. Thus, the proposition from which extrapolation will be made asserts that the ratio of human somatic-cell damage (A) to human germ-cell damage (A') will be proportional to the ratio of animal somatic-cell damage (B) to that of animal germ-cell damage (B'). Because A and B can be obtained directly from test data and B' can be obtained directly in some cases or estimated, it will be possible to predict the A' value.

Estimates for mutagen-induced chromosome damage in mammalian germ-cell stages will probably be obtained more readily than for gene mutational damage because reasonably large samples of germ cells can be screened using a small number of animals. Even mature human sperm cells treated outside the male can be screened with the very recently developed techniques of Jacobs et al. (1978), and while this is not usually the stage of major interest in risk assessment, there will be situations (see discussion) where these data can provide information for these purposes.

What is not often appreciated, even by geneticists, is that induced mutation data in existing experimental systems do not directly translate into increased incidence of genetic disease in human populations. What is needed is a way of determining what the relative mutational risk will be for a given dose or exposure of that agent. The methods by which the relative mutational risk values are applied to the human disease burden are briefly described by Abrahamson. This methodology has been used by a variety of national and international agencies since 1956 to prepare risk estimates for radiation-induced genetic damage in humans. Revisions based on new data are prepared every five years. These estimates have been used by regulatory agencies to set population exposure limits, and it therefore seems obvious that evaluating chemical mutagens could involve equating a given dose of mutagen to a dose of radiation that produce the equivalent level of genetic damage. This rad-equivalent chemical value provides a prediction of induced genetic disease for the specific end point analyzed. This approach is utilized by Ehrenberg in his presentation. A number of participants describe pitfalls and limitations. Nevertheless, such approaches may provide upper limits of risk when more direct assessments are not available.

From extensive data on radiation-induced gene mutation in a variety of organisms--bacteria through animals and plants--a simplifying concept has emerged. This concept states that the amount of mutational damage in a given organism (i.e., the average gene mutation rate) induced by a given dose of irradiation (mutagen) will be proportional to the amount of DNA in that organism (Abrahamson et al., 1973).   Although there are certain apparent exceptions to this rule, it may have heuristic value in predicting chemical mutagen responses.   Indeed, Heddle and Athanasiou have suggested (1975) that a parallel relationship was found for the mutagen EMS, although data were less extensive.   It would be amazing, indeed, if such a simplified model could be used to extrapolate to humans, considering the wide difference in physiology and metabolism and the different potential repair capacities of the various organisms employed in test systems.   Nevertheless, it may turn out that a particular experimental test system or systems will more effectively and inexpensively represent the human induced mutation   rate   than   the   present   expensive   mammalian germ-cell tests available.   The plant Tradescantia emerges as a candidate because of its greater amount of DNA per cell (at least an order of magnitude) than the human cell. Tradescantia has been an extremely sensitive monitoring indicator   of   chemical   and   irradiation   mutagenesis   (as demonstrated by Sparrow and his colleagues, 1972).

RESEARCH NEEDS

The   attendees   at   this   workshop   agreed   that   existing methodology can be utilized to derive risk estimates for human   exposure   to   chemical   mutagens.   The   current scientific basis is, in fact, much stronger than the one that existed for regulatory measures taken decades ago to limit human exposure to radiation.   It is emphasized, however, that   such   estimates,   like   all   extrapolations,   consist   of certain unavoidable assumptions and undefined levels of uncertainty that can be reduced with better understanding of mutational phenomena in eukaryotes and more information regarding   the   genetic   disease   mechanisms   of   humans. Several areas of research needs were identified as neces-sary to increase the level of confidence in the risk equa-tion.

Clearly, a heightened effort is required to establish a more accurate estimate of the spontaneous human mutation rate.   Some   useful   techniques   are   available,   and   Neel presents   others   that   appear   to   have   merit.   Accurate determination of the effect of newly arising mutations on genetic diseases of complex origin will have an impact on risk-assessment conclusions.

Population subgroups whose genetic constitution leads to abnormally heightened responses to low-level mutagen exposure should be identified.   A promising approach for the identification of such subgroups would involve screening somatic cells in culture from a wide variety of people. Additional efforts required to understand any differences in susceptibility are investigations of repair processes and metabolic conversion capabilities relevant to mutagen activation.

The development of in vivo eukaryotic systems that discriminate intragenic from intergenic mutations will facilitate the extrapolation of genetic harm to humans, especially if some of the systems being developed use the same enzymes for detection of mutational change utilized in Neel's human population studies.

Among the major needs recognized and discussed in detail at the meeting was a coordinated approach to determine the dose at the target cells. Baseline data do exist for a few chemicals; however, carefully selected "type" compounds from various structural classes should be studied in detail.

Information on differential sensitivity of mammalian germ-cell stages should be increased--especially with regard to the female. Additional areas of research that would be helpful are: improved methodology for detecting nondisjunctional effects; the role of DNA repair in eukaryotic mutagenesis; and increased information on the already detailed molecular mechanisms of mutation in eukaryotes.

REFERENCES

Aaron, C.S. 1976. Molecular dosimetry of chemical mutagens: Selection of appropriate target molecules for
determining molecular dose to the germ line. Mutat.
Res. 38:303.
Aaron, C.S. and W.R. Lee. 1978. Molecular dosimetry
of the mutagen ethyl methanesulfonate in Drosophila
melanogaster spermatozoa: Linear relation of DNA
alkylation per sperm cell (dose) to sex-linked recessive
lethals. Mutat. Res. 49:27.
Abrahamson, S. 1961. Chromosome rearrangement induced
by X-rays in immature germs of Drosophila. Nature
191:323.
Abrahamson, S., M.A. Bender, A.D. Conger, and S. Wolff.
1973. Uniformity of radiation-induced mutation rates
among different species. Nature 245:460.
Adetugbo, K., C. Milstein, and D.S. Secher. 1977. Molecular analysis of spontaneous somatic mutants. Nature
265:299.
Allen, R.C., H. Meier, and W.G. Hoag. 1962. Ethylene
glycol produced by ethylene oxide sterilization and its
effects in an inbred strain of mice. Nature 193:387.
Amacher, D.E., J.A. Elliott, and M.W. Lieberman. 1977.
Differences in removal of acetylaminofluorene and
pyrimidine dimers from the DNA of cultured mammalian
cells. Proc. Natl. Acad. Sci. USA. 74:1553.
Ames, B.N. and K. Hooper. 1978. Does carcinogenesis
potency correspond with mutagenesis in the Ames
assay? Nature 274:19.
Ames, B.N., F.D. Lee, and W.E. Durston. 1973. An
improved bacterial test system for the detection and
classification of mutagens and carcinogens. Proc.
Natl. Acad. Sci. USA 70:782.
Ames, B.N., J. McCann and E. Yamasaki. 1975. Methods
for detecting carcinogens and mutagens with the
Salmonella/mammalian-microsome mutagenicity test.
Mutat. Res. 31: 347.
Ames, B.N., W.E. Durston, E. Yamasaki, and F.D. Lee.
1973. Carcinogens and mutagens: A simple test system
combining liver homogenates for activation and bacteria
for detection. Proc. Natl. Acad. Sci. USA 70:2281.
Anderson, L. and N.G. Anderson. 1977. High resolution
two-dimensional electrophoresis of human plasma proteins. Proc. Natl. Acad. Sci. USA 74:5421.
Appelgren, L.E., G. Eneroth, and C. Grant. 1977. Studies
on ethylene oxide: Whole-body autoradiography and
dominant lethal test in mice. Proc. Eur. Soc. Toxicol.
18:315.
Attardi, B. and S. Ohno. 1974. Cytosol androgen receptor from kidney of normal and testicular feminized
(Tfm) mice. Cell 2:205.

Baum, J.W. 1973. Population heterogeneity hypothesis on radiation-induced cancer. Health Phys. 25:97.
————. 1976. Multiple simultaneous event model for radiation carcinogenesis. Health Phys. 30:85.
Bernstine, E.G., L.B. Russell, and C.S. Cain. 1978. Effect of gene dosage on expression of mitochondrial malic enzyme activity in the mouse. Nature 271:748.
Blum, H.F. 1959. Carcinogenesis by ultraviolet light. Princeton University Press, Princeton, New Jersey.
Brewen, J.G. 1977. The application of mammalian cytogenetics to mutagenicity studies. In Progress in genetic toxicology (ed. D. Scott, B.A. Bridges, and F.H. Sobels), vol. 2, p. 165. Elsevier/North-Holland Biomedical Press, Amsterdam.
Brewen, J.G. and H.S. Payne. 1976. Studies on chemically induced dominant lethality. II. Cytogenetic studies of MMS-induced dominant lethality in maturing dictyate mouse oocytes. Mutat. Res. 37:77.
————. 1978. Studies on chemically induced dominant lethality. III. Cytogenetic analysis of TEM effects on maturing dictyate mouse oocytes. Mutat. Res. 50:85.
Brewen, J.G. and W.J. Peacock. 1969. Restricted rejoining of chromosomal subunits in aberration formation: A test for subunit dissimilarity. Proc. Natl. Acad. Sci. USA 62:389.
Brewen, J.G. and R.J. Preston. 1978. Radiation-induced chromosome aberration in somatic and germ cells of the male marmoset. In Marmosets in experimental medicine. Primates in medicine series (ed. N. Genzogian, F. Deinhardt) vol. 10, p. 199. Karger, Basel.
Brewen, J.G., R.J. Preston, and N. Gengozian. 1975. Analysis of X-ray induced chromosomal translocations in human and marmoset spermatogonial stem cells. Nature 253:468.
Brewen, J.G., H.S. Payne, K.P. Jones, and R.J. Preston. 1975. Studies on chemically induced dominant lethality. I. The cytogenetic basis of MMS-induced dominant lethality in post-meiotic male germ cells. Mutat. Res. 33:239.
Bridges, B.A. 1974. The three-tier approach to mutagenicity screening and the concept of radiation-equivalent dose. Mutat. Res. 26: 335.
Brock, R.D. 1965. Induced mutations affecting quantitative characters. Radiat. Bot. (Suppl.) 5:451.
Brown, J.M. 1976. Linearity vs. nonlinearity of dose response for radiation carcinogenesis. Health Phys. 31:231.
Bryan, W.R. and M.B. Shimkin. 1943. Quantitative analysis of dose-response data obtained with three carcinogenic hydrocarbons in strain C3H male mice. J. Natl. Cancer Inst. 3:503.

Burnet, B. and J.H. Sang. 1964. Physiological genetics of melanotic tumors in Drosophila melanogaster. II. The genetic basis of response to tumorigenic treatments in the tuK and tu bw; st su-tu strains. Genetics 49:223.

Burns, F.J., R.E. Albert, and R.D. Heimbach. 1968. The RBE for skin tumors and hair follicle damage in the rat following irradiation with alpha particles and electrons. Radiat. Res. 36:225.

Burtis, C.A., J.C. Mailen, W.F. Johnson, C.D. Scott, and T.O. Tiffany. 1972. Development of a miniature fast analyzer. Clin. Chem. 18:753.

Burtis, C.A., W.F. Johnson, J.C. Mailen, J.B. Overton, T.O. Tiffany, and M.D. Watsky. 1973. Development of an analytical system based around a miniature fast analyzer. Clin. Chem. 19:895.

Calleman, C.J., L. Ehrenberg, B. Jansson, S. Osterman-Golkar, D. Segerbäck, K. Svenson, and C.A. Wachtmeister. 1978. Monitoring and risk assessment by means of alkyl groups in hemoglobin in persons occupationally exposed to ethylene oxide. J. Environ. Pathol. Toxicol. 2: 427.

Carr, D.J. and M. Gedeon. 1977. Population cytogenetics of human abortuses. In Population cytogenetics (ed. E.B. Hook and I.H. Porter), p. 1. Academic Press, New York.

Carter, T.C. 1958. Radiation-induced gene mutations in adult female and foetal male mice. Br. J. Radiol. 31:407.

Cattanach, B.M. 1975. Comparison of the mutagenic effect of chemicals and ionizing radiation in the spermiogenic cells of the mouse. In Radiation research: Biomedical, chemical, and physical perspectives (ed. O.F. Nygaard, H.I. Adler, and W.K. Sinclair), p. 984. Academic Press, New York.

Cattanach, B.M. and H. Mosely. 1974. Sterile period, translocation, and specific locus mutation in the mouse following fractionated X-ray treatment with different fractionation intervals. Mutat. Res. 25:63.

Cattanach, B.M., C.E. Pollard, and J.H. Isaacson. 1968. Ethyl methanesulfonate-induced chromosome breakage in the mouse. Mutat. Res. 6:297.

Chand, N. and D.G. Hoel. 1974. A comparison of the models for determining safe levels of environmental agents. In Reliability and biometry (ed. F. Proschan and R.J. Serfling), p. 382. Siam, Philadelphia, Pennsylvania.

Childs, B., S.M. Miller, and A.G. Bearn. 1972. Gene mutation as a cause of human disease. In Mutagenic effects of environmental contaminants (ed. H.E. Sutton and M.I. Harris), p. 3. Academic Press, New York.

Chu, E.H.Y. and H.V. Malling. 1968. Mammalian cell genetics. II. Chemical induction of specific locus mutations in Chinese hamster cells in vitro. Proc. Natl. Acad. Sci. USA 61:1306.

Cleaver, J.E. 1968. Defective repair replication of DNA in xeroderma pigmentosum. Nature 218:652.

Clive, D., W.G. Flamm, and J.B. Patterson. 1973. Specific-locus mutational assay systems for mouse lymphoma cells. In Chemical mutagens: Principles and methods for their detection. (ed. A. Hollaender), vol. 3, p. 73. Academic Press, New York.

Clive, D., W.G. Flamm, M.R. Machesko, and N.J. Bernheim. 1972. A mutational assay system using the thymidine kinase locus in mouse lymphoma cells. Mutat. Res. 16:77.

Committee 17. 1975. Environmental mutagenic hazards. Science 187:503.

Conner, T.H., M. Stoeckel, J. Evrard, and M.S. Legator. 1977. The contribution of metronidazole and two metabolites to the mutagenic activity detected in urine of treated humans and mice. Cancer Res. 37:629.

Cornfield, J. 1977. Carcinogenic risk assessment. Science 198:693.

Coulondre, C. and J.H. Miller. 1977. Genetic studies of the lac repressor. IV. Mutagenic specificity in the lacI gene of Escherichia coli. J. Mol. Biol. 117:577.

Crump, K.S., D.G. Hoel, C.H. Langley, and R. Peto. 1976. Fundamental carcinogenic processes and their implications for low dose risk assessment. Cancer Res. 36:2973.

Day, N. and L.D. Holmes. 1973. The incidence of genetic disease in a university hospital population. Am. J. Hum. Genet. 25:237.

Dean, B.J. 1978. Reviews in genetic toxicology. Mut. Res. 47:75.

Defais, M., P. Caillet-Fauquet, M.S. Fox, and M. Radman. 1976. Induction kinetics of mutagenic DNA repair activity in E. coli following ultraviolet irradiation. Mol. Gen. Genet. 148:125.

Denic, M., J. Dumanovic, and L. Ehrenberg. 1969. Induced variation of protein content and composition in wheat. Contemp. Agric. 11:85.

Department of Health, Education and Welfare (DHEW). 1970. Vital Statistics of the United States, vol. 2, Mortality, part A. U. S. Government Printing Office, Washington, D.C.

Drake, J.W. 1970. The molecular basis of mutation. Holden-Day, San Francisco.

Druckrey, H. 1967. Quantitative aspects of chemical carcinogenesis. In UICC Monograph Series: Potential carcinogenic hazards from drugs (Evaluation of risks) (ed. R. Truhart), vol. 7, p.60. Springer-Verlag, New York.

Edwards, J.H. 1974. The mutation rate in man. In Progress in medical genetics (ed. A.G. Steinberg and A.G. Bearn), vol. X, p. 1. Grune & Stratton, New York.

Ehling, U.H. 1971. Comparison of radiation- and chemically induced dominant lethal mutations in male mice. Mutat. Res. 11:35.

————. 1977. Dominant lethal mutations in male mice. Arch. Toxicol. 38:1.

Ehling, U.H., R.B. Cumming, and H.V. Malling. 1968. Induction of dominant lethal mutations by alkylating agents in male mice. Mutat. Res. 5:417.

Ehrenberg, L. 1971. Higher plants. In Chemical mutagens: Principles and methods for their detection (ed. A. Hollaender), vol. 2, p. 365. Plenum Press, New York.

————. 1974. Genetic toxicity of environmental chemicals. Acta Biol. Iugosl. Ser. F Genet. 6:367.

————. 1977. Aspects of statistical inference in testing for genetic toxicity. In Handbook of mutagenicity test procedures (ed. B. Kilbey et al.), p. 419. Elsevier/North-Holland Biomedical Press, Amsterdam.

————. 1978. Dose response relationships for biological effects of ionizing radiation. In Report to the Swedish Energy Commission, Ds I:24 (see summary and references).

————. 1979. Methods of comparing risks of radiation and chemicals: The rad-equivalence of stochastic effects of chemicals. In IAEA Reports. Vienna. (In press)

Ehrenberg, L. and G. Eriksson. 1966. The dose dependence of mutation rates in the rad range, in the light of experiments with higher plants. Acta Radiol. Suppl. 254:73.

Ehrenberg, L. and T. Hällström. 1967. Haematologic studies on persons occupationally exposed to ethylene oxide. In Radiosterilization of medical products, p. 327. IAEA, Vienna.

Ehrenberg, L. and S. Osterman-Golkar. 1977. Reaction kinetics of chemical pollutants as a basis of risk estimates in terms of rad-equivalence. In First European Symposium on Rad-Equivalence, EUR. 5725E, p. 199. Commission of the European Communities, Luxemborg.

Ehrenberg, L. and S. Hussain. 1979. Genetic toxicity of some important epoxides. Heriditas (in press).

Ehrenberg, L., K.D. Hiesche, S. Osterman-Golkar, and I. Wennberg. 1974. Evaluation of genetic risks of alkylating agents: Tissue doses in the mouse from air contaminated with ethylene oxide. Mutat. Res. 24: 83.

Ehrenberg, L., S. Osterman-Golkar, D. Segerbäck, K. Svensson, and C.J. Calleman. 1977. Evaluation of genetic risks of alkylating agents. III. Alkylation of haemoglobin after metabolic conversion of ethene to ethene oxide in vivo. Mutat. Res. 45:175.

Eisenstadt, E. and A. Gold. 1978. Cyclopenta /c,d/pyrene: Highly mutagenic polycyclic aromatic hydrocarbon. Proc. Natl. Acad. Sci. USA 75:1667.

Embree, J.W. 1976. "Mutagenicity of ethylene oxide and associated health hazard." Ph.D. thesis, University of California, San Francisco.

Embree, J.W., J.P. Lyon, and C.H. Hine. 1977. The mutagenic potential of ethylene oxide using the dominant lethal assay in rats. Toxicol. Appl. Pharmacol. 40:261.

Environmental Protection Agency (EPA), Pesticide Programs. Proposed guidelines for registering pesticides in the United States; Hazard evaluation: Humans and domestic animals. Fed. Reg. 43:37336.

Erickson, R.P., E.M. Eicher, and S. Gluecksohn-Waelsch. 1974. Demonstration in mouse of X-ray induced deletions for a known enzyme structural locus. Nature 248:416.

Evans, H.J. and D. Scott. 1964. Influence of DNA synthesis on the production of chromatid aberrations by X-rays and maleic hydrazide in Vicia faba. Genetics 49:17.

————. 1969. The induction of chromosome aberration by nitrogen mustard and its dependence on DNA synthesis. Proc. R. Soc. Lond. B 173:491.

Evans, R.D., A.T. Keane, and M.M. Shanahan. 1972. Radiogenic effects in man of long-term skeletal alpha-irradiation. J. W. Press, Salt Lake City, Utah.

Felton, J.S. and D.W. Nebert. 1975. Mutagenesis of certain activated carcinogens in vitro associated with genetically mediated increases in monooxygenase activity and cytochrome P1-450. J. Biol. Chem. 250:6769.

Fielek, S. and H.W. Mohrenweiser. 1979. Assays for erythrocyte enzyme deficiencies utilizing a miniature centrifugal fast analyzer. Clin. Chem. Acta (in press).

Finkel, M. 1959. Induction of tumors with internally administered isotopes. In Radiation biology and cancer, p. 322. University of Texas Press, Austin.

Flamm, W.G., Chairman. 1977. DHEW Report on approaches to determining the mutagenic properties of chemicals: Risk to future generations. Prepared for DHEW by the DHEW Committee to coordinate Toxicology and Related Programs (Working Group of the Subcommittee on Environmental Mutagenesis.) J. Environ. Path. Toxicol. 1:301.

Ford, C.E., A.G. Searle, E.P. Evans, and B.J. West. 1969. Differential transmission of translocations induced in spermatogonia of mice by irradiation. Cytogenetics 8:447.

Frost, D.V. 1975. Is selenium depletion the answer to the "arsenic cancer" mystery? Feedstuffs 47/14 (see references).

Gabridge, M.G. and M.S. Legator. 1969. A host-mediated microbial assay for the detection of mutagenic compounds. Proc. Soc. Exp. and Biol. Med. 130:831.

Generoso, W.M. and W.L. Russell. 1969. Strain and six variations in the sensitivity of mice to dominant lethal induction with ethyl methanesulfonate. Mutat. Res. 8:589.

Generoso, W.M., S.W. Huff, and S.K. Stout. 1971. Chemically induced dominant lethal mutations and cell killing in mouse oocytes in the advanced stage of follicular development. Mutat. Res. 11:411.

Generoso, W.M., M. Krishna, R.E. Sotomayer, and N.L.A. Cacheiro. 1977. Delayed formation of chromosome aberrations in mouse pachytene spermatocytes treated with triethylenemelamine (TEM). Genetics 85:65.

Generoso, W.M., K.T. Cain, M. Krishna, and S.W. Huff. 1979. Genetic lesions by chemicals and spermatozoa and spermatids of mice are repaired in the egg. Proc. Natl. Acad. Sci. USA 76:435.

Generoso, W.M., W.L. Russell, S.W. Huff, S.K. Stout, and D.G. Gosslee. 1974. Effects of dose on the induction of dominant-lethal mutations and heritable translocations with ethyl methanesulfonate in male mice. Genetics 77:741.

Gibson, R., S. Graham, A. Lilienfeld, L. Schuman, J.E. Dowd, and M.L. Levin. 1972. Irradiation in the epidemiology of leukemia among adults. J. Natl. Cancer Inst. 48:301.

Giudotti, G. 1967. Studies on the chemistry of hemoglobin. J. Biol. Chem. 242:3673.

Gluecksohn-Waelsch, S., M.B. Schiffman, J. Thorndike, and C.F. Cori. 1974. Complementation studies of lethal alleles in the mouse causing deficiencies of glucose-6-phosphate, tyrosine-aminotransferase, and serine dehydratase. Proc. Natl. Acad. Sci. USA 71:825.

Goldstein, J.L. and M.S. Brown. 1977. The low-density lipoprotein pathway and its relation to atherosclerosis. Annu. Rev. Biochem. 46:897.

Göthe, R., C.J. Calleman, L. Ehrenberg, and C.A. Wacht-meister. 1974. Trapping with 3,4-dichlorobenzenethiol of reactive metabolites formed in vitro from the carcinogen vinyl chloride. Ambio 3:234.

Green, E.L. 1968a. Body weights and embryonic mortality in an irradiated population of mice. Mutat. Res. 6:437.

————. 1968b. Reproductive fitness of descendents of mice exposed to spermatogonial irradiation. Radiat. Res. 35:263.

Green, S. and J.A. Springer. 1973. The dominant-lethal test: Potential limitations and statistical considerations for safety evaluation. Environ. Health Perspect. 6:37.

Griggs, H.G. and M.A. Bender. 1973. Photoreactivation of ultraviolet-induced chromosomal aberrations. Science 179:86.

Guess, H. and K.S. Crump. 1978. Best-estimate low-dose extrapolation of carcinogenicity data. Environ. Health Perspect. 22:149.

Guess, H., K. Crump, and R. Peto. 1977. Uncertainty estimates for low-dose rate extrapolations of animal carcinogenicity data. Cancer Res. 37:3475.

Harris, H. 1963. Garrod's inborn errors of metabolism (see pp. xi and 207). Oxford University Press, London.

Haynes, R.H. 1964. Role of DNA repair mechanism in microbial inactivation and recovery phenomena. Photochem. Photobiol. 3:429.

Heddle, J.A. 1978. Extrapolation of mutation rate data from experimental organisms to man. In Proceedings of IAEA. Consultants Meeting on the "Radiobiological Equivalents of Chemical Pollutants." IAEA, Vienna. (In press).

Heddle, J.A. and K. Athanasiou. 1975. Mutation rate, genome size and their relation to the rec concept. Nature 258: 359.

Hieger, I. 1959. Carcinogenicity by cholesterol. Br. J. Cancer 13:439.

Hogstedt, C., N. Malmqvist, and B. Wadman. 1979. Leukemia in ethylene oxide exposed personnel. J. Am. Med. Assoc. (In press).

Hogstedt, C., O. Rohlen, S.S. Berntsson, O. Axelson, and L. Ehrenberg. 1978. A cohort study on mortality among employees in ethylene oxide production. Lakartidningen 75:3285.

———— . 2nd ref. English version: British Journal of Industrial Medicine. (In press).

Hsu, T.C., W.C. Dewey, and R.M. Humphrey. 1962. Radiosensitivity of cells of Chinese hamster in vitro in relation to the cell cycle. Exp. Cell Res. 27:441.

Hunt, V.R. 1973. Polonium 210 concentrations measured in human semen. Health Phys. 25:336.

Hussain, S. and L. Ehrenberg. 1975. Prophage inductive efficiency of alkylating agents and radiations. Int. J. Radiat. Biol. 27:355.

―――. 1977. Gene mutations: Dose-response relationships and their significance for extrapolation to man. Abh. Akad. Wiss. DDR abt. Math.-Naturwiss.-Techn. N9:95.

Hussain, S. and S. Osterman-Golkar. 1976. Comment on the mutagenic effectiveness of vinyl chloride metabolites (addendum to a paper by U. Rannug et al.). Chemico-Biological Interactions 12:265.

IARC (Int. Agency Res. Cancer). 1973. Certain polycyclic aromatic hydrocarbons and heterocyclic compounds. In On the evaluation of carcinogenic risk of the chemical to man, vol. 3, IARC Monographs, Lyon, France.

International Commission on Radiological Protection. 1977. Recommendations of the international commission on radiological protection. In Annals of the ICRP, Publ. 26. Pergamon Press, Oxford.

Ivankovic, S. 1969. Erzeugung von genitalkrebs beiträchtigen ratten. Arzneimittelforsch. 19:1040.

Jacobs, P.A. 1975. The load due to chromosome abnormalities in man. In The role of natural selection in human evolution (ed. F.M. Salzano), p. 337. North-Holland, Amsterdam.

Jacobs, P.A., A. Frackiewicz, and P. Law. 1972. Incidence and mutation rates of structural rearrangements of the autosomes in man. Ann. Hum. Genet. 35:301.

Jacobs, P.S., Melville, and S. Ratcliffe. 1974. A cytogenetic survey of 11,680 newborn infants. Ann. Hum. Genet. 37:359.

Janca, F.C. 1977. Stability of induced DNA alkylations in sperm and embryos of Drosophila melanogaster. Abstracts of the 8th Annual meeting of the Environmental Mutagen Society, Colorado Springs, Colorado, p. 59.

Jerina, D.M., R. Lehr, M. Schaefer-Ridder, H. Yagi, J. M. Karle, D.R. Thakker, A.W. Wood, A.Y. H. Lu, D. Ryan, S. West, W. Levin, and A.H. Conney. 1977. Bay-region epoxides of dihydrodiols: A concept explaining the mutagenic and carcinogenic activity of benzo(a)pyrene and benzo(a)anthracene. Cold Spring Harbor Conf. Cell Proliferation 4:639.

Kato, T. and Y. Shinoura. 1977. Isolation and characterization of mutants of Escherichia coli deficient in induction of mutations by ultraviolet light. Mol. Gen. Genet. 156: 121.

Kazazian, H., S. Cho, and J.S. Phillips. 1977. The mutational basis of the thalassemia syndromes. Prog. Med. Genet. (new series) II:165.

Kimura, M. 1968. Genetic variability maintained in a finite population due to mutational pressure of neutral and nearly neutral isoalleles. Genet. Res. 11:247.

King, J. L. 1967. Continuously distributed factors affecting fitness. Genetics 55:483.

Kirkman, H.N. 1972. Enzyme defects. Prog. Med. Genet. VIII:125.

Klose, J. 1975. Protein mapping by combined isoelectric focusing and electrophoresis of mouse tissue. A novel approach to testing for induced point mutations in mammals. Humangenetik 26:231.

———. 1977. The protein-mapping method employed to test for chemically induced point mutations in mice. Arch. Toxicol. 38:53.

Knudson, A.G. 1971. Mutation and cancer: Statistical study of retinoblastoma. Proc. Natl. Acad. Sci. USA 68:820.

Lambert, B., A. Lundblad, M. Nordenskjöld, and B. Werelis. 1978. Increased frequency of sister-chromatid exchanges in cigarette smokers. Hereditas 88:147.

Lawley, P.D. 1976. Carcinogenesis by alkylating agents. In Chemical carcinogens (ed. C. E. Searle), monogr. 173, p. 83. American Chemical Society, Washington, D.C.

Lawley, P.D., D.J. Orr, and S.A. Shah. 1971/72. Reaction of alkylating mutagens and carcinogens with nucleic acids: N-3 of guanine as a site of alkylation by N-methyl-N-nitrosourea and dimethyl sulphate. Chem. Biol. Interact. 4:431.

Lebowitz, H., D. Brusick, D. Matheson, M. Reed, S. Goode, and G. Roy. 1978. The genetic activity of benzene in various short-term in vitro and in vivo assays for mutagenicity. Abstracts of the 9th Annual meeting of the Environmental Mutagen Society, San Francisco, California. p. 81.

Lee, W.R. 1975. Comparison of the mutagenic effects of chemicals and ionizing radiation using Drosophila melanogaster test systems. In Radiation research, biomedical, chemical, and physical perspectives (ed. O.F. Nygaard, H.I. Adler, and W.K. Sinclair), p. 976. Academic Press, New York.

Lee, W.R., 1976. Molecular dosimetry of chemical mutagens: Determination of molecular dose to the germ line. Mutat. Res. 38:311.

————. 1978. Dosimetry of chemical mutagens in eukaryote germ cells. In Chemical mutagens: Principles and methods for their detection. (ed. A. Hollaender and F.J. deSerres), vol. 5, p. 177. Plenum Press, New York.

Legator, M., L. Truong, T.H. Connor. 1978. Analysis of body fluids including alkylation of macromolecules for determination of mutagenic agents. In Chemical mutagens: Principles and methods for their detection (ed. A. Hollaender and F.J. deSerres), vol. 5, p. 1. Plenum Press, New York.

Leonard, A. and G.H. DeKnudt. 1967. Relation between the X-ray dose and the rate of chromosome rearrangements in spermatogonia of mice. Radiat. Res. 32:35.

Lindahl, T., P. Karran, and S. Riazuddin. 1978. DNA glycosylases of Escherichia coli. J. Supramol. Struct., Suppl. 2, p. 12.

Lindgren, K. 1971. "The mutagenic effects of ethylene oxide in air." Ph.D. thesis, Stockholm University, Sweden.

Linn, S., W.S. Linsley, V. Kuhnlein, E.H. Penhoet, and W.A. Deutsch. 1978. Enzymes for the repair of apurinic/apyrimidine sites in human cells. J. Supramol. Struct., Suppl. 2, p. 11.

Luippold, H.E., P.C. Gooch, and J.G. Brewen. 1978. The production of chromosome aberrations in various mammalian cells by triethylenemelamine. Genetics 88:317.

Lyon, M.F., D.G. Papworth, and R.J. Phillips. 1972. Dose-rate and mutation frequency after irradiation of mouse spermatogonia. Nat. New Biol. 238:101.

Magee, P.N. 1977. The relationship between mutagenesis, carcinogenesis, and teratogenesis. In Progress in genetic toxicology (ed. D. Scott, B.A. Bridges, and F.H. Sobels), p. 15. Elsevier/North-Holland Biomedical Press, Amsterdam.

Maher, V.M. and J.J. McCormick. 1976. Effect of DNA-repair on cytoxicity and mutagenicity of polycyclic hydrocarbon derivatives in normal and xeroderma pigmentosum cells. In Biology of radiation carcinogenesis (ed. J.M. Yuhas, R.W. Tennant, and J.D. Regan), p. 129. Raven Press, New York.

Maldague, P. 1969. Comparative study of experimentally induced cancer of the kidney in mice and rats with X-rays. In Radiation-induced cancer, p. 439. IAEA, Vienna.

Malling, H.V. 1967. The mutagenicity of the acridine mustard (ICR-70) and the structurally related compounds in Neurospora. Mutat. Res. 4:265.

————. 1972. Mutation induction in Neurospora crassa incubated in mice and rats. Mol. Gen. Genet. 116:211.

Malling, H.V. and F.J. de Serres. 1973. Genetic alterations at the molecular level in X-ray induced ad-3B mutants of Neurospora crassa. Radiat. Res. 53:77.

Malling, H.V. and L.R. Valcovic. 1977a. A biochemical specific locus mutation system in mice. Arch. Toxicol. 38:45.

Malling, H.V. and L.R. Valcovic. 1977b. Gene mutations in mammals. In Progress in genetic toxicology (ed., D. Scott, B.A. Bridges, and F.H. Sobels), p. 155. Elsevier/ North-Holland Biomedical Press, Amsterdam).

Mantel, N. and W.R. Bryan. 1961. Safety testing of carcinogenic agents. J. Natl. Cancer Inst. 27:455.

Mantel, N. and M.A. Schneiderman. 1975. Estimating "safe" levels. A hazardous undertaking. Cancer Res. 35:1379.

Matter, B.E. and I. Jaeger. 1975. Premature chromosome condensation, structural chromosome aberrations and micronuclei in early mouse embryos after treatment of paternal post-meiotic germ cells with triethylenemelamine. A possible mechanism for chemically induced dominant lethal mutations. Mutat. Res. 33:251.

McCann, J. and B.N. Ames. 1976. Detection of carcinogens as mutagens in the Samonella/microsome test: Assay of 300 chemicals. Discussion. Proc. Natl. Acad. Sci. USA 73:950.

McCann, J., E. Choi, E. Yamasaki, and B.N. Ames. 1975a. Detection of carcinogens as mutagens in the Salmonella/microsome test: assay of 300 chemicals. Proc. Natl. Acad. Sci. USA 72:5135.

McCann, J., N.E. Spingarn, J. Kobori, and B.N. Ames. 1975. Detection of carcinogens as mutagens: Bacterial tester strains with R factor plasmids. Proc. Natl. Acad. Sci. USA 72:979.

McCoy, E.C., R. Hankel, K. Robbins, H. Rosenkranz, J. G. Giuffrida, and D.V. Bizzari. 1978. Abstracts from the 8th Annual Meeting of the Environmental Mutagen Society. Mutat. Res. 53:71.

Meier, H. and W.G. Hoag. 1966. Blood coagulation. In Biology of the laboratory mouse, Jackson Laboratory (ed. E. L. Green), p. 373. McGraw-Hill, New York.

Meselson, M. and K. Russell. 1977. Comparisons of carcinogenic and mutagenic potency. In Origins of human cancer. Book A. Incidence of cancer in humans. (ed., H.H. Hiatt, J.D. Watson, and J.A. Winsten) Vol. 4, p. 1473. Cold Spring Harbor Laboratory, New York.

Meyer, W.J. III, B.R. Migeon, and C.J. Migeon. 1975.
Locus on human X chromosome for dihydro-testosterone
receptor and androgen insensitivity. Proc. Natl.
Acad. Sci. USA 72:1469.

Milkman, R.D. 1967. Heterosis as a major cause of heterozygosity in nature. Genetics 55:493.

Miwa, S. 1973. Hereditary hemolytic anemia due to erythrocyte enzyme deficiency. Acta. Haematol. Jpn.
36:573.

Mohn, G. 1977. In Proceedings of the IAEA Consultants
Meeting on the "Radiobiological Equivalents of Chemical
Pollutants". IAEA, Vienna. (In press).

Moreau, P. and R. Devoret. 1977. Potential carcinogens
tested by induction and mutagenesis of prophage λ in
Escherichia coli K12. Cold Spring Harbor Conf. Cell
Proliferation 4:1451.

Moreau, P., A. Bailone, and R. Devoret. 1975. Prophage
lambda induction in Escherichia coli K12 envA uvrB: A
highly sensitive test for potential carcinogens. Proc.
Natl. Acad. Sci. USA 73:3700.

Morton, N.E., J.F. Crow, and H.J. Muller. 1956. An estimate of the mutational damage in man from consan-
quineous marriages. Proc. Natl. Acad. Sci. USA
42:855.

Moutschen, J. 1961. Differential sensitivity of mouse spermatogenesis to alkylating agents. Genetics 46:291.

Mrak, M. 1969. Report of the Secretary's Commission on
Pesticides and their relationship to environmental
health. U.S. Government Printing Office, Washington,
D.C.

Mukai, T. and C.C. Cockerham. 1977. Spontaneous mutation rates at enzyme loci in Drosophila melanogaster.
Proc. Natl. Acad. Sci. USA 74:2514.

Muller, H.J. 1950. Our load of mutations. Am. J. Hum.
Genet. 2:111.

National Academy of Sciences (NAS). 1956-1960. The
biological effects of atomic radiation. (BEAR report)
Summary reports. National Research Council,
Washington, D.C.

———— . 1972. The effects on populations of exposure to
low-levels of ionizing radiation. Report of the
Advisory Committee on the Biological Effects of
Ionizing Radiation (BEIR report). National Research
Council, Washington, D.C.

———— . 1972. Report of the consultative panel on the
health effects of chemical pesticides (M. Meselson,
chairman), vol. 1, p. 67. National Academy of
Sciences, Washington, D.C.

Neel, J.V. 1978. Mutation and disease in man. Can.
J. Genet. Cytol. 20: 295.

Neel, J.V. and E.D. Rothman. 1978. Indirect estimates of mutation rates in tribal Amerindians. Proc. Natl. Acad. Sci. USA 75:5585.

Neel, J.V., H. Mohrenweiser, C. Satoh, and H.B. Hamilton. 1978. A consideration of two biochemical approaches to monitoring human populations for a change in germ cell mutation rates. In Proceedings of the Conference on the Detection of Genetic Damage Caused by Environmental Factors. Ottawa, Canada. (In press).

O'Brien, S.J. 1973. On estimating functional gene number in eukaryotes. Nat. New Biol. 242:52.

O'Farrell, P.H. 1975. High resolution two-dimensional electrophoresis of proteins. J. Biol. Chem. 250:4007.

Osterman-Golkar, S. 1974. Reaction kinetics of N-methyl-N'-nitro-N-nitrosoguanidine and N-ethyl-N'-nitronitrosoguanidine. Mutat. Res. 24:219.

————. 1975. "Studies on the reaction kinetics of biologically active electrophile reagents as a basis for risk estimates." Ph.D. thesis, Stockholm University, Sweden.

Osterman-Golkar, S. and C.A. Wachtmeister. 1976. On the reaction kinetics in water of 1,3-propane sultone and 1,4-butane sultone: A comparison of reaction rates and mutagenic activities of some alkylating agents. Chem. Biol. Interact. 14:195.

Osterman-Golkar, S., L. Ehrenberg, and C.A. Wachtmeister. 1970. Reaction kinetics and biological action in barley of monofunctional methanesulfonic esters. Radiat. Bot. 10:303.

Osterman-Golkar, S., L. Ehrenberg, D. Segerbäck, and I. Hällström. 1976. Evaluation of genetic risks of alkylating agents. II. Haemoglobin as a dose monitor. Mutat. Res. 34:1.

Osterman-Golkar, S., D. Hultmark, D. Segerbäck, C.J. Calleman, R. Göthe, L. Ehrenberg, and C.A. Wachtmeister. 1977. Alkylation of DNA and proteins in mice exposed to vinyl chloride. Biochem. Biophys. Res. Commun. 76:259.

Paterson, M.C., B.P. Smith, P.A. Knight, and A.K. Anderson. 1977. Ataxia telangiectasia--Inherited human disease involving radiosensitivity, malignancy, and defective DNA repair. In Research in photobiology (ed. A. Castellani), p. 207. Plenum Press, New York.

Parker, D.R. and A.E. Hammond. 1958. The production of translocations in Drosophila oocytes. Gen 43: 92.

Parker, D.R. and J. McCrone. 1958. The genetic analysis of some rearrangements induced in oocytes of Drosophila. Gen. 43: 172.

Payne, H.S. and K.P. Jones. 1975. Technique for mass isolation and culture of mouse ova for cytogenetic analysis of the first cleavage mitosis. Mutat. Res. 33:247.

Pegg, A.E. 1978a. Dimethylnitrosamine inhibits enzymatic removal of O-6-methylguanine from DNA. Nature 274:182.

―――. 1978b. In Proceedings of the International Conference on Defective DNA Repair, Mutation and Human Ill Health, Ottawa, Canada. (In press).

Peto, R. and P.N. Lee. 1973. Weibull distributions for continuous-carcinogenesis experiments. Biometrics 29: 457.

Pomerantzeva, M.D., G.A. Vilkina, and V.N. Svanov. 1975. Mutagenic effect of different types of irradiation on germ cells of male mice. VIII. The frequency of reciprocal translocations in spermatogonia after chronic gamma irradiation. Genetika 11:8.

Popp, R.A., G.P. Hirsch, and R.A. Conard. 1975. Errors in synthesis of human hemoglobin. Gerontologist 15:33. (Abstr.)

Preston, R.J. and J.G. Brewen. 1973. X-ray-induced translocations in spermatogonia. I. Dose and fractionation responses in mice. Mutat. Res. 19:215.

―――. 1976. X-ray-induced translocations in spermatogonia. II. Fractionation responses in mice. Mutat. Res. 25:63.

Radford, E.P. and V.R. Hunt. 1964. Polonium 210: A volatile radioelement in cigarettes. Science 143:247.

Radman, M. 1975. SOS repair hypothesis: Phenomenology of an inducible DNA repair which is accompanied by mutagenesis. In Molecular mechanism for repair of DNA (ed. P.C. Hanawalt and R.B. Setlow), p. 283. Plenum Press, New York.

Rapoport, I.A. 1948. The effect of ethylene oxide, glycide, and glycol on genic mutations. Dokl. Akad. Nauk SSSR 60(3):467.

Ray, V.A. and M.L. Hyneck. 1973. Some primary considerations in the interpretation of the dominant-lethal assay. Environ. Health Perspect. 6:27.

Regan, J.D. and R.B. Setlow. 1974. Two forms of repair in the DNA of human cells damaged by chemical carcinogens and mutagens. Cancer Res. 34:3318.

Robbins, J.H., K.H. Kraemer, M. A. Lutzner, B.W. Festoff, and H.G. Coon. 1974. Xeroderma pigmentosum--inherited disease with some sensitivity, multiple cutaneous neoplasms, and abnormal DNA-repair. Ann. Intern. Med. 80:221.

Rossi, H.H. and A.M. Kellerer. 1972. Radiation carcinogenesis at low doses. Science 175:200.

Rowland, R.E., P.M. Failia, A.T. Keane, and A.F. Stehney. 1971. The use of the initial radium burden for dose response relationships, Report ANL-7860, Part II. Argonne National Laboratory, Argonne, Illinois.

Russell, L.B. 1963. The effect of radiation dose rate and fractionation on mutation in mice. In Repair from genetic radiation damage and differential radiosensitivity in germ cells (ed. F.H. Sobels), p. 205. Macmillan, New York.

————. 1965. Effect of the interval between irradiation and conception on mutation frequency in female mice. Proc. Natl. Acad. Sci. USA 54:1551.

————. 1971. Definition of functional units in a small chromosomal segment of the mouse and its use in interpreting the nature of radiation-induced mutations. Mutat. Res. 11:107.

————. 1972a. The genetic effects of radiation. In Peaceful use of atomic energy, vol. 13, p. 487. IAEA, Vienna.

————. 1972b. Radiation and chemical mutagenesis and repair in mice. In Proceedings Miles Fifth International Symposium on Molecular Biology: Molecular and Cellular Repair Processes (ed. R.F. Beers, R.M. Herriot, and R.C. Tilghman), p. 239. Johns Hopkins University Press, Baltimore, Maryland.

————. 1977. Mutation frequencies in female mice and the estimation of genetic hazards of radiation in women. Proc. Natl. Acad. Sci. USA 74:3523.

Russell, W.L. and E.M. Kelly. 1976. Specific-locus mutation frequencies in mouse spermatogonia at very low radiation dose rates. Genetics 83:s66.

Russell, L.B. and N.L.A. Cacheiro. 1977. The c-locus region of the mouse: Genetic and cytological studies of small and intermediate deficiencies. Genetics 86: 553.

Russell, L.B., W.L. Russell, R.A. Popp, C. Vaughan, and K.B. Jacobson. 1976. Radiation-induced mutations at mouse hemoglobin loci. Proc. Natl. Acad. Sci. USA 73:2843.

Sasaki, M.S. 1973. DNA repair capacity and susceptibility to chromosome breakage in xeroderma pigmentosum cells. Mutat. Res. 20:291.

Schalet, A.P. and K. Sankaranarayanan. 1976. Evaluation and re-evaluation of genetic radiation hazards in man. I. Interspecific comparison of estimates of mutation rates. Mutat. Res. 35: 341.

Schalet, A.P. 1978. Interspecific comparison of ethyl methanesulfonate-induced mutation rates in relation to genome size. Mutat. Res. 49: 313.

Schendel, P., M. Defais, P. Jeggo, L. Samson, and J.

Cairns. 1978. An inducible error-free repair pathway involved in the repair of alkylation damage in E. coli. J. Supramol. Struct., Suppl. 2, p. 25.

Schrauzer, G.N. 1976. Selenium and cancer: A review. Bioinorg. Chem. 5:275.

Scriver, C.R. 1973. Genetics defects in membrane transport mechanisms. In Medical genetics (ed. V. A. McKusick and R. Claiborne), p. 80. Hospital Practice Publishing, New York.

Scudiero, D., A. Norin, P. Karren, and B. Strauss. 1976. DNA excision-repair deficiency of human peripheral blood lymphocytes treated with chemical carcinogens. Cancer Res. 36:1397.

Searle, A.G. 1974. Mutation induction in mice. In Advances in radiation biology. (ed., Lett, J.T., H. Adler, and M. Zelle), vol. 4, p. 131. Academic Press, New York.

Searle, A.G., C.V. Beechey, D. Green, and E.R. Humphreys. 1976. Cytogenetic effects of protracted exposures to alpha particles from plutonium-239 and to gamma rays from cobalt-60 gamma rays compared in male mice. Mutat. Res. 41:297.

Searle, A.G., C.V. Beechey, E.P. Evans, C.E. Ford, and D.G. Papworth. 1971. Studies on the induction of translocations in mouse spermatogonia. IV. Effects on acute γ-irradiation. Mutat. Res. 12:411.

Searle, A.G., E.P. Evans, C.E. Ford, B.J. West, and D.G. Papworth. 1968. Studies on the induction of translocation in mouse spermatogonia. I. The effect of dose rate. Mutat. Res. 6: 427.

Seiler, J.P. 1977. Apparent and real thresholds: A study on two mutagens. In Progress in genetic toxicology. (ed., D. Scott, B.A. Bridges, and F.H. Sobels), p. 233. Elsevier/North-Holland Biomedical Press, Amsterdam.

Sega, G.A. 1974. Unscheduled DNA synthesis in the germ cells of male mice exposed in vivo to the chemical mutagen ethane methanesulfonate. Proc. Natl. Acad. Sci. USA 71:4955.

———— 1976. Molecular dosimetry of chemical mutagens: measurement of molecular dose and DNA repair in mammalian germ cells. Mut. Res. 38: 317.

Sega, G.A., and R.B. Cumming. 1975. Ethylation pattern in mouse sperm as a function of developmental stage and time after exposure to ethyl methanesulfonate. Mut. Res. 26:448.

Sega, G.A. and J.G. Owens. 1978. Ethylation of DNA and protamine by ethyl methanesulfonate in the germ cells of male mice and relevancy of these molecular targets to the induction of dominant lethals. Mut. Res. 52: 87.

Sega, G.A., R.B. Cumming, and M.F. Walton. 1974. Dosimetry studies on the ethylation of mouse sperm DNA after in vivo exposure to [³H]ethyl methanesulfonate. Mutat. Res. 24:317.

Sega, G.A., R.E. Sotomayor, and J.G. Owens. 1978. A study of unscheduled DNA synthesis induced by X-rays in the germ cells of male mice. Mutat. Res. 49:239.

Segerbäck, D., C.J. Calleman, L. Ehrenberg, G. Lofroth, and S. Osterman-Golkar. 1978. Evaluation of genetic risks of alkylating agents. IV. Quantitative determination of alkylated amino acids in hemoglobin as a measure of the dose after treatment of mice with methyl methanesulfonate. Mutat. Res. 49:71.

Setlow, R.B. 1978. Repair-deficient human disorders and cancer. Nature 271:713.

Setlow, R. and J.K. Setlow. 1972. Effects of radiation on polynucleotides. Annu. Rev. Biophys. Bioeng. 1:293.

Shellabarger, C.J. 1978. Rat mammary carcinogenesis following neutron- or X-radiation. In IAEA symposium on late biological effects of ionizing radiation. IAEA, Vienna. (In press).

Shellabarger, C.J., A.M. Kellerer, H.H. Rossi, L.J. Goodman, R.D. Brown, R.E. Mills, A.R. Rao, M.P. Shavley, and V.P. Bond. 1974. Rat mammary carcinogenesis following neutron or X-radiation. In Biological effects of neutron irradiation, p. 391. IAEA, Vienna.

Sheu, C.W., F.M. Moreland, E.J. Oswald, S. Green, and W.G. Flamm. 1978. Heritable translocation test on random-bred mice after prolonged triethenemalamine treatment. Mutat. Res. 50:241.

Shimkin, M.B., J.H. Weisburger, E.K. Weisburger, N. Gubaref, and V. Suntzeff. 1966. Bioassay of 29 alkylating chemicals by the pulmonary-tumor response in strain A mice. J. Natl. Cancer Inst. 36:915.

Shore, F.J., J.S. Robertson, and J.L. Bateman. 1973. Childhood cancer following obstetric radiography. Health Phys. 24:259.

Siciliano, M.J., M.R. Bordelon, and P.O. Kohler. 1978. Expression of human adenosine deaminase after fusion of adenosine deaminase-deficient cells with mouse fibroblasts. Proc. Natl. Acad. Sci. USA 75:936.

Slater, E.E., M.D. Anderson, and H.S. Rosenkranz. 1971. Rapid detection of mutagens and carcinogens. Cancer Res. 31:970.

Slizynska, H. 1973. Cytological analysis of storage effects on various types of complete and mosaic change induced in Drosophila chromosomes by some chemical mutagens. Mutat. Res. 19:199.

Sobels, F.H. 1977. Extrapolation from experimental test systems for evaluation of genetic risks in man. In Progress in genetic toxicology (ed. D. Scott, B.A. Bridges, and F.H. Sobels), p. 175. Elsevier/North-Holland Biomedical Press, Amsterdam.

Sotomayor, R.E., G.A. Sega, and R.B. Cumming. 1978. Unscheduled DNA synthesis in spermatogenic cells of mice treated in vivo with the indirect alkylating agents cyclophosphamide and mitomen. Mut. Res. 5: 229.

Spalding, J.F. and M.R. Brooks. 1972. Comparative litter and reproduction characteristics of mouse populations with X-ray exposure, including 45 generations of male progenitors. Proc. Soc. Exp. Biol. Med. 141/2:445.

Sparrow, A.H., H. Price, and A. Underbrink. 1972. A survey of DNA content per cell and per chromosome of prokaryotic and eukaryotic organisms: Some evolutionary considerations. Brookhaven Symp. Biol. 23:451.

Sparrow, A.H., A.G. Underbrink, and H.H. Rossi. 1972. Mutations induced in Tradescantia by small doses of X-rays and neutrons: Analysis of dose-response curves. Science 176:916.

Spiess, H. and C.W. Mays. 1970. Bone cancers induced by ^{224}Ra (Th X) in children and adults. Health Phys. 19:713.

Sporn, M.B., C.W. Dingman, H.L. Phelps, and G.N. Wogan. 1966. Aflatoxin B$_1$: Binding to DNA in vitro and alteration of RNA metabolism in vivo. Science 151: 1539.

Stanbury, J.B. 1974. Inborn errors of thyroid. Prog. Med. Genet. X:55.

Stevenson, A.C. 1959. The load of hereditary defects in human populations. Radiat. Res. Suppl. 1:306.

Stewart, A. and G.W. Kneale. 1970. Radiation dose effects in relation to obstetric X-rays and childhood cancers. Lancet 6:1185.

Sved, J.A., T.E. Reed, and W.F. Bodmer. 1967. The number of balanced polymorphisms that can be maintained in a natural population. Genetics 55:469.

Swain, C.G. and C.B. Scott. 1953. Quantitative correlation of relative rates. Comparison of hydroxide ion with other nucleophilic reagents toward alkyl halides, esters, epoxides, and acyl halides. J. Am. Chem. Soc. 75:141.

Swift, M. 1971. Fanconi's anemia in the genetics of neoplasia. Nature 230:370.

Swift, M., L. Sholman, M. Perry, and C. Chase. 1976. Malignant neoplasms in the families of patients with ataxia-telangiectasia. Cancer Res. 36:209.

Szybalski, W., G. Ragni, and N.K. Cohn. 1964. Mutagenic response of human somatic cell lines. Symp. Int. Soc. Cell Biol. 3:209.

Taylor, J.H., P.S. Woods, and W.L. Hughes. 1957. The organization and duplication of chromosomes as revealed by autoradiographic studies using tritium-labeled thymidine. Proc. Natl. Acad. Sci. USA 43:122.

Timoféeff-Ressovsky, N.W. and K.G. Zimmer. 1947. Biophysik I. Das Trefferprinzip in der Biologie. S. Hirzel Verlag, Leipzig.

Tomatis, L., J. Hilfrich, and V. Turusov. 1975. The occurrence of tumours in F_1, F_2 and F_3 descendants of BD rats exposed to N-nitrosomethylurea during pregnancy. Int. J. Cancer 15:385.

Trimble, B.K. and J.H. Doughty. 1974. The amount of hereditary disease in human populations. Ann. Hum. Genet. 38:199.

Trimble, B.K., and M.E. Smith. 1977. The incidence of genetic disease and the impact on man of an altered mutation rate. Can. J. Genet. Cytol. 19:375.

Turtóczky, I. and L. Ehrenberg. 1969. Reaction rates and biological action of alkylating agents: Preliminary report on bactericidal and mutagenic action in E. coli. Mutat. Res. 8:229.

Uchida, I.A. and C.P.V. Freeman. 1977. Radiation-induced nondisjunction in oocytes of aged mice. Nature 265:186.

United Nations. 1962. Report of the Scientific Committee on the Effects of Atomic Radiation (UNSCEAR). Supplement no. 16 (A/5216) New York.

———. 1966. Supplement no. 14 (A/6314). New York.

———. 1972. Ionizing radiation: Levels and effects, vol. II. New York.

———. 1977. Sources and effects of ionizing radiation, pp. 588, 725. New York.

Upton, A.C., M.L. Randolph, and J.W. Conklin. 1970. Late effects of fast neutrons and gamma rays in mice as influenced by the dose rate of irradiation; induction of neoplasia. Radiat. Res. 41:467.

Valcovic, L.R. and H.V. Malling. 1973. An approach to measuring germinal mutations in the mouse. Environ. Health Perspect. 6:201.

van Duuren, B.L., N. Nelson, L. Orris, E.D. Palmes, and F.L. Schmitt. 1963. Carcinogenicity of epoxides, lactones and peroxy compounds. J. Natl. Cancer Inst. 31:41.

van Duuren, B.L., L. Orris, and N. Nelson. 1965. Carcinogenicity of epoxides, lactones and peroxy compounds. II. J. Natl. Cancer Inst. 35:707.

van Duuren, B.L., L. Langseth, B.M. Goldschmidt, and L. Orris. 1967. Carcinogenicity of epoxides, lactones and peroxy compounds. VI. Structure and carcinogenic activity. J. Natl. Cancer Inst. 39:1217.

Veleminsky, J., S. Osterman-Golkar, and L. Ehrenberg. 1970. Reaction rates and biological action of N-methyl- and N-ethyl-N-nitrosourea. Mutat. Res. 10:169.

Vogel, F. 1975. Spontaneous mutation in man. Adv. Hum. Genet. 5:223.

Vogel, H.H., Jr. and R. Zaldivar. 1969. Experimental mammary neoplasms: A comparison of effectiveness between neutrons, X- and gamma-radiation. In Neutrons in radiobiology, p. 207. Agricultural Research Laboratory, Oak Ridge National Laboratory, and United States Atomic Energy Commission.

Vogel, F. and F.H. Sobels. 1976. The function of Drosophila in genetic toxicology testing. In Chemical mutagens: Principles and methods for their detection (ed. A. Hollaender), vol. 4, p. 93. Plenum Press, New York.

Walker, G.C. 1977. Plasmid (pKM101)-mediated enhancement of repair and mutagenesis: Dependence on chromosomal genes in Escherichia coli K-12. Mol. Gen. Genet. 152:93.

————. 1978a. Isolation and characterization of mutants of the plasmid pKM101 deficient in their ability to enhance mutagenesis and repair. J. Bacteriol. 133:1203.

————. 1978b. Inducible reactivation and mutagenesis of UV-irradiated bacteriophage CPP in Salmonella typhimurium LT2 containing the plasmid pKM101. J. Bacteriol. 135: 415.

Walpole, A.L. 1957. Carcinogenic action of alkylating agents. Ann. N. Y. Acad. Sci. 68:750.

Williams, M.H.C. 1958. Occupational tumors of the bladder. In Cancer (ed. R. W. Raven), vol. 3, p. 337. Butterworth, London.

Witkin, E.M. 1976. Ultraviolet mutagenesis and inducible DNA repair in Escherichia coli. Bacteriol. Rev. 40:869.

Yakubova, Z.N., N.A. Shamova, F.A. Miftakhova, and L.F. Shilova. 1976. Gynecological sickness of female workers at an ethylene oxide factory. Kazan. Med. Zh. 57:558.

Yamasaki, E. and B.N. Ames. 1977. Concentration of mutagens from urine by adsorption with the non-polar resin XAD-2: Cigarette smokers have mutagenic urine. Proc. Natl. Acad. Sci. USA 74:3555.

Yanagimachi, R., H. Yanagimachi, and B.J. Rogers. 1976. The use of zone-free animal ova as a test-system for the assessment of the fertilizing capacity of human spermatozoa. Biol. Reprod. 15:471.

Yanysheva, N. Ya. 1971. Substantiation of the threshold limit of benzo(a)pyrene in the atmosphere of populated areas. Gig. Sanit. 37:87.

Yuhas, J.M. 1976. Dose-response curves and their modification by specific mechanisms. In Biology of radiation carcinogenesis (ed. J.M. Yuhas, K.W. Tennant, and J.D. Regan), p. 51. Raven Press, New York.

Yuhas, J.M. and A.E. Walker. 1973. Exposure-response curve for radiation-induced lung tumours in the mouse. Radiat. Res. 54:261.

APPENDIX

Reprinted from Cancer Research, Vol. 36, pp. 2973-2979, September 1976

[CANCER RESEARCH 36, 2973-2979, September 1976]

Fundamental Carcinogenic Processes and Their Implications for Low Dose Risk Assessment

K. S. Crump,[1] D. G. Hoel,[2] C. H. Langley, and R. Peto

National Institute of Environmental Health Sciences, National Institutes of Health, Research Triangle Park, North Carolina 27709 [K. S. C., D. G. H., C. H. L.], and University of Oxford, Oxford, England [R. P.]

Summary

Various possible models of carcinogenesis are analyzed with respect to low dose kinetics. The importance of background carcinogenesis upon the shape of the dose-response curve at low dose is emphasized. It is shown that, if carcinogenesis by an external agent acts additively with any already ongoing process, then under almost any model the response will be linear at low dose. Measures of the degree of linearity are obtained for multistage models of carcinogenesis, where it is shown that throughout the dose range where the extra risk is less than the spontaneous risk linear extrapolation must be quite accurate.

Introduction

The presence of carcinogenic agents in the environment is an accepted fact. Although most agents can be avoided once they are identified as carcinogenic, some may be avoided only at great expense or alternative risk, in which case "risk *versus* benefit" must be evaluated. One important aspect of the determination of risk is the estimation from animal experiments conducted at high doses on small to moderate numbers of animals of the risks to such animals of cancer associated with very low levels of exposure. This is likely to be a principal element in risk estimation for the myriad of chemicals that must be evaluated. Relevant human data are usually not available.

The estimation of attributable risk at a dose very much lower (say 1/1000th) than the smallest practical experimental dose involves the interpolation between 2 dose levels: the control and the experimental dose levels. Interpolation necessitates an assumption about the behavior of the risk with increasing dose. The assumption can be specified arbitrarily or it can be deduced from reasonable models of the carcinogenic process. An "estimate" of risk is as arbitrary as the interpolation scheme that produced it. We will attempt in what follows to relate the properties of various risk estimation procedures to several observations and assumptions about carcinogenesis.

Two properties of carcinogenesis are critical to low dose risk estimation.

[1] Present address: Louisiana Tech University, Ruston, La. 71270.
[2] To whom requests for reprints should be addressed, at National Institute of Environmental Health Sciences, P. O. Box 12233, Research Triangle Park, N. C., 27709.
Received September 25, 1975; accepted June 1, 1976.

1. Cancers are believed to be single cell in origin (6, 7). Of a large number of cells at risk in the individual organism, 1 undergoes certain changes that allow it to divide and grow into a tumor. Thus we can view the carcinogenic process as mechanistically single cell in origin even though, by the time a cancer is pathologically recognizable, very extensive changes may have developed.

2. It will be shown that it is important to know whether the causal processes associated with the particular carcinogen of interest are common to those involved in carcinogenesis due to other causes, either "spontaneous" or from other carcinogens. In other words, we need to know whether or not carcinogenesis due to a particular carcinogen is independent of other modes of carcinogenesis.

In the 1st section of this paper, the consequences of the manner of combining "spontaneous" and "induced" carcinogenesis will be explored. We will show that, if the addition of the test carcinogen merely increases the rates of processes that were occurring anyway, then dose-response relationships will be linear at low dose levels. In the 2nd section several models will be considered and their low-dose properties will be identified. We will find that every reasonable model of carcinogenesis is linear or sublinear at low dose. Finally, in the 3rd section we will look more closely at this linearity and determine the accuracy of linear approximations in "multistage" models of cancer.

It should be recognized that there may be agents that indirectly affect the carcinogenic process. An example might be some dietary alteration that led to a modification of gut flora that may change the carcinogenic process in a qualitative way. Although our analysis and conclusions might be appropriate for some of these indirect carcinogenic processes as well, we are chiefly discussing direct carcinogenic processes in which the compound or its metabolite acts at the cellular level to produce an irreversible and heritable (genetic or epigenetic) change.

Significance of the Relation of a Carcinogen to Occurrence of Cancer due to Other Causes

Throughout this paper we shall concentrate upon the case of a population chronically exposed to carcinogens at constant dose rates. We are interested in the individual response when the population is exposed to a particular carcinogen at an approximately constant dose rate d per unit time. This response can be described by the age-specific cancer incidence rate $I(t,d)$ which is the expected rate per unit time at which cancer will be discovered in individ-

K. S. Crump et al.

uals of age *t* who were previously cancer free. In considering this response, it is important to keep in mind that individuals at risk will ordinarily be exposed to a large number of carcinogens, and we are interested in the effect upon the response of a single one of these which we shall for convenience call the primary carcinogen. As we shall see, the independence or equivalence of the mechanism(s) of action of the primary carcinogen and the other carcinogens can be important in determining the response due to a low dose rate of the primary carcinogen.

We can reasonably divide the totality of carcinogens into 2 groups: Group 1, containing all of those carcinogens that cause a response of cancer in a way that is completely independent of the mechanisms by which the primary carcinogen causes a response; and Group 2, consisting of those carcinogens (including spontaneous biochemical accidents) that somehow act in conjunction with the primary carcinogen in causing cancer. Let I_1 be the incidence rate of new cancers at a fixed time *t* due to a carcinogen in Group 1 or via an inherent spontaneous phenomenon that is mechanistically related to the effects of the carcinogens of Group 1. Let I_2 be the incidence rate of new cancers at time *t* due either to a carcinogen in Group 2 or to an inherent spontaneous phenomenon that is mechanistically related to the effects of the carcinogens of Group 2. Then, because of the assumed independence, we can write

$$I(d) = I_1 + I_2 \qquad (A)$$

where, as shall be done throughout the paper when convenient, the argument *t* has been omitted.

Now suppose that Group 2 consists of *m* carcinogens at dose levels $d^{(1)}, \ldots, d^{(m)}$ in addition to the primary carcinogen at a dose level *d*. The simplest assumption with regard to the interactive effect of these carcinogens would be to suppose that the effect is additive, *i.e.*, the rate I_2 at which cancer occurs due to a carcinogen in Group 2 is a function of an effective dose rate

$$D = D_0 + \beta d \qquad (B)$$

where D_0 is some function of $d^{(1)}, \ldots, d^{(m)}$. Now we can write

$$I_2 = H(D)$$

and we will assume that *H* is a nondecreasing analytical function. (This merely implies that any increase in the dose rate does not decrease the age-specific cancer incidence rate.) Now we can write

$$I(d) = I_1 + H(D_0 + \beta d) \qquad (C)$$
$$= I_1 + H(D_0) + \beta H'(D_0)d + o(d)$$

as the dose rate *d* approaches zero where o(*d*) denotes a function with the property o(*d*)/*d* approaches zero as *d* approaches zero. Thus we see that *I*(*d*) will be a linear function of the dose rate *d* at low dose rates provided $H'(D_0) > 0$.

Other authors (11) have allowed for cancers in the models due to causes other than the primary carcinogen of interest

by using the formula of Abbott (1) for correcting for response due to extraneous causes. In terms of the above formulation, this is equivalent to supposing that the 2nd group of carcinogens contains only the primary one, or, in other words, the carcinogen of interest acts in some manner completely independent of the mechanism by which all other cancers are formed. If this does, in fact, turn out to be the true biological situation, then the response function *I*(*d*) is still represented by Equation C except now $D_0 = 0$. Thus we see that even in this case *I*(*d*) can still be linear at low dose provided the slope of the function *H* is positive at zero. This turns out to be true for some models of carcinogenesis, *e.g.*, 1-hit models (2), but not for others, *e.g.*, some multihit models (15) and the Mantel-Bryan model (11). However, when other carcinogens act in conjunction with the primary one ($D_0 > 0$), the linearity of the response merely depends upon *H* having a positive slope at the point D_0. This seems intuitively likely and, in fact, is the case in all models of carcinogenesis with which we are familiar.

There are, of course, a number of questions about the biological validity of the assumptions.

1. Do all carcinogens act independently or do certain subgroups act in conjunction with each other? It should not be difficult to answer this question experimentally with regard to the effects of specific carcinogens on specific cancers.

2. Given that at least some carcinogens act in conjunction with the primary carcinogen, is it reasonable to assume that their individual effects are additive in the sense of Equation B? This question is probably much more difficult than the 1st one. However, the idea of complete additivity of effects is not essential to our arguments, and a variety of other assumptions would lead to effectively the same conclusion.

3. Is the assumption that $H'(D_0)$ is positive valid? For example, if there were some type of threshold effect operating so that $H(D) = 0$ for *D* less than some threshold value D_{th}, then if D_0 were less than D_{th}, the argument would break down and *I*(*d*) would, in fact, not be linear at the lowest dose rates. On the other hand, if cancer is single cell in origin, then the threshold D_{th} is a property of a single cell rather than of the whole organism. Viewed in this light, it is entirely plausible that, even if a threshold effect does exist for each cell, nevertheless in the entire organism the probability of response may be linear at low dose rates. These cellular thresholds will not all be constant but will be distributed over some range of doses. If this range includes D_0, the organismic response will, generally speaking, be linear at $D_0 + 0$. (The same conclusion would follow from postulating that each person in a large population has a particular threshold but that individual thresholds have a random distribution.)

4. Even if one is willing to accept the fact that the response curve is linear for low dose rates, this in itself may be of little value unless there is some knowledge about "how" linear and "how" low the dose rates must be. To answer such quantitative questions as these, one must make more specific assumptions than are incorporated into the very general discussion presented here. We shall return to this question in the light of some particular models for carcinogenesis.

Particular Models for Carcinogenesis

Experimental evidence (6, 7) indicates that cancers originate from a single cell. The models we shall look at will be based upon this premise. First, consider the time to response of a single cell, where the response might possibly be detection of or death due to a cancer originating with this cell. This time to response can be written as the sum of the period of genetic and/or epigenetic alteration of the cell to a malignant phenotype, plus the growth period from the time at which the cell is completely altered to the time of the observed response. The time to cell alteration is presumably dependent upon the dose rate d. This may also be true for the growth time, but we shall assume that the latter effect is negligible. If these 2 times are independent of each other, we can in general write

$$I_r(t,d) = \int_0^t I_a (t - u,d)f(u)du \qquad (D)$$

where $I_a (t,d)$ is the incidence rate of the alteration of a single cell, $f(t)$ is the density of cancer growth time, and $I_r(t,d)$ is the observed incidence rate for cancer response. The approximation in Equation D is valid because $I_a(t,d)$ applies to a single cell and will be very small. Now the observed incidence rate is for an entire tissue and, as pointed out by Armitage and Doll (4), insufficient attention has been given in some earlier models to the distinction between cell response and tissue response. If a tissue is composed of n cells, then the time to response of a tissue is the minimum of the associated n cell response times. If we suppose that these n cells all respond in the same manner but independently, then we arrive at the formula

$$I(t,d) = nI_r(t,d) \qquad (E)$$

1. Multihit and Multistage Models. Suppose $k \geq 1$ different events (hits) must occur in a cell before it is sufficiently altered and suppose the ith event occurs at a constant rate λ_i, $i = 1,2,\ldots,k$. Suppose further that cells that have suffered some, but not all, of the relevant events have no selective advantage or disadvantage relative to normal cells. Nordling (15) used the multihit model for the total response time, time to alteration, plus growth time, but here we generalize his approach by using the multihit process to model only the time to cellular alteration. The effect of dose rate is introduced in the manner of Neyman and Scott (14) by taking $\lambda_i = \alpha_i + \beta_i d$ (subject to $\alpha_i \geq 0$ and $\beta_i \geq 0$). The incidence rate of the alteration of a single cell is [see Armitage and Doll (4)]

$$I_a(t,d) \doteq kt^{k-1} \left\{ \prod_{i=1}^{k} (\alpha_i + \beta_i d) \right\} = kt^{k-1} Q_k(d) \qquad (F)$$

where $Q_k(d)$ is a kth degree polynomial in d with constant coefficients. For the observed incidence rate of cancer we obtain, using Equations D, E, and F,

$$I(t,d) \doteq Q_k(d)S_k(t) \qquad (G)$$

where

$$S_k(t) = nk \int_0^t f(t - u)u^{k-1}du \qquad (H)$$

At low dose rates this response is linear in the dose rate. To see this, we note that it is possible to write

$$I(t,d) = S_k(t)Q_k(d) = S_k(t) \{A + Bd + o(d)\}$$

where

$$A = \prod_{i=1}^{k} \alpha_i \text{ and } B = \sum_{i=1}^{k} \beta_i \prod_{j \neq i} \alpha_j$$

The incidence rate will be linear in dose rate at low dose rates whenever the constant B is positive. In order that there be both background carcinogenesis and also some effect of the dose rate d, it is necessary that all of the α_i's and at least 1 of the β_i's be positive. However, under these conditions the constant B is seen to be positive, and thus the incidence rate is linear at low dose.

If $k = 1$ (1-hit model) then

$$I(d) = (\alpha_1 + \beta_1 d)S_1(t) \qquad (I)$$

and the incidence rate is exactly linear in dose for all dose rates.

Alternatively, one could consider the time to cellular alteration to be the result of a multistage process. This process has been applied to carcinogenesis by Armitage and Doll (5). As in the multihit process, k events must occur in a cell to initiate cancer, these events occurring with fixed rate constants. The only difference between the multistage and the multihit processes is that the k-initiating events in a multistage process must occur in some particular time sequence. It can be shown (3) that Expression G still holds provided the right side of this equation is divided by k. Consequently, the comments on the linearity of the response for the multihit model hold true for the multistage model also. Our comments would, of course, also hold for intermediate models in which some stages must occur in a fixed sequence while others may occur in various orders.

2. Generalized Multievent Model. More generally, a large number of events related to the initiation of cancer could occur in a cell. However, rather than its being necessary for all of the events to occur to initiate cancer, there could be a (possibly quite large) number of subcollections $A_1, \ldots, A_n$ of these events so that cancer is initiated as soon as all of the events in any 1 of these subcollections occur. Thus, in this model there are many paths through which cancer can be initiated, a single path corresponding to a particular subcollection A_i of events. A path containing k events can be called a k-hit path. The subcollections need not be disjoint so that 1 particular event could be included in a number of different paths. The general consequences of this model are readily understood without going through all of the details. It makes no difference for our purposes whether or not some of the events must occur in a specified order since adjustments necessary to go from one case to

K. S. Crump et al.

the other are quite like the adjustment necessary for going from a multihit to a multistage model. It is again supposed that the ith event occurs at a constant rate $\alpha_i + \beta_i d$ where the α_i's may be functions of dose rates of other carcinogens but are not functions of d. In the terminology of the previous section, all of the paths in which the rates are not functions of d (that is in which the β_i's are all zero) represent the "1st-group" mechanisms, which are independent of the mechanisms by which the primary carcinogen causes cancer. The incidence rate associated with the union of these paths represents I_1 of Equation A, and the incidence rate associated with the union of those paths in which at least 1 of the rates is a function of d represents I_2. It can be shown that the response will be linear in d for small dose rate d unless all paths depending upon d contain at least 2 events that occur only in the presence of the specific primary carcinogen.

How Linear Is "Linear"?

In this section we attempt to describe quantitatively the range of dose rates for which the linear approximations are valid. To do this one must obviously be somewhat model specific, and we will assume the hit models. Two different approaches to the question of "how linear?" will be considered.

For a k-hit model with an arbitrary distribution for cancer induction time, we found (Equation G) that $I(t,d)$ can be expressed as the product of a function of age t only, and the polynomial $\overset{k}{\underset{i=1}{\pi}} (\alpha_i + \beta_i d)$ in the dose rate d. It is of interest to compare this exact expression with its linear approximation

$$I_1(d) = I(o) + dI'(o) \quad (J)$$

where $I(d)$ is given exactly by Equation G. To do this we shall consider the ratio r of $I(d)$ to the linear approximation $I_1(d)$ when $I(d)$ is a certain prescribed proportional excess p of $I(o)$, the age-specific incidence rate at a zero dose rate. Symbolically, we have

$$r = \frac{I(d_p)}{I_1(d_p)} = \frac{I(o)(1 + p)}{I(o) + I'(o)d_p} \quad (K)$$

$$= \frac{1 + p}{1 + \dfrac{I'(o)d_p}{I(o)}}$$

where d_p satisfies $I(d_p) = (1 + p)/(o)$.

It is easily seen that $r \geq 1$ is independent of t. Moreover, it can be shown using the method of Lagrange multipliers that r assumes its largest value when $\alpha_1/\beta_1 = \alpha_2/\beta_2 = \ldots = \alpha_k/\beta_k$. When this condition holds, we find that

$$r = \frac{1 + p}{1 + k\{(1 + p)^{1/k} - 1\}} \quad (L)$$

This is an appealing result in that r depends only on the number of stages k and the proportion of background p, parameters that are easily interpretable. This expression is increasing in k and approaches

$$\frac{1 + p}{1 + \log(1 + p)}$$

as $k \to \infty$. Thus, we have the bounds

$$1 \leq r \leq (1 + p)/\{1 + \log(1 + p)\} \quad (M)$$

This upper bound for r holds for any k, and for any multipath model with different values of k for different paths. The upper bound for the ratio is increasing in p. For a "doubling dose" $p = 1$ we have $r \leq 1.18$ regardless of the value of k, and if $k = 2$ we have $r \leq 1.09$. For a 10% increase in incidence over background, we set $p = 0.1$ and find that $r \leq 1.004$. These results are quite interesting and useful for 2 reasons: (a) they indicate the closeness to linearity for a very general class of models; (b) the results depend only on the proportion over background. If a finer bound is desired, the number of stages of the carcinogenic process or an upper bound to the number of stages is needed.

Our next approach to the question "how linear?" could be of interest in the following situation. Suppose estimates for $I(d)$ and $I(o)$ are available from experiments where d is a known experimental dose and information is desired about the incidence rate curve at dose rates much lower than d. There are 2 possible problems to consider. First of all, one might ask what dose rate d_a would yield a prescribed incidence rate I_a which may represent "a given acceptable" increase in the incidence rate over the background incidence rate $I(o)$. It should be expected that, if d is so small as to be on the linear portion of the dose-response curve, then d_a can be approximated by fitting a straight line through the points $[o,I(o)]$ and $[d,I(d)]$ and using the dose rate corresponding to I_a on the line. The dose computed using this linearization process is

$$d_L = \frac{I_a - I(o)}{I(d) - I(o)} d \quad (N)$$

Since $I_a - I(o)$ will usually be very small, $d_L \doteq d_a I'(o)d/\{I(d) - I(o)\}$, and thus the ratio of the true dose d_a and the approximation d_L is

$$\frac{d_a}{d_L} \doteq \frac{I(d) - I(o)}{I'(o)d} \equiv R \quad (O)$$

On the other hand, one may be interested in estimating the incidence rate I_E which corresponds to a very small environmental dose d_E. If I_E is approximated by I_L, the incidence rate corresponding to d_E on the line joining $[o,I(o)]$ and $[d,I(d)]$, then the ratio of the approximation $I_L - I(o)$ of the increase over background incidence to the true value $I_E - I(o)$, is the same R, since

$$\frac{I_L - I(o)}{I_E - I(o)} \doteq \frac{I(d) - I(o)}{dI'(o)} = R \quad (P)$$

Let us now consider the k-hit model and express R in

terms of p, the excess response over background, determined by $1 + p = I(d)/I(o)$. It can be shown that

$$1 \leq R \leq \frac{p}{k\{(1 + p)^{1/k} - 1\}} \qquad (Q)$$

the upper bound being attained when all β_i/α_i are equal. This upper bound increases steadily from 1 for a 1-hit model $(k = 1)$ to $\dfrac{p}{\log(1 + p)}$ as $k \to \infty$. We have tabulated the upper bound for R for different values of p and k in Table 1. We see that the linear approximations are reasonable over a wide range of values of k and p. The only circumstances in which linear approximation might be inappropriate are seen to be those where the background rate is vanishingly small and thus p is very large. An example of this might be the induction of angiosarcomas by vinyl chloride; however, if recent evidence (13) that common tumors are also caused by vinyl chloride is confirmed, p will not be extreme, and linear approximation will be adequate even in this case. The excess p of experimental incidence rate over background incidence $I(o)$ thus plays a key role in the accuracy of the linear approximations. In particular, the linear approximations improve as p decreases towards zero.

DISCUSSION

We have shown under some reasonable assumptions about carcinogenic mechanisms and processes that dose responses will be approximately linear at low doses. Let us examine the evidence in favor of these assumptions and review the generality of models considered.

Single-Cell Origin. If individual cancers arise from an original, single, "transformed" cell, then the statistical nature of the carcinogenic dose response will be governed by the extreme tail of the "transformation" response distribution. The effect of this is to make virtually any process of discrete events approximately linear at low dose.

Two primary observations indicate the single-cell origin of cancers. In women who are heterozygous for electrophoretic variants of X-linked glucose-6-phosphate dehydrogenase, cancers are uniformly of one phenotype or the other (6), whereas a comparable amount of normal tissue is composed of a mixture of cells of the 2 phenotypic classes. Further evidence for the single-cell origin of cancers comes from experimental efforts in which "transformed" cells are transplanted into whole animals. Although there is much controversy associated with various aspects of this line of research, it seems that the ability of a single cell to give rise to a cancer is well demonstrated (7). Thus, 2 lines of evidence indicate that cancer can be most reasonably as-

sumed to arise from events associated with or occurring inside single cells.

We note again here that this analysis is appropriate only for those agents that affect cancer incidence through the alteration of single cells in an irreversible and hereditable manner (e.g., chronic exposure to low-level ionizing radiation). Those agents that increase cancer by anatomical and/or physiological alteration of whole tissues and organs (e.g., dietary modification of gut flora) may or may not be described by these models. Since we do not know the relative proportion of these 2 types of carcinogens and often do not know into which category a particular agent falls, we must stress the importance of understanding basic carcinogenic mechanisms.

Relationship between "Spontaneous" and Induced Carcinogenesis. As we have shown, the independence or dependence of "spontaneous" and "induced" carcinogenesis is critical to the shape of the low dose-response curve. Two types of evidence indicate that these 2 processes share many common mechanistic steps if they are not identical.

Cancers thought to be induced are generally indistinguishable from "spontaneous" cancers. This obviously does not demonstrate that the cancers arise by a common mechanism, but it is consistent with a common pathway to "induced" and "spontaneous" carcinogenesis.

The view of carcinogenesis as a fundamentally mutational phenomenon, as recently reviewed by Knudson (8, 9), supports the assumption that induced and spontaneous steps are mechanistically identical. That is, experimental induction of cancer is the speeding up or the increasing of the probability of the various steps.

The most important observation relevant to the relationship between "induced" and "spontaneous" is that humans demonstrate a high background incidence of cancer. Whether these are due totally to "induction" by environmental agents or also to some truly spontaneous process is immaterial when considering the effects of a small amount of increased human exposure to a particular carcinogen.

Approximately 1 of 5 Americans develops a cancer, and for any particular environmental carcinogen we are interested in a very small associated increase in risk. This 20% background must surely provide some significant "spontaneous" processes that are shared with carcinogenesis by the carcinogen in question; from a public health standpoint the assumption that "induced" and "spontaneous" are not independent is conservative, as well as being biologically plausible. Small extra doses of a carcinogen will therefore elicit linear increases in risk for virtually any response model.

One practical implication of the fact that different carcinogens share many mechanistic steps is that enhancement of certain carcinogenic processes may have a more readily detectable effect on cancer incidence in animals with high background levels of all other carcinogenic processes. Therefore carcinogenicity tests of various substances should possibly include tests on high-spontaneous-incidence strains or experiments to see whether the test substance enhances the carcinogenic effect of a standard carcinogen.

Induction Time and Dose. In our discussion of stochastic models, we assumed that induction time is variable but

Table 1
Values of the upper bound of the ratio R from Equation Q

k \ p	0.1	0.5	1	4	10	100
1	1	1	1	1	1	1
2	1.02	1.11	1.21	1.62	2.16	5.52
5	1.04	1.18	1.35	2.11	3.25	13.18
∞	1.05	1.23	1.44	2.49	4.17	21.67

K. S. Crump et al.

independent of dose. This assumption is unfortunately weak in that high doses could well affect induction time. This, then, is an area of research that is in need of further effort. If we consider the low doses at which individual environmental carcinogens are experienced, however, it seems reasonable to us to assume relatively little effect on induction times.

Now let us examine the generality of the result: linear dose response at low dose. Given the uncertainties and complexities of carcinogenesis, it is conceivable that several distinct mechanistic phenomena will eventually be discovered to contribute to the appearance of cancer. Thus, we must have an open mind about our modelling and attempt to present the least model-dependent result that we can. This we have done.

Virtually all models of carcinogenesis that depict the exposure as affecting an already ongoing process will lead to linearity at low dose. We have discussed the validity of this assumption above. This result then implies that, no matter what the biological mechanism we might imagine, if the carcinogen increases some part of the already ongoing process, then we should expect the response to be approximately linear at low dose.

As pointed out above, this assumption of dependence or common mechanism is not trivial. It can make orders of magnitude differences in the estimated risk associated with low dose exposure.

If we conceive of the cell alteration process as a series of discrete single-cellular events that can occur in sequence or randomly in any given cell and that a dose-independent induction period follows, then we should expect dose response over background to be linear. We have required neither that all steps be affected by the carcinogen (only some) nor that these steps be all mechanistically similar in quantity or quality. This general class incorporates most of the reasonable models that have been proposed. The keys to this result are the assumptions of the single-cell origin and the lack of any appreciable dose dependence in the induction period.

A further extension of this group of models allows the incorporation of threshold models into the class of "linear at low dose." We have indicated that, if we conceive of single cells as the biological unit at risk and that the initiation response is a threshold phenomenon, then by assuming that the threshold is randomly distributed in dose we find that the low dose response of the whole tissue over background will be approximately linear. If, rather implausibly, we do suppose that some sort of cellular thresholds exists, then clearly all cells do not have the same threshold since all cells do not all become cancers simultaneously. Here again, we have assumed that the carcinogen acts in conjunction with the "spontaneous" or background effects.

The Mantel-Bryan procedure (11) may be interpreted as a random threshold model (albeit without our assumption that substances equivalent to the suspect carcinogen are already present in the environment), although this interpretation was not made by Mantel and Bryan. This requires that the whole organism or tissue be interpreted as the biological unit with a threshold. However, if the single cell is the unit at risk, it must be tentatively accepted that even the threshold concept of carcinogenesis (if it were appropriate)

might not be excluded from the class of "linear at low dose."

We have also attempted to answer the question of how linear is "linear at low dose" for particular models. For the multihit and multistage models, linearity is dependent on background incidence. If the background is within a typically observable range, then the linear model provides a reasonable estimate of the true state of nature, while approaching this estimate from the conservative side.

All these considerations clearly demonstrate the importance of explicit and realistic modelling in the development of low-dose extrapolation schemes. Many may feel that we have not considered certain biological observations or hypotheses in the models presented above. We have tried to embrace as much relevant information about carcinogenesis as possible and to obtain results that were the least model dependent.

The weight of these results for human risk assessment is difficult to judge. It is likely that the error in the acceptable dose associated with simple linear extrapolation will be much less than that associated with the species-to-species extrapolation to man from the laboratory animal data. The BEIR report (16) recommended linear extrapolation on pragmatic grounds. The theoretical conclusions of the present paper are that linear extrapolation to low dose levels is generally valid as a realistic yet slightly conservative procedure.

Practical Implications. Our results may be crudely summarized by the observation that, in environments already containing appreciable amounts of carcinogenic processes, the effects of any slight addition to these processes will be proportional to the amount added. Both control laboratory animals and wild humans already suffer a considerable incidence of cancer; thus the extra incidence caused by a small amount of a new carcinogen will be proportional to the dose rate of that carcinogen. This thought is not particularly remarkable, but its implications are that much previous investigation of the form of the dose-response relationship at infinitesimal doses is irrelevant to the interpretation of animal studies for the formulation of social policy.

Unfortunately, the implications of linear extrapolation are bleak. Mantel et al. (10–12) have proposed that safe doses be defined on the basis of "probit" extrapolation from upper confidence limits defined by the experimental results, arguing that such a procedure would reward good experimental investigations (by allowing industry bigger permitted doses) while enabling regulators to guarantee to the public that permitted doses were so small that they would cause cancer in less than 1 person in 10^8. Probit extrapolation may be scientifically valid for a few very special "indirect" carcinogenic processes, but our arguments suggest that in general it is not correct. The social implications of our results are best understood by considering, as an extreme case, the use of linear extrapolation to define a "safe" level after doing a large experiment in which no carcinogenic effects were observed. The most definite such negative experiment that is practical might compare animals fed with the order of 10% of the test substance in their diet with a control group and might conclude that the extra risk of cancer was less than something like 1%. Linear extrapolation, even from

Carcinogenic Processes and Low Dose Risk Assessment

such ideal results as these, implies that a dose level below 100 ppb is needed for the risk to be less than 10^{-8}, and in real experiments dose levels below 10 or even 1 ppb are likely to be indicated by linear extrapolation in order to guarantee a risk below 10^{-8}. Our arguments that linear extrapolation is generally appropriate at least suffice to demonstrate that linear extrapolation may be appropriate; thus dietary concentrations as low as a few ppb or less will always be needed to guarantee a risk below 10^{-8}.[3]

These levels are of little practical use for the regulatory control of deliberate food additives, although they might occasionally be of practical value for the legislative control of certain special contaminants. Our investigations have thus led us, reluctantly, away from Mantel's hopes and back to the familiar ground where the discovery of an apparently relevant carcinogenic effect of a putative food additive in animals is likely to cause its rapid withdrawal rather than merely a slight reduction of the permitted dose level, unless there are compelling reasons otherwise. This does encourage any carcinogenicity testing sponsored by the industrial users of an additive to be as bad as possible. Moreover, it also means that essentially absolute human safety (e.g., a risk of 10^{-8}) in general cannot be guaranteed by extrapolation from the results of animal carcinogenicity tests. This makes rational public action more difficult than it would be if we lived in a universe where probit extrapolation was true, but it is not a step towards rationality to adopt probit extrapolation because of this. In our opinion, linear dose-response relationships are likely to be approximately correct for many environmental carcinogens, and this should be

publicly agreed for such substances, as it was for radiation 20 years ago.

REFERENCES

1. Abbott, W. S. A Method of Computing the Effectiveness of an Insecticide. J. Econ. Ent., 18: 265–267, 1952.
2. Arley, N., and Iversen, N. On the Mechanism of Experimental Carcinogenesis. Acta Pathol. Microbiol. Scand., 31: 164–171, 1952.
3. Armitage, P. A Note on the Time-homogenous Birth Process. J. Roy. Statist. Soc. Ser. B, 15: 90–91, 1953.
4. Armitage, P., and Doll, R. Stochastic Models for Carcinogenesis. In: Proceedings of the Fourth Berkeley Symposium on Mathematical Statistics and Probability, Vol. 4, pp. 19–38. Berkeley and Los Angeles: University of California Press, 1961.
5. Armitage, P., and Doll, R. The Age Distribution of Cancer and a Multistage Theory of Carcinogenesis. Brit. J. Cancer, 18: 1–12, 1954.
6. Fiaklow, P. J. The Origin and Development of Human Tumors Studied with Cell Markers. New Engl. J. Med., 219: 26–35, 1974.
7. Gartler, S. M. Utilization of Mosaic Systems in the Study of the Origin and Progression of Tumors. In: J. German (ed.), Chromosomes and Cancer, pp. 313–334, New York, Wiley/Interscience, 1974.
8. Knudson, A. G. Mutation and Human Cancer. Advan. Cancer Res., 17: 317–352, 1974.
9. Knudson, A. G. Heredity and Cancer. Am. J. Pathol., 77: 77–84, 1974.
10. Mantel, N., Bohidar, N., Brown, C., Ciminera, J., and Tukey, J. An Improved "Mantel-Bryan" Procedure for "Safety" Testing of Carcinogens. Cancer Res., 35: 865–872, 1975.
11. Mantel, N., and Bryan, W. R. Safety Testing of Carcinogenic Agents. J. Natl. Cancer Inst., 27: 455–470, 1961.
12. Mantel, N., and Schneiderman, M. Estimating "Safe" Levels, a Hazardous Undertaking. Cancer Res., 35: 1379–1386, 1975.
13. Monson, R. R., Peters, J. M., and Johnson, M. N. Proportional Mortality among Vinyl Chloride Workers. Environmental Health Perspectives, 11: 75–77, 1975.
14. Neyman, J., and Scott, E. G. Statistical Aspect of the Problem of Carcinogenesis. In: Proceedings of the Fifth Berkeley Symposium on Mathematical Statistics and Probability, Vol. 4, pp. 745–776. Berkeley and Los Angeles: University of California Press, 1965.
15. Nordling, C. O. A New Theory on the Cancer-inducing Mechanism. Brit. J. Cancer, 7: 68–72, 1953.
16. The Effect on Populations of Exposure to Low Levels of Ionizing Radiation (BEIR Report). In: Report of the Advisory Committee of the Biological Effects of Ionizing Radiations, National Academy of Sciences, National Research Council. Publication No. 0-489-797, p. 217. Washington, D. C., U. S. Government Printing Office, 1972.

---

[3] There is no compelling reason why the guarantee should be of an extra risk of 10^{-8} or less; if, for example, we merely wanted to guarantee an extra risk of less than 10^{-5}, a few ppm might be permitted, and, since human cancer death rates in middle age exceed 10^{-3} per annum anyway, a limit substantially greater than 10^{-8} might be considered for substances that are particularly valuable.

Uniformity of Radiation-induced Mutation Rates among Different Species

ONE of the major difficulties in estimating the genetic hazards of ionising radiation to human populations has been our inability to extrapolate with confidence from mutation rate data in lower organisms to man[1,2]. Experimentally observed mutation rates per locus per rad extend over an enormous range of three orders of magnitude. For instance, the forward mutation rate per locus per rad is 1×10^{-9} in *Escherichia coli* B/r at two loci for phage T1 resistance, 2.7×10^{-9} in *Neurospora* at the *ad3* locus, 1.4×10^{-8} in *Drosophila* for eight specific loci (averaged), 1.7×10^{-7} in the mouse for twelve specific loci (averaged), and 1×10^{-6} in barley for three loci.

Reprinted from *Nature*,
Vol. 245, pp. 460-462,
October 26, 1973

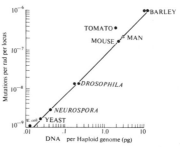

Fig. 1 Relation between forward mutation rate per locus per rad and the DNA content per haploid genome. Line drawn with slope of one through the mouse point. Point for man estimated from DNA content.

The development of target theory in radiobiology and the recognition that the genetic material is the target for many radiobiological endpoints led to the demonstration that the mean lethal dose for survival of irradiated single cells is related to the nuclear DNA content[3,4]. Sparrow *et al.*[5] have noted that in plants, radiosensitivity is closely related to several nuclear parameters such as nuclear volume and interphase chromosome volume and thus to the DNA content per nucleus. In amphibians, too, it has been shown that the mean lethal dose for survival of whole-body irradiated animals is directly related to the amount of DNA per nucleus and per chromosome[6]. The work of Sparrow and his coworkers[7-9] has demonstrated that the relation between nuclear parameters and radiosensitivity is not entirely simple, however, for although the organisms studied do fall into a series of 'radiotaxa' within which a simple linear relation holds, the sensitivities of the radiotaxa differ from one another.

We re-examined the data for radiation-induced forward mutation rates from organisms as disparate as bacteria, fungi, higher plants, insects, and mammals for which we also know the amounts of DNA per nucleus. As seen in Table 1, and as noted above, the mutation rates per locus per rad vary over three orders of magnitude. Nonetheless, when these rates are adjusted for the amount of DNA per nucleus and thus normalised to a common biological baseline, the mutation rates obtained are all essentially the same, varying by a mere factor of three instead of 1,000.

of the functional genetic unit would fail to complement mutations in any of the other components[14].

Models can also be postulated in which the repair processes vary quantitatively in the different species.

Whatever the basic explanation might be, we conclude that, empirically, the radiation-induced mutation rate is proportional to the total genome size (DNA content) for the species. This correspondence, which is shown graphically in Fig. 1, allows us to extrapolate from mutation rates obtained in experimental organisms to man with greater confidence.

This work was performed under the auspices of the US Atomic Energy Commission and supported in part by a

Table 1 Specific Locus Mutation Rates Normalized for Amount of DNA per Nucleus

Organism	DNA per haploid genome (pg)	Relative amount of DNA as compared with human A	Specific locus mutations per locus per rad B	Normalised specific locus mutations per locus per rad B/A	References
E. coli B/r (Bacterium)	0.013 *	4.5×10^{-3}	1×10^{-9}†	2.2×10^{-7}	*[15], †[16]
Saccharomyces cerevisiae (Yeast)	0.024 *	8.3×10^{-3}	1.6×10^{-9}†	1.9×10^{-7}	*[17] †R. Mortimer, personal communication
Neurospora crassa (Fungus)	0.042 *	1.4×10^{-2}	2.7×10^{-9}†	1.9×10^{-7}	*[17], †[18]
Drosophila melanogaster (Fruit fly)	0.17 * 0.22	0.058 0.076	1.4×10^{-8} † (Spermatogonia)	2.4×10^{-7} 1.8×10^{-7}	*[19] †[20,21]
Lycopersicon esculentum (Tomato)	1.95 *	0.67	3.75×10^{-7} †	5.6×10^{-7}	*[22] †[23]
Mus musculus (Mouse)	2.26 *	0.78	1.7×10^{-7} * (Spermatogonia)	2.2×10^{-7}	*[2]
Hordeum vulgare (Barley)	10 * 11.5 †	3.45 3.97	1×10^{-6} ‡	2.9×10^{-7} 2.5×10^{-7}	*[24], †[17], ‡[25]
Homo sapiens (Man)	2.9	1	—	2.6×10^{-7} (unweighted average)	

This remarkable consistency in normalised mutation rates in such a wide variety of organisms strongly suggests that extrapolation directly from experimental organisms to man can be done with confidence. For all the species listed in the table, the unweighted average of the mutation rates normalised to the human DNA value is 2.6×10^{-7} per locus per rad. (These rates are all for forward mutations induced by acute irradiation. With chronic radiation or with germ cells irradiated during different cell stages, the mutation rates often vary by a factor of three to four. These differences are conventionally attributed to differential repair. Back mutations, which are often the result of base changes in suppressor loci, are usually lower by a factor of ten.)

The consistency that obtains when the data are adjusted for the amount of DNA per nucleus for each species indicates either that it is the nucleus, and not the locus, that determines target size, or that, on the average, the size of a (radiation-mutable) locus is proportional to the total genome size (DNA content) for the species.

Although the latter conclusion is contrary to the usual genetic expectation that structural genes should be the same size in bacteria as in man, we note that the functional genetic unit in Drosophila corresponds to a band in the salivary gland polytene chromosomes[10]. This indicates that complementation groups in higher forms contain much more DNA than is necessary for specification of a protein. It has been postulated that the extra DNA has a regulatory function[11–13] and that mutations in any of the components

Public Health research grant, and a Research Career award, to A. D. C.

SEYMOUR ABRAHAMSON

Departments of Zoology and Genetics,
University of Wisconsin,
Madison, Wisconsin 43713

MICHAEL A. BENDER

Department of Radiology,
The Johns Hopkins University School of Medicine,
Baltimore, Maryland 21205

ALAN D. CONGER

Department of Radiobiology,
Temple University School of Medicine,
Philadelphia, Pennsylvania 19140

SHELDON WOLFF

Laboratory of Radiobiology and Department of Anatomy,
University of California,
San Francisco, California 94143

Received August 30, 1973.

[1] Biological Effects of Ionizing Radiation Advisory Committee, *The Effects on Populations of Exposure to Low Levels of Ionizing Radiation* (National Academy of Sciences, National Research Council, Washington, DC, 1972).

[2] United Nations Scientific Committee on the Effects of Atomic Radiation, *Ionizing Radiation: Levels and Effects, Vol. II, Effects. A/8725: General Assembly Official Records, 27th Session, Supplement No. 25* (United Nations, New York, 1972).

[3] Terzi, M., *Nature*, **191**, 461 (1961).

[4] Terzi, M., *J. theor. Biol.*, **8**, 233 (1965).

[5] Sparrow, A. H., Sparrow, R. C., Thompson, K. H., and Schairer, L. A., *Radiat. Bot. Suppl.*, **5**, 101 (1965).

[6] Conger, A. D., and Clinton, J. H., *Radiat. Res.*, **54**, 69 (1973).

[7] Sparrow, A. H., Underbrink, A. G., and Sparrow, R. C., *Radiat. Res.*, **32**, 915 (1967).

[8] Sparrow, A. H., Rogers, A. F., and Schwemmer, S. S., *Radiat. Bot.*, **8**, 149 (1968).

[9] Underbrink, A. G., Sparrow, A. H., and Pond, V., *Radiat. Bot.*, **8**, 205 (1968).

[10] Judd, B. H., Shen, M. W., and Kaufman, T. C., *Genetics*, **71**, 139 (1972).

[11] Britten, R. J., and Davidson, E. H., *Science, N.Y.*, **165**, 349 (1969).

[12] Georgiev, G. P., *J. theor. Biol.*, **25**, 473 (1969).

[13] Crick, F., *Nature*, **234**, 25 (1971).

[14] Shannon, M. P., Kaufman, T. C., Shen, M. W., and Judd, B. H., *Genetics*, **72**, 615 (1972).

[15] Gillies, N. E., and Alper, T., *Biochim. biophys. Acta*, **43**, 182 (1960).

[16] Demerec, M., and Latarjet, R., *Cold Spring Harb. Symp. quant. Biol.*, **11**, 38 (1946).

[17] Sparrow, A. H., Price, H. J., and Underbrink, A. G., in *Evolution of Genetic Systems, Brookhaven Symp. Biol.*, **23**, 451 (Gordon and Breach, New York, 1972).

[18] Webber, B. B., and deSerres, F. J., *Proc. natn. Acad. Sci., U.S.A.*, **53**, 430 (1965).

[19] Tates, A. D., thesis. Univ. Leiden.

[20] Alexander, M. L., *Genetics*, **39**, 409 (1954).

[21] Alexander, M. L., *Genetics*, **45**, 1019 (1960).

[22] Rees, H., and Jones, R. N., *Int. Rev. Cytol.*, **32**, 53 (1972).

[23] Brock, R. D., and Franklin, I. R., *Radiat. Bot.*, **6**, 171 (1966).

[24] Bennett, M. D., *Proc. R. Soc., B.*, **181**, 109 (1972).

[25] Ehrenberg, L., and Eriksson, G., *Mutat. Res.*, **1**, 139 (1964).

Reprinted from Nature,
Vol. 258, pp. 359-361,
November 27, 1975

Mutation rate, genome size and their relation to the rec concept

ORGANISMS vary greatly in genome size, that is, in the amount of DNA comprising the haploid genome. Rates of radiation-induced mutation expressed as mutations per locus per rad, also differ widely among organisms, but it is surprising that mutation rates and genome size are correlated[1]. This correlation is unexpected because proteins are of a similar size in all organisms, implying that structural genes must also be of a similar size. Accordingly, one would expect that, although the overall mutation rate would be proportional to the overall number of genes, the mutation rate per locus would be similar in all organisms or, at least,

bear no relation to genome size. Surveying published data, however, Abrahamson et al.[1] found a direct correlation between rate of radiation-induced mutation and size of the haploid genome from Escherichia coli to Hordeum vulgare (the ABCW relationship). We wondered whether rates of chemically induced mutation would also be related to genome size, both because of the practical importance of being able to extrapolate to the genetic effect of a chemical on the human population and because the information might help to elucidate the mechanism underlying the ABCW relationship.

We therefore undertook a similar survey of the literature for ethyl methane sulphonate (EMS), the most widely used chemical mutagen. We were limited to studies for which we could determine the number of mutations per survivor, the number of loci at risk, the actual applied dose, and the haploid DNA content of the test organism. Dose estimation for EMS posed problems because we do not know how much EMS reached the DNA in active form: the chemical might have penetrated to the DNA in different ways in different organisms or might have been differently metabolised. Furthermore, the duration of EMS treatment varied as did the methods and conditions of the exposure. For our purposes, therefore, we assumed a uniform distribution of the chemical within the organism at the applied dose. In the case of the mouse, the injected dose of $200 \, mg \, kg^{-1}$ became $200 \, mg \, l^{-1}$ or $1.6 \times 10^{-3} \, M$. To provide a consistent measure of dose, it was necessary to use only concentration in all cases, rather than the product of concentration and the duration of exposure which was often unknown. The data are shown in Table 1.

To obtain the best fit of a curve representing the relationship between mutation rate and genome size, we used the method of least squares on the unweighted data or the unweighted logarithms of the data. In the former case the line of fit deviates markedly from the points for organisms with smaller genomes. Thus the logarithmic values are the only ones reported. This represents a fit to the equation $y = mx^b$ where y is the mutation rate and x is the genome size. The

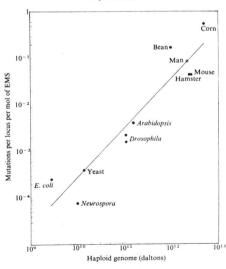

Fig. 1 Rate of X-ray-induced mutation in organisms with different haploid genome sizes. The human point is not experimental.

lines shown in Figs 1 and 2 were obtained in this way. Figure 1 shows the data of Abrahamson *et al.,* for rates of X-ray-induced mutation, except that a few points have been replotted at DNA values we believe to be more accurate. The line has the parameters of $m=1.20\times10^{-14}$ mutations per locus per rad per dalton and $b=0.82$ ($r=0.97$). The EMS results are given in Fig. 2. In this case the line has the parameters $m=2.24\times10^{-14}$ mutations per locus per M per dalton and $b=1.03$ ($r=0.94$). We do not regard either of the values of b as being significantly different from 1.0 given the inhomogeneity of the data.

The relationship between mutation rate and genome size is as striking for EMS as it is for radiation, thus confirming the reality of the ABCW relation. This relation was so unexpected that we could not exclude the possibility that it was coincidence. Since the EMS data involve several organisms, loci and investigators not associated with the radiation data (although there are some of each in common), it seems most unlikely that the relationship is a statistical artefact. Accordingly it is proper to consider both the possible mechanisms that may underlie the relation and its significance for estimating human risk from chemical mutagens.

There are at least three possible ways of explaining the ABCW relationship, in which we include now EMS as well as X rays (and, presumably, many or all mutagens). These possibilities, which are not mutually exclusive, are : (1) that the target for mutation is roughly proportional to genome size, (2) that the efficiency of repair of genetic damage is inversely proportional to genome size, and (3) that the size of the mutational event is proportional to genome size. We assume, of course, that the initial lesion (for example, an alkylation) is the same but that the fate of the lesion might differ. It is conceivable, for example, that the average size of interstitial chromosomal deletions could bear some relation to genome size because two different parts of the same chromosome must be in close proximity. Thus if the condensation pattern of chromosomes resulted in proportionately longer folds or gyres in organisms with larger genomes, then the effectiveness of each lesion at producing forward mutations would increase in proportion to genome size and could account for the ABCW relationship.

The second possibility is that the effectiveness of repair is inversely proportional to genome size. This would arise if, for example, the absolute amount of repair were the same

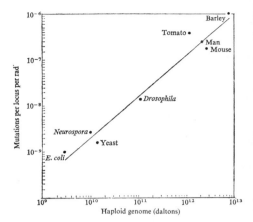

Fig. 2 Rate of ethyl methane sulphonate induced mutation rate in organisms with different haploid genome sizes. The human point is not experimental.

in all organisms (even though the total amount of damage is directly proportional to DNA content).

The remaining possibility that we have considered is that gene size differs systematically. A similar possibility has been raised, for example, from the correlation between the number and location of salivary gland chromosome bands and gene loci in *Drosophila*[2]. Various models for the organisational and control of genes in higher organisms fit rather well with such a model in those cases where each structural gene is part of a larger genetic unit that includes controlling DNA[2-4]. Others have concluded that among higher organisms, specifically man and chimpanzee, the differences cannot be accounted for primarily by differences in structural genes but that differences in the controlling genes are involved[5]. Such models predict an increase in forward mutation rates with genome size since hits on controlling DNA could lead to loss of function. One test of this

Table 1 Data used to calculate the values in Fig. 2

Organism	DNA per haploid genome (daltons)	Specific locus mutation rate	Genes mutated	Dose of EMS	Duration of treatment	Specific locus mutations per mol of EMS	References
E. coli (bacterium)	$2.8\times10^{9*}$	3.12×10^{-5}† 3.8×10^{-5}†	*tsx* (resistance to phage T$_6$)	0.1 M 0.2 M	8–15 min 10 min	3.1×10^{-4} 1.9×10^{-4}	*8, †9
Neurospora crassa (fungus)	$1\times10^{10*}$	7.25×10^{-6}†	*ad-3A* and *ad-3B*	9.5×10^{-2} M	60 min	7.6×10^{-5}	*10, †11
Schizosaccharomyces pombe (yeast)	$1.4\times10^{10*}$	3.9×10^{-4}†	*ad$_6$* and *ad$_7$*	1 M	2 h	3.9×10^{-4}	*12, †13
Drosophila melanogaster (fruit fly)	$1.1\times10^{11*}$	5.7×10^{-5}†	10^3 loci for sex-linked recessive lethals‡	2.5×10^{-2} M	Mutagen injected	2.3×10^{-3}	*1, †14, ‡3, 15
Arabidopsis thaliana	$1.6\times10^{11*}$	7.8×10^{-5}†	Four loci for thiamine auxotrophy	4.1×10^{-3} M	15 h	2.0×10^{-2}	*16, †17
Phaseolus vulgaris (bean)	$1\times10^{12*}$	1.10^{-2}†	Gene for white seed-coat colour	0.04 M	6 h	2.5×10^{-1}	*16, 18
Homo sapiens (man)	$2.16\times10^{12*}$						*19
Cricetulus griseus (Chinese hamster cell cultures)	$2.51\times10^{12*}$	4.46×10^{-4}†	*azg^5*	1×10^{-2} M	2 h	4.4×10^{-2}	*19, †20
Mus musculus (mouse)	$2.57\times10^{12*}$	7.1×10^{-5}§	Eight specific loci	200 mg kg^{-1} or 1.6×10^{-3} M	Mutagen injected	4.4×10^{-2}	*19
Zea mays (corn)	$5\times10^{12*}$	1.53×10^{-2}†	*C, sh* and *wx*	0.028 M	5 h–5 d	5.5×10^{-1}	*16, †21

Within each line asterisks, daggers and double daggers identify the appropriate references.
§ Personal communication from R. B. Cumming.

Table 2 Forward mutation rates induced in prokaryotic organisms

Organism	Genome size (daltons)	Radiation		EMS		References
		Observed values	Extrapolated values	Observed values	Extrapolated values	
E. coli	$2.8 \times 10^{8*}$	1×10^{-9}†	6.74×10^{-10}	2.5×10^{-4}	6.75×10^{-5}	*8, †9
T₂	$1.2 \times 10^{8*}$	7.8×10^{-13}†	3.2×10^{-11}	7×10^{-3}‡	1.8×10^{-6}	*22, †23, ‡24
T₄	$1.5 \times 10^{8*}$	1.08×10^{-8}†	4.5×10^{-11}	–	3×10^{-6}	*22, †25
φX174 and S13	$1.7 \times 10^{8*}$	–	7.91×10^{-13}	2.91×10^{-16}†	2.38×10^{-8}	*26, †27

Asterisks, daggers and double daggers apply as in Table 1.

explanation would be to measure mutation rates in conditions such that only changes in the structural gene are detected in organisms of different genome size. Another prediction from these models is that the mutation rate will be determined mostly by the size of the structural gene when the proportion of controlling DNA is small. Thus one would expect that organisms with most of their genomes consisting of structural genes would have similar mutation rates, presumably much like that of *E. coli*. Although we have not been able to find much data on this matter, Table 2 shows that neither this prediction nor an extrapolation of the ABCW relation seems satisfactory.

The correlations, regardless of the nature of the mechanism underlying them, provide support for the proposal to express the exposure to chemical mutagens as an equivalent radiation dose. One of the major difficulties in the regulation of human exposure to mutagens is the quantitative estimation of the genetic risk. The most thorough assessment of mutagenicity has been carried out for ionising radiation and maximum population exposure limits have been laid down. On this basis a unit which could be used to quantify human exposure has been suggested, the rem-equivalent-chemical (rec or "radequiv.") which is defined as that concentration of a chemical mutagen that produces an amount of genetic damage equal to that produced by 1 rem of chronic irradiation[6,7]. For such a unit to be meaningful the ratio of mutagenicity of the chemical to radiation must be the same for man and the test organisms. The curves in Figs 1 and 2 indicate that there is a remarkably constant relationship over several orders of magnitude of mutation rate, although there is some uncertainty in the data for any one organism. Since the lines of best fit have somewhat different slopes (1.1 and 0.9) we have used the ratio of the fitted values at the geometric mean (*Arabidopsis*) to calculate the rec value of 4×10^{-6} M. Expressed in terms of rads, therefore, treatment by a 1-M solution is equivalent to about 2.5×10^{5} rad.

There are, of course, other problems in estimating the human risk and there is the problem of assessing the benefit of the chemical also. Nevertheless, if similar correlations are found for other mutagens, rough extrapolations from the simple, rapid microbiological screens to human risk can be made to provide a quantitative evaluation. This would be useful in planning mammalian experiments and evaluating the results. Mammalian systems will still be important because of the potential influence of uniquely mammalian aspects of metabolism, absorption, and excretion of compounds and the possibility of classes of damage that do not occur in prokaryotes, such as chromosome breakage and non-disjunction. Nevertheless, the rec concept has many possible uses in the light of the data presented here which suggest that there is a relatively constant value of rec for all organisms.

The work in our laboratory is supported by grants from the National Research Council and the National Cancer Institute. Dr R. D. Benz has been helpful to us in numerous discussions.

JOHN A. HEDDLE
K. ATHANASIOU

Departments of Natural Science and Biology,
York University, Downsview, Ontario, Canada M3J 1P3

Received August 5; accepted October 1, 1975.

[1] Abrahamson, S., Bender, M. A., Conger, A. D., and Wolff, S., *Nature*, 245, 460–462 (1973).
[2] Judd, B. H., Shen, M. W., and Kaufman, T. C., *Genetics*, 71, 139–156 (1972).
[3] Bishop, J. O., *Cell*, 2, 81–86 (1974).
[4] Britten, R. J., and Davidson, E. H., *Science*, 165, 349–357 (1969).
[5] King, M. C., and Wilson, A. C., *Science*, 188, 107–116 (1975).
[6] Bridges, B. A., *Environ. Hlth Perspect.*, 6, 221–227 (1973).
[7] Crow, F., *Environ. Hlth Perspect.*, 6, 1–5 (1973).
[8] Lethbak, A., Christiansen, C., and Stenderup, A., *J. gen. Microbiol.*, 64, 377–380 (1970).
[9] Loveless, A., and Howarth, S., *Nature*, 184, 1780–1782 (1959).
[10] Minagawa, T., Wagner, B., and Strauss, B., *Archs Biochem. Biophys.*, 80, 442–445 (1959).
[11] de Serres, F. J., Brockman, H. E., Barnett, W. E., and Kølmark, H. C., *Mutat. Res.*, 12, 129–142 (1971).
[12] Ogur, M., Minckler, S., Lindegren, G., and Lindegren, C. C., *Archs Biochem. Biophys.*, 40, 175–184 (1952).
[13] Loprieno, N., *Mutat. Res.*, 3, 486–493 (1966).
[14] Lim, J. K., and Snyder, L. A., *Mutat. Res.*, 6, 129–137 (1968).
[15] Alikhanian, S. J., *Zool. Zhur.*, 16 (1937).
[16] Bennett, M. D., *Proc. R. Soc.*, B181, 109–135 (1972).
[17] Rédei, G. P., and Li, S. L., *Genetics*, 61, 453–459 (1969).
[18] Moh, C. C., *Mutat. Res.*, 7, 469–471 (1969).
[19] Bachmann, K., *Chromosoma*, 37, 85–93 (1972).
[20] Chu, E. H. Y., and Malling, H. V., *Genetics*, 61, 1306–1312 (1968).
[21] Amano, E., and Smith, H. H., *Mutat. Res.*, 2, 344–351 (1965).
[22] Rees, H., and Jones, R. N., *Int. Rev. Cytol.*, 32, 53 (1972).
[23] Ardashnikov, S. N., Soyfer, V. N., and Goldfarb, D. M., *Biochem. biophys. Res. Commun.*, 16, 455–459 (1964).
[24] Strauss, B. S., *Nature*, 191, 730–731 (1961).
[25] Brown, D. F., *Mutat. Res.*, 3, 365–373 (1966).
[26] Sinsheimer, R. L., *Procedures in Nucleic Acid Research* (edit. by Cantoni, and Davies), 559–576 (Harper and Row, New York, 1966).
[27] Tessman, I., Poddar, R. K., and Kumar, S., *J. molec. Biol.*, 9, 352–363 (1964).